CARDIOLOGY RESEARCH AND CLINICAL DEVELOPMENTS

CURRENT ADVANCES IN CARDIOVASCULAR RISK

VOLUME 2

CARDIOLOGY RESEARCH AND CLINICAL DEVELOPMENTS

Additional books in this series can be found on Nova's website under the Series tab.

Additional E-books in this series can be found on Nova's website under the E-book tab.

CARDIOLOGY RESEARCH AND CLINICAL DEVELOPMENTS

CURRENT ADVANCES IN CARDIOVASCULAR RISK

VOLUME 2

SANDEEP AJOY SAHA

EDITOR

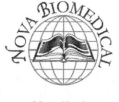

New York

For permission to use material from this book please contact us:
Telephone 631-231-7269; Fax 631-231-8175
Web Site: http://www.novapublishers.com

NOTICE TO THE READER

The Publisher has taken reasonable care in the preparation of this book, but makes no expressed or implied warranty of any kind and assumes no responsibility for any errors or omissions. No liability is assumed for incidental or consequential damages in connection with or arising out of information contained in this book. The Publisher shall not be liable for any special, consequential, or exemplary damages resulting, in whole or in part, from the readers' use of, or reliance upon, this material. Any parts of this book based on government reports are so indicated and copyright is claimed for those parts to the extent applicable to compilations of such works.

Independent verification should be sought for any data, advice or recommendations contained in this book. In addition, no responsibility is assumed by the publisher for any injury and/or damage to persons or property arising from any methods, products, instructions, ideas or otherwise contained in this publication.

This publication is designed to provide accurate and authoritative information with regard to the subject matter covered herein. It is sold with the clear understanding that the Publisher is not engaged in rendering legal or any other professional services. If legal or any other expert assistance is required, the services of a competent person should be sought. FROM A DECLARATION OF PARTICIPANTS JOINTLY ADOPTED BY A COMMITTEE OF THE AMERICAN BAR ASSOCIATION AND A COMMITTEE OF PUBLISHERS.

Additional color graphics may be available in the e-book version of this book.

Library of Congress Cataloging-in-Publication Data

Library of Congress Control Number: 2012936879

ISBN: 978-1-62081-746-9

Published by Nova Science Publishers, Inc. † *New York*

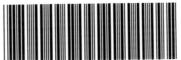

Contents

In: Current Advances in Cardiovascular Risk. Volume 2   ISBN: 978-1-62081-746-9
Editor: Sandeep Ajoy Saha   © 2012 Nova Science Publishers, Inc.

Chapter XIV

Cardiovascular Risk in Patients with Type 2 Diabetes Mellitus

Kleopatra Alexiadou and Nicholas Tentolouris[*]

First Department of Propaedeutic and Internal Medicine, Athens University Medical
School, Laiko General Hospital, Athens, Greece

Abstract

Cardiovascular disease affects >50% of all people with diabetes and is the major
cause of death. Macroangiopathy is one of the complications of diabetes and
atherosclerotic manifestations tend to be more frequent and their progression faster in
diabetic compared to non-diabetic patients. These manifestations involve the coronary
arteries, the arteries of the lower extremities as well as the carotid and cerebral arteries.

The increased risk of macroangiopathy and therefore cardiovascular disease in
diabetes seems to be present from the stage of impaired glucose tolerance or even earlier
at the stage of insulin resistance and hyperinsulinemia.

Multiple risk factors contribute to the occurrence of cardiac episodes, strokes and
peripheral vascular disease in diabetic patients. Among them are the classic
atherosclerotic risk factors like smoking, hypertension and dyslipidemia (high
triglyceride levels, low HDL-cholesterol, high LDL-cholesterol). Other risk factors
include platelet disorders, insulin resistance, central body fat distribution, autonomic
neuropathy and hyperglycemia itself. Insulin resistance accompanied by a condition of
chronic inflammation seems to play a central role. Adipocytes, monocytes, endothelial
cells and smooth muscle cells produce cytokines which contribute to this inflammatory
state. Furthermore, the oxidative stress as a consequence of hyperglycemia and increased
free fatty acid levels promotes the production of various mediators as well as oxidized
LDL-cholesterol. Oxidized LDL is taken up by the macrophages leading to the formation
of foam cells and thus aggravating the atherosclerotic lesions.

Strict control of all the risk factors is necessary along with glycemic control, weight
control and physical activity in order to diminish cardiovascular risk and therefore
prevent cardiovascular disease.

[*] Correspondence: N. Tentolouris, 33 Lakonias Street, 11523 Athens, Greece. Tel: 0030 201 745 6448, Fax: 0030
210 746 2640, E-mail: ntentol@med.uoa.gr.

Abbreviations

CVD	cardiovascular disease;
BMI	body mass index;
HDL	high density lipoprotein;
NCEP ATPIII	National Cholesterol Education Program Adult Treatment Panel III;
TNF-α	tumor necrosis factor α;
SNP	single nucleotide polymorphism;
MAGIC	Meta-Analysis of Glucose and Insulin-related traits Consortium;
LDL	low density lipoprotein;
NF-κB	Nuclear Factor κB;
FFAs	free fatty acids;
NO	nitric oxide;
ET-1	endothelin-1;
ANG II	angiotensin II;
t-PA	tissue-type plasminogen activator;
PAI-1	plasminogen activator inhibitor-1;
VWF	von Willebrand factor;
UKPDS	United Kingdom Prospective Diabetes Study;
DCCT	Diabetes Control and Complications Trial;
OGTT	Oral Glucose Tolerance Test;
eNOS	endothelial NO synthase ;
PKC	protein kinase C;
ROS	reactive oxygen species;
AGEs	Advanced glycation end products;
ATP	adenosine triphosphate;
VLDL	very low density lipoprotein: PI-3: Phosphoinositide-3;
ICAM-1	Inter-Cellular Adhesion Molecule 1;
VCAM-1	vascular cell adhesion molecule 1;
IR	insulin receptor;
IRS-1	insulin receptor substrate;
MAPK	Mitogen activated protein kinase;
CRP	C-reactive protein;
IL	interleukin;
MCP-1	Monocyte chemotactic protein-1;
RAS	renin angiotensin system;
AT1Rs	angiotensin type 1 receptors;
AT2Rs	angiotensin type 2 receptors;
ACE	Angiotensing Converting Enzyme;
TG	triglycerides;
apo B	apolipoprotein B;
CETP	Cholestrol ester transfer protein;
apo A1	apolipoprotein A1;
DPP	Diabetes Prevention Program;
DASH	Dietary Approaches to Stop Hypertension;

IGT	impaired glucose tolerance;
NHANES	National Health and Nutrition Examination Survey;
IFG	impaired fasting glucose;
ADA	American Diabetes Association;
AACE/ACE	American Association of Clinical Endocrinologists/American College of Endocrinology;
CHD	coronary heart disease;
EPIC-Norfolk	Norfolk cohort of the European Prospective Investigation of Cancer and Nutrition;
CV	cardiovascular;
ACCORD	Action to Control Cardiovascular Risk in Diabetes;
ADVANCE study	the Diabetes and Vascular Disease: Preterax and Diamicron Modified Release Controlled Evaluation study;
VADT	Veterans Affairs Diabetes Trial;
ARBs	angiotensin receptor blockers;
CARDS	Collaborative Atorvastatin Diabetes Study;
MI	myocardial infarction;
CTTC	Cholesterol Treatment Trialist Collaborators;
PPARalpha	peroxisome proliferator-activated receptor-alpha;
LPL	lipoprotein lipase;
ABCA1	ATP binding cassette A1;
HHS	Helsinki heart study;
T2DM	type 2 diabetes mellitus;
VA-HIT	Veterans affairs HDL-C intervention trial;
FIELD	Fenofibrate intervention and event lowering in diabetes.

Epidemiology

The incidence and prevalence of diabetes has increased dramatically affecting about 3-5% of Western populations and representing a major health issue in the 21st century. This may be attributed to environmental, behavioral and lifestyle changes. Chronic hyperglycemia leads to diabetic macro- and microvascular complications which have an impact on the function of many organs, such us heart, blood vessels, eyes, nerves and kidneys.

Obesity, type 2 diabetes and cardiovascular disease (CVD) have long been recognized as conditions which are intimately linked. In his landmark book, Epidemiology of Diabetes and Its Vascular Lesions published in 1978 [1], Kelly West reviewed and summarized the scientific knowledge about the distribution and causes of type 1 and 2 diabetes mellitus. He pointed out that the state of prediabetes is identifiable and that type 2 diabetes should be preventable. He also hypothesized that new biochemical and genetic markers of diabetes risk would emerge and reveal the mechanisms linking obesity, type 2 diabetes and CVD.

The Framingham Heart Study, a longitudinal, multigenerational cohort study of CVD and its risk factors has provided a rich source to address the points raised by West. The prevalence of obesity (BMI$\geq$30 kg/m^2) in the study has risen in both men and women over the past 30 years from just a few percent among men in the 1970s to 25-30% among men in the 1990s

[2]. A similar trend occurred in women. Over the same time frame, the prevalence of type 2 diabetes in the study rose steadily [3]. The entire rise in type 2 diabetes has occurred in individuals with obesity, from about 6% in the 1970s to over 12% in the 1990s. Although the absolute risk of CVD in the Framingham Heart Study (defined by fatal and nonfatal myocardial infarction, stroke and intermittent claudication) has declined between the 1950s and the 1990s by 35% in people without diabetes and by 49% in those with diabetes, the relative risk among those with diabetes to develop CVD has persistently remained about twofold higher compared to those without diabetes [4]. The rising prevalence of type 2 diabetes, combined with a constant relative risk for CVD, has translated into a 60% increase in the attributable risk ratio for CVD associated with diabetes, even though the attributable risk for CVD associated with other risk factors like hypertension and smoking has held constant or fallen [5]. The experience of the Framingham Heart Study shows that the rising tide of obesity leads to a rise in the prevalence of type 2 diabetes which in turn leads to increased risk for CVD and death.

From the clinical point of view, CVD is often considered as a consequence of diagnosed type 2 diabetes. However, the experience of the Framingham Heart Study and other cohorts has shown that prediabetes is also associated with risk for CVD [6]. This observation has formed the notion that type 2 diabetes and CVD may share a common pathogenesis. These diseases share many common risk factors including central obesity, hyperinsulinemia and insulin resistance, hyperglycemia, dyslipidemia characterized by low levels of HDL cholesterol and elevated levels of triglycerides and elevated blood pressure. These parameters are intercorrelated and often coexist, forming an entity in the centre of which lays obesity and insulin resistance [7, 8].

This phenomenon of risk factor clustering is called metabolic syndrome. The definition the most often studied is the one proposed by the National Cholesterol Education Program Adult Treatment Panel III (NCEP ATPIII) [9]. The concept of the metabolic syndrome raises the hypothesis that its presence increases future risks for both type 2 diabetes and CVD. In the Framingham Heart Study, metabolic syndrome increases the 7- to 11-year risk for CVD in men by about threefold compared to those without metabolic syndrome and for type 2 diabetes the increase is about sevenfold. Associations among women are similar. Data suggest that beyond the specific risk factors, it is something about their clustering that appears to account, at least in part, for subsequent disease risk. Metabolic syndrome also explains part of the heterogeneity for future disease risk observed in individuals with obesity. Among the Framingham Heart Study individuals with BMI <25 kg/m^2 who meet the criteria for metabolic syndrome, the 7-year cumulative incidence of type 2 diabetes was about 7%, while among those with BMI ≥30 kg/m^2 but without metabolic syndrome, the rate was only about 3% [11]. Similar but less dramatic patterns were seen for risk of CVD. This may lead to the conclusion that metabolic syndrome is far more powerful risk factor for type 2 diabetes than for CVD.

Several research efforts have aimed to identify molecular and physiological mechanisms in order to explain the phenomenon of risk factor clustering. Abnormal adipocyte signaling, impaired endothelial function and systemic subclinical inflammation have been proposed to play a role that unifies excess adiposity with insulin resistance, impaired β-cell function and small and large vessel disease [12]. The adipokines adiponectin, resistin and tumor necrosis factor α (TNF-α) are all associated with obesity and insulin resistance [13]. However, the interrelationships of adipokine biomarkers with incident diabetes and CVD have been difficult to elucidate.

After the introduction and use in the research field of high-density single nucleotide polymorphism (SNP) arrays, a new era in genetic discovery was opened. The Meta-Analysis of Glucose and Insulin-related traits Consortium (MAGIC) has pooled data including over 120,000 individuals of European ancestry without clinical diabetes from over 50 cohort studies. MAGIC has identified 16 common SNPs associated with levels of fasting glucose, fasting insulin and levels of glucose 2 h after an oral glucose tolerance test [14-16]. Several loci have revealed or confirmed novel mechanistic pathways underlying diabetes physiology, including variants localized in or near genes involved in the Circadian and alpha-adrenergic systems, fatty acid metabolism and the incretin system. In the Framingham Heart Study, a genetic score comprised of 18 confirmed type 2 diabetes risk SNPs was higher among individuals who developed type 2 diabetes over 28 years compared with those who remained free of diabetes [17]. Interestingly, both parental history of type 2 diabetes and the genetic risk score were independently associated with type 2 diabetes risk. This implies both that our genetic understanding of type 2 diabetes remains incomplete and that family history, which is considered to represent inherited genetic risk, also represents behaviors that are learned and transmitted in families.

The last decades of epidemiology and clinical trials resulted in remarkable progress in the biochemical and genetic understanding of the importance of type 2 diabetes as risk factor for CVD. This is considered as a valuable tool in order to reverse the steadily rising tide of both diabetes and CVD and to optimize therapeutic management of cardiovascular risk in this high-risk patient population.

Pathophysiological Mechanisms

All major risk factors (elevated high total and LDL cholesterol, low HDL cholesterol, elevated blood pressure and smoking) are similar in patients with type 2 diabetes and nondiabetic individuals [18]. However, at every level for each of the cardiovascular risk factors, diabetic subjects have at least two-fold higher risk than nondiabetic individuals. This indicates that although classic risk factors are very important determinants of increased risk of CVD in type 2 diabetic subjects, they do not explain the higher risk of CVD events in these individuals. Therefore, in order to understand the excess risk of CVD in type 2 diabetes, other risk factors have to be considered.

The primary event in the process of atherosclerosis is the accumulation of LDL cholesterol in the subendothelial matrix in diabetic and nondiabetic individuals [19]. Small and dense LDL particles are likely to enhance atherogenesis and CVD risk in type 2 diabetes. In vitro studies show that small LDL particles rapidly enter the arterial wall, cause greater production of procoagulant factors and are more readily oxidized [20]. Activation of Nuclear Factor κB (NF-κB) signaling cascade leads to the production of E-selectin, ICAM-1, VCAM-1, as well as chemoattractant cytokines [19]. Increased concentrations of free fatty acids (FFAs) may also induce inflammation, worsen insulin resistance and impair endothelium-dependent vasodilatation [21]. Low HDL cholesterol and apolipoprotein A1 levels are likely to contribute to impaired removal of excess cholesterol from atherosclerotic plaques [22].

Dysfunction of the endothelium is regarded as an important factor in the pathogenesis of vascular disease in diabetes mellitus [23-25]. The endothelium is the active inner monolayer of the blood vessels, forming a barrier between circulating blood in the lumen and the rest of the vessel wall, playing a critical role in vascular homeostasis. It actively regulates vascular tone and permeability, the balance between coagulation and fibrinolysis, the inflammatory activity and cell proliferation. The endothelium even affects the function of other cell types, such us vascular smooth muscle cells, platelets, leukocytes, retinal pericytes, renal mesangial cells and macrophages through the production of several chemical mediators [23-28].

To maintain vascular homeostasis, the endothelium produces components of the extracellular matrix such as collagen and a variety of regulatory chemical mediators, including nitric oxide (NO), prostanoids (prostacycline), endothelin-1 (ET-1), angiotensin II (ANG-II), tissue-type plasminogen activator (t-PA), plasminogen activator inhibitor-1 (PAI-1), von Willebrand factor (VWF), adhesion molecules (VCAM, LAM, ICAM) and cytokines, among them Tumor Necrosis Factor α (TNFα) [29].

Under physiological circumstances, there is a balanced release of endothelial-derived relaxing factors such as NO and prostacyclin (PGI2) and contracting factors such as ET-1, prostaglandins and ANG-II. In endothelial dysfunction, this balance is altered, predisposing the onset and progression of atherosclerosis [30]. Risk factors such as hypercholesterolemia, dyslipidemia, smoking and diabetes initiate atherosclerosis through endothelial activation and therefore through endothelial dysfunction. Endothelial dysfunction is expressed in increased interactions with leykocytes, smooth muscle growth, vasoconstriction, impaired coagulation, vascular inflammation, thrombosis and atherosclerosis [31].

The role of endothelial dysfunction in type 2 diabetes is very complicated due to many independent factors involved including ageing, obesity, hyperlipidemia, hypertension, low grade inflammation, insulin resistance and hyperglycemia [32].

Hyperglycemia

Several prospective studies including a large number of patients with type 2 diabetes have shown that glycemic control is important for the risk of CVD [33-35]. However the risk was not particularly strong for coronary heart disease. The United Kingdom Prospective Diabetes Study (UKPDS) [36] and a 7-year follow up study conducted in Finland on 1059 patients with type 2 diabetes [33] showed that the most important risk factors for coronary heart disease were classic risk factors, particularly dyslipidemia (high total and LDL cholesterol, high total triglycerides and low HDL cholesterol). However, in both these studies poor glycemic control predicted coronary events but the association was much weaker than for classic risk factors.

Epidemiological analysis of the UKPDS [37] demonstrated that rising HbA1c was associated with increased risk of myocardial infarction and stroke. However, the increased hazard ratio was modest and reduction in HbA1c following insulin or sulfonylurea therapy did not significantly decrease the incidence of myocardial infarction or stroke [38], although long-term follow up demonstrated a significant reduction in atherosclerotic cardiovascular events [39]. The latter suggests a 'memory effect' of improved glycemic control, reminiscent of the Diabetes Control and Complications Trial (DCCT) in type 1 diabetic patients [40].

Hyperglycemia, in order to be considered a CV risk factor must contribute to processes leading to early atherosclerosis. The CATHAY study [41] has shown that, even in nondiabetic individuals, modest increments of plasma glucose concentration within the normal range are associated with impaired flow-mediated dilatation and increase of the intima-media thickness. Moreover, in prediabetic individuals both fasting and 2-h Oral Glucose Tolerance Test (OGTT) plasma glucose are inversely correlated with the number of circulating endothelial progenitor cells [42].

Several in vivo and in vitro studies have demonstrated the direct effect of hyperglycemia on endothelial cells. The endothelium plays an important role in the regulation of the vessel tone and in ensuring the integrity of the arterial wall. Under physiological conditions, the production of antiatherogenic factors (endothelin-1, angiotensin II, thromboxane) increases [43]. In diabetes, NO availability drops, while the activity of proatherogenic factors increases [43]. Exposure of endothelial cells to high glucose concentrations causes upregulation of endothelial NO synthase (eNOS) with accelerated production of free radicals and peroxynitrate with reduction of NO availability [44]. Moreover, hyperglycemia activates transcription factors such us the NF-κB that modulates the expression of genes coding for adhesion molecules and the activation of protein kinase C (PKC) [45]. The latter can phosphorylate p66Shc, allowing translocation of the protein from the cytosol into the mitochondrion resulting in activation of the respiratory chain and production of reactive oxygen species (ROS) [45]. As a consequence of increased ROS generation, the permeability of the mitochondrion increases with release of proapoptotic factors.

The arterial wall is also a critical target for the glycemic insult. Advanced glycation end products (AGEs) induce vascular stiffness, increase vascular permeability, initiate inflammation-mediated proliferative processes and propagate inflammation [46], modify low-density lipoproteins limiting their clearance and promote uptake by macrophages [47]. High glucose concentrations can also stimulate the proliferation of vascular smooth muscle cells and smooth muscle cell migration to the intima, where they participate in the formation of a fibrous cap. Alterations of glucose metabolism may affect the energy status of the heart. Glucose metabolism is a major myocardial energy source, but FFAs oxidation is a preferred source of energy in the resting aerobic state. Myocardial ischemia increases the rate of glucogen breakdown and glucose uptake via translocation of GLUT-4 to the sarcolemma [48]. This adaptive mechanism is important because glucose oxidation requires less oxygen than FFAs oxidation to maintain adenosine triphosphate (ATP) production. With relative insulin deficiency, as it may occur under conditions of insulin resistance or overt diabetes, such an adaptation in energy metabolism in response to acute ischemia is unlikely to occur. Thus, despite acute hyperglycemia, FFAs oxidation will remain the main source of energy with fewer ATP molecules generated. Catecholamine release in response to ischemia will result in a further release of FFAs, which may contribute to myocardial damage and risk of arrhythmia [49, 50].

Insulin Resistance

Insulin resistance is a characteristic abnormality in glucose metabolism in patients with prediabetes and type 2 diabetes. It is defined as the decreased ability of insulin to promote glucose uptake in skeletal muscle and adipose tissue and the decreased hepatic output of glucose. This may be present years before the development of abnormal plasma glucose levels becomes evident [51, 52]. Insulin resistance often coexists with elevated blood pressure, obesity, central obesity, elevated levels of total triglycerides, low levels of HDL cholesterol and hemostatic abnormalities. This clustering of CVD factors exists in nondiabetic individuals and patients with type 2 diabetes and predicts coronary heart disease [53, 54]. Whether hyperinsulinemia itself is a predictor of CVD has been debated [55]. A meta-analysis of published studies [56] showed that a weak positive association was found between high insulin levels and CVD events.

Insulin resistance and diabetes cause accelerated atherosclerosis via several mechanisms affecting endothelium, vascular wall, smooth muscle cells and platelets. Insulin resistance is associated with impaired vasodilatation, increased oxidative stress and high concentration of FFAs, vasoconstrictors, cellular adhesion molecules, PAI-1, cytokines and other mediators of low-grade inflammation and thrombosis formation. Type 2 diabetes further enhances these abnormalities and induces multiple adverse changes in the function and structure of vessel wall including excess formation of AGEs [57].

Insulin resistance is associated with an increased FFAs release from adipose tissue, which results in dyslipidemia, including VLDL-hypertriglyceridemia, high plasma FFAs and low HDL-cholesterol concentrations. High FFAs levels and hypertriglyceridemia are associated with endothelial dysfunction. FFA-mediated endothelial dysfunction is probably caused by reduced availability of L-arginine and/or NO and oxidative stress [58].

Insulin is a vasoactive hormone and enhances muscle blood flow and vasodilatation via stimulation of NO production. Insulin can also redirect blood flow in skeletal muscles so that more glucose can be uptaken by muscle cells. This is called capillary recruitment. In type 2 diabetes, hypertension and obesity, insulin's vasodilatating actions are impaired, probably because of low NO availability and action. Normally, stimulation of NO production by insulin is mediated by signaling pathways involving activation of Phosphoinositide-3 (PI-3) kinase leading to phosphorylation of eNOS. It is suggested that endothelial dysfunction and impaired capillary recruitment can cause insulin resistance because the microvascular endothelium cannot react properly to insulin and glucose disposal is decreased. This is called endothelial insulin resistance. The exact relationship between metabolic and endothelial insulin resistance is not fully understood. Both can be caused by TNFα and FFAs. Inflammatory cytokines like TNF-α can act as mediators of insulin resistance by impairing the tyrosine kinase activity of both the insulin receptor (IR) and insulin receptor substrate (IRS-1), thus inhibiting insulin signaling. It is suggested that hyperinsulinemia can lead to vascular inflammation which in turn causes insulin resistance and finally compensatory hyperinsulinemia. At physiological concentrations insulin exerts anti-inflammatory effects, while hyperinsulinemia increases levels of oxidative stress and inflammation.

A very important effect of insulin resistance is the fact that the normal route for insulin to activate the PI-3 kinase and Akt-dependent signaling pathways is impaired, whereas hyperinsulinemia overactivates Mitogen activated protein kinases (MAPK)-pathways, creating an imbalance between PI-3 kinase and MAP-kinase-dependent functions of insulin. This probably leads to decreased NO production and increased ET-1 secretion, characteristics of endothelial dysfunction. Through activation of the MAP-kinase signaling pathways, hyperinsulinemia promotes secretion of ET-1 and increases expression of VCAM-1 and E-selectin [59]. ET-1, a strong vasoconstrictor, can increase serine phosphorylation of IRS-1, causing a decreased activity of PI-3 kinase in vascular smooth muscle cells. Moreover, ET-1 may also impair insulin-stimulated translocation of GLUT-4 in adipocytes [60, 61].

Inflammation

Nowadays atherosclerosis is considered as an inflammatory disease. Inflammation is regarded as an important independent cardiovascular risk factor and is associated with endothelial dysfunction. The existence of chronic inflammation in diabetes is mainly based on the increased plasma concentrations of C-reactive protein (CRP), fibrinogen, interleukin-6, interleukin-1 and TNFα [62-64]. Inflammatory cytokines increase vascular permeability, change vasoregulatory responses, increase leukocyte adhesion to endothelium and facilitate thrombus formation by inducing procoagulant activity, inhibiting anticoagulant pathways and impairing fibrinolysis via stimulation of PAI-1. NF-κB consists of a family of transcription factors, which regulate the inflammatory response of vascular cells, by transcription of various cytokines which causes an increased adhesion of monocytes, neutrophils and macrophages, resulting in cell damage. NF-κB is activated by TNFα and IL-1 next to hyperglycemia, AGEs, ANG-II, oxidized lipids and insulin. Genes regulated by NF-κB are VCAM-1, E-selectin, ICAM-1, IL-1, IL-6, IL-8, tissue factor, PAI-1 and NOS.

The TNF family of cytokines plays an important role in regulating the immune response, inflammation and apoptosis. The first cytokine discovered was TNFα, which is produced by neutrophils, macrophages and adipocytes and can induce other cytokines such us IL-6 which in turn regulates the expression of CRP. CRP increases the expression of endothelial ICAM-1, VCAM-1, E-selectin, and MCP-1 and increases the secretion of ET-1. Moreover, CRP increases eNOS expression and elevates the expression of angiotensin receptor type 1 in the vessel wall [65, 66].

TNFα can induce insulin resistance and this is probably a part of the explanation why insulin resistance, endothelial dysfunction and athcrothrombosis are interrelated. Recent studies indicate that TNFα is likely involved in the pathogenesis of diabetic nephropathy and retinopathy.

Plasma levels of CRP are increased in both type 1 and type 2 diabetes. CRP plays a significant role in atherogenesis in endothelial cells, next to vascular smooth muscle cells and macrophages and several studies have shown that CRP levels predict cardiovascular disease [67]. CRP causes numerous proinflammatory and proatherogenic effects in endothelial cells such us decreased NO and prostacyclin, increased ET-1, cell adhesion molecules, MCP-1, IL-8 and PAI-1 [25].

Concommitant Metabolic Perturbations

Obesity

Obesity is a proatherogenic condition that predisposes to CVD via its major associated risk factors such as dyslipidemia, hypertension, insulin resistance and type 2 diabetes mellitus. Obesity represents a state of enlarged adipose tissue, low-grade inflammation and insulin resistance; hence it shares with diabetes common soil. There is a strong correlation between obesity and type 2 diabetes, with 80-95% diabetic patients being overweight or obese. Studies have shown that the risk of developing diabetes increases in proportion to BMI [68]. In addition, obesity exacerbates the metabolic abnormalities of type 2 diabetes, in particular hyperglycemia, dyslipidemia and hypertension [69]. Obese individuals are at higher risk of developing cardiovascular disease and the risk is even higher in those with type 2 diabetes who are obese [70]. In overweight and obese individuals with type 2 diabetes, weight loss is associated with improvements in risk factors. In fact, small amounts of weight loss (~ 5%) can improve glycemic control in type 2 diabetes [71, 72]. Longitudinal cohort studies indicate that changes in BMI in patients with type 2 diabetes are significant predictors of changes in HbA1c and blood pressure [73]. Similarly, lifestyle intervention trials in type 2 diabetic patients have shown that weight loss improves glycemic control, reduces blood pressure and improves lipid levels [74] and even a modest weight loss can result in an improved cardiovascular risk profile [75]. In patients with type 2 diabetes, intentional weight loss has been associated with a 28% reduction in cardiovascular disease and diabetes-related mortality [72]. The adipose tissue has become known to be a highly active endocrine organ, releasing hormones, cytokines and enzymes with the tendency to impair insulin sensitivity. It is an important modulator of endothelial function via secretion of several hormones including adiponectin, resistin, leptin, PAI-1, angiotensin, estradiol and the cytokines TNFα and IL-6. Several studies suggest that TNFα and IL-6 are both involved in obesity-related insulin resistance and that TNF is one of the most important mediators of inflammation [76]. In contrast to IL-6, TNFα is not secreted by adipocytes but by infiltrating macrophages in the adipose tissue and functions as a paracrine/autocrine factor [77, 78]. Adipose tissue is a significant source of circulating IL-6 and its secretion is related to BMI and adipocyte size [79]. TNFα and IL-6 are known to promote lipolysis and the secretion of FFAs, which contribute to an increase in hepatic glucose production and insulin resistance [80]. Both cytokines impair adipocyte differentiation and promote inflammation [81]. Moreover, IL-6 promotes inflammation not only in adipose tissue but in endothelial cells and liver cells [82]. It also promotes insulin resistance by interfering with the insulin signaling in adipose tissue [83]. Large adipocytes are more frequently found in subjects with impaired glucose tolerance and type 2 diabetes than those with a similar degree of adiposity but with normal glucose tolerance. Impaired adipocyte differentiation appears to be one of the most important factors in the progression of type 2 diabetes [84]. Elevated levels of intracellular FFAs can blunt the response to insulin leading to subsequent metabolic effects [85]. Ectopic lipid accumulation in the pancreas combined with diminished activation of the insulin receptor in adipocytes results in an impairment of insulin-stimulated glucose transport, a reduced anti-lipolytic effect, an increase in the amount of FFAs released, impaired preadipocyte differentiation and a decrease in lipoprotein lipase production and activity. These effects lead to the development of insulin resistance, type 2 diabetes and cardiovascular disease.

Hypertension

Patients with type 2 diabetes tend to develop hypertension, which is a major determinant of cardiovascular morbidity and mortality in this patient population. The UKPDS has shown that tight blood pressure control in diabetes patients significantly reduces the risks of macrovascular and microvascular complications. Though the mechanisms underlying the relationship among diabetes, hypertension, and cardiovascular events remain to be defined, microvascular insulin resistance and dysfunction have been implicated as a major culprit.

In healthy humans, insulin acts on the vascular endothelium to maintain vascular tone and integrity and thus adequate tissue perfusion. Insulin resistance causes endothelial dysfunction and impairs insulin-mediated increases in total muscle blood flow. In insulin resistant states, insulin action through the PI3-K/Akt/eNOS pathway is blunted but its signals through the MAPK pathway remain intact or are even enhanced, a phenomenon referred to as selective insulin resistance [86, 87]. This leads to decreased NO availability and same or enhanced ET-1 production, tilting the balance between ET-1 and NO production and resulting in increased vasoconstriction [88, 89].

Patients with diabetes tend to develop hypertension, which is an independent risk factor for cardiovascular events and contributes significantly to morbidity and mortality in patients with diabetes. Though the exact mechanisms underlying the propensity remain to be clarified, microvascular insulin resistance and dysfunction and microvascular structural abnormalities, together with renal damage, may play major role.

The renin angiotensin system (RAS) along with its role in the regulation of fluid and electrolyte balance and blood pressure, has also a major role in modulating vascular insulin sensitivity and endothelial function. The RAS is present both systemically and locally in many tissues, including the cardiovascular system [90, 91]. The major biologically active end-product of RAS is angiotensin II, which acts on both angiotensin type 1 receptors (AT1Rs) and type 2 receptors (AT2Rs) [90, 92]. The AT1R mediates the vast majority of the cardiovascular, renal and adrenal actions of angiotensin II, resulting in arterial vasoconstriction, aldosterone secretion, dipsogenic responses, sympathetic nervous system stimulation and renal sodium reabsorption. The cardiovascular RAS is upregulated in diabetes, a state that has been implicated in the development of many diabetic cardiovascular complications [90, 93, 94]. Hyperglycemia increases transcription of angiotensinogen and angiotensin II production from the local Angiotensing Converting Enzyme (ACE). The enhanced AT1R effects are particularly important in patients with pre-existing insulin resistance, as insulin resistance and RAS activation aggravate each other and facilitate vasoconstriction by reducing NO bioavailability and enhancing ET-1 production. These findings provide an explanation for the clinical observations that RAS inhibition improves endothelial dysfunction, slows the progression of microalbuminuria (which reflects endothelial dysfunction) and of early renal damage from diabetes and reduces cardiovascular morbidity and mortality in patients with diabetes [93].

Mixed Dyslipidemia

Diabetic dyslipidemia is characterized by high triglycerides (TG), low HDL-C and increased small dense LDL [95-99]. This atherogenic lipid profile contributes to the excess risk of CVD in people with type 2 diabetes mellitus. The dyslipidemia is partially corrected by the control of hyperglycemia, but abnormalities persist partly due to the effects of insulin resistance on lipoprotein metabolism [96, 99].

Increased hepatic production of VLDL, apolipoprotein B (apo B) and TG results from insulin resistance. Insulin deficiency increases mobilization of fatty acids from adipose tissue resulting in increased lipid availability in the liver for triglyceride synthesis and assembly with apo B into VLDL. Reduced ability of insulin to degrade newly synthesized apo B may also be important. Impaired lipolysis of circulating VLDL-TG results from decreased activity of the enzyme lipoprotein lipase, which is due to insulin deficiency. Hypertriglyceridemia in turn contributes to lower HDL-C levels and smaller cholesterol depleted LDL.

LDL-C levels in type 2 diabetic patients are usually the same or modestly elevated compared to non-diabetic individuals of similar age and sex. However, these LDL particles have abnormal composition (small, dense LDL particles) resulting in increased number of LDL particles that are cholesterol depleted [97].

Cholestrol ester transfer protein (CETP) mediates the exchange of VLDL-TG for LDL cholesterol. Increased levels of VLDL-TG in the presence of CETP promote the transfer of TG to LDL in exchange for LDL cholesterol. The TG-rich LDL undergoes hydrolysis by hepatic lipase (increased in insulin resistance), which produces small, dense cholesterol-depleted LDL. These small dense LDL particles are more atherogenic and more susceptible to oxidation of glycated LDL-cholesterol.

Low levels of HDL-C and apo A1 are also characteristic of type 2 diabetes. This is due largely to the interaction between HDL, TG-rich lipoproteins and the enzyme CETP, which transfers cholesterol esters from HDL to TG-rich lipoproteins. HDL-TG in turn is hydrolyzed by hepatic lipase which leads to smaller dense particles. Apo A1 is then rapidly cleared from the circulation due to these compositional changes, leading to fewer HDL particles.

Over the last century, the role of LDL cholesterol in atherosclerotic cardiovascular disease has become well established. A curvilinear relationship between levels of LDL cholesterol and prospective risk of coronary heart disease has been consistently demonstrated in population studies [100]. Lowering LDL cholesterol with lifestyle and pharmacological interventions in large placebo-controlled trials of both primary and secondary prevention [101-107] has shown significant benefits in terms of risk reduction.

Therapeutic Management of Cardiovascular Risk

Lifestyle Modification

It is well established that weight loss is beneficial for treating excessive adiposity, dyslipidemia, hypertension, insulin resistance and hyperglycemia [108] and the magnitude of weight loss doesn't need to be drastic. The Finnish Diabetes Prevention Study [109] and the Diabetes Prevention Program (DPP) [110] in the US both showed that lifestyle intervention with increased physical activity and reduction in dietary fat/calories, resulting in modest weight loss, significantly reduced the incidence of type 2 diabetes compared with the control groups. In addition, a weight loss of a small as a 5-10% of body weight can significantly reduce triglycerides and increase HDL cholesterol as well as improve blood pressure, fasting blood glucose, insulin and HbA1c.

Notably, the DPP demonstrated that weight loss was the number one predictor of reduction in the incidence of diabetes. In fact, for every kilogram of weight loss, the risk of diabetes development was decreased by 16%.

Diet

A decrease in caloric intake promotes a chronic negative energy balance resulting in weight loss. The macronutrient classification of the consumed calories may play a role in terms of the health benefits for patients with metabolic risk factors. Currently, most guidelines recommend a low-fat diet, which is associated with a fairly high carbohydrate intake. Due to the rise in popularity of low-carbohydrate diets, there has been interest in the effect of carbohydrate intake on serum lipid levels. Carbohydrate intake is positively associated with plasma TGs and negatively associated with HDL cholesterol. In addition, lower-carbohydrate diets have been associated with improved carbohydrate metabolism in patients with insulin resistance and/or type 2 diabetes. Although weight loss has been shown to be greater with lower carbohydrate diets in the short term, the effects on long term weight loss have been controversial. A diet high in complex, unrefined carbohydrates with an emphasis on fiber and low in added sugars is recommended for individuals with metabolic risk factors. This type of diet was recommended for participants in the lifestyle intervention group of the DPP (i.e. high carbohydrate, low fat), which contributed to weight loss and to a decrease in diabetes incidence.

The effects of total fat consumption on insulin sensitivity are variable. Nevertheless, evidence suggests that the type of fat consumed influences insulin sensitivity, with saturated fat being associated with insulin resistance and fasting insulin levels. Because saturated fat also increases LDL cholesterol and CVD risk, it is prudent to recommend a reduction in saturated fat intake (<7% of caloric intake) and an increase in the unsaturated fatty acids, specifically linoleic (5-10% of caloric intake) and α-linolenic (0.7-1.6% of caloric intake), as it is promoted by the US department of Agriculture guidelines [111]. Trans-fat consumption also relates to insulin resistance, CVD and type 2 diabetes. Thus, the intake of trans-fat should be restricted to <1% of total calories. Both serum cholesterol and overall CVD risk have been shown to be improved after a reduction in saturated fat and an increase in unsaturated fat consumption. The Nurses' Health Study reported that a 5% increase in saturated fat intake was associated with a 17% increase in coronary risk, whereas monounsaturated and polyunsaturated fat intake was inversely related to coronary disease.

In addition to the effects of diet on weight loss, other diet-related lifestyle modifications can have significant impact on blood pressure regulation. A clear positive association has been shown between sodium intake and blood pressure, with excessive sodium intake associated with hypertension. In addition, sodium restriction has been proven to be an important strategy in the prevention and treatment of hypertension and its associated comorbidities. The Dietary Approaches to Stop Hypertension (DASH) diet showed that lower sodium intake reduced blood pressure in patients with high-normal blood pressure and mild hypertension [112]. Guidelines therefore recommend that daily sodium intake should be restricted to no more than 1.5-2.3 g (65-100 mmol). In addition to sodium restriction, increased potassium intake has also been shown to improve blood pressure, especially in the setting of high sodium intake. Guidelines have recommended the intake of foods enriched with potassium, such as fruit and vegetables, with a goal of 3.5-4.7 g (90-120 mmol) of potassium pre day.

Summarizing, it is prudent to recommend a diet absent in trans-fat, low in saturated fat, higher in unsaturated fat, high in complex carbohydrates and low in sodium.

Physical Activity

A lifestyle intervention designed to increase physical activity and decrease body weight is another important approach for CVD risk modification. Higher cardiorespiratory fitness and increased self-reported physical activity have been shown to be inversely related to CVD mortality and to the incidence of IGT and type 2 diabetes. Even in the absence of weight loss, exercise has been shown to reduce visceral adipose tissue [113]. Exercise is also particularly effective at reducing insulin resistance and has also been shown to improve dyslipidemia and hypertension. Clinically, it may seem more difficult to elicit changes in physical activity in normally sedentary individuals than to prescribe insulin-sensitizing, antihypertensive and lipid-lowering medications, but exercise may be the best option for addressing each of these conditions without the added polypharmacy risk.

Glycemic Control

Most patients who have type 2 diabetes develop vascular complications despite a variety of available anti-diabetes medications and improved methods of assessing disease progression. The current disease model supports more aggressive treatment later in the course of the disorder and less aggressive treatment in its earlier stages. However, there is a growing argument to invert this treatment paradigm and aggressively identify and treat type 2 diabetes earlier in order to reduce the morbidity and mortality associated with advanced disease.

Approximately 24 million persons in the United States have diabetes, of which type 2 accounts for the vast majority of cases [114]. Based on the National Health and Nutrition Examination Survey (NHANES) 1999 to 2002 data, ~73 million Americans have diabetes or impaired fasting glucose (IFG), a condition that increases the risk for diabetes [115].

The present goal of type 2 diabetes therapy is to reduce HbA1c to <7% or ≤6.5%, according to guidelines set by the ADA and the American Association of Clinical Endocrinologists/American College of Endocrinology (AACE/ACE) respectively [116, 117].

Although many patients with type 2 diabetes are aware of HbA1c goals and are receiving therapy to lower their HbA1c, data from NHANES indicate that greater improvement in glycemic control is possible. NHANES data for 1999 to 2000 showed glycemic control rates (defined as the proportion of patients with HbA1c <7%) of 35.8% [118]. In NHANES 2003 to 2004, ~57% of patients diagnosed with diabetes achieved the HbA1c goal of <7% [119]. Thus, despite the abundance of available antidiabetes therapies, a considerable number of patients continue to have relatively poor glycemic control and are at risk for macrovascular and microvascular disease [118, 119]. It is important to consider that these guidelines do not represent a normalization of metabolic risk, but rather a consensus target for adequacy of risk management of glycemia related complications.

The incidence and prevalence of neuropathy, retinopathy and nephropathy increase with the duration of diabetes [120]. The UKPDS demonstrated that HbA1c is strongly related to microvascular effects in patients with type 2 diabetes. Over a mean follow-up of 10 years, which was equivalent to the duration of type 2 diabetes in the study, a 1% reduction in HbA1c was associated with a 37% reduction in microvascular complications and a 43% reduction in amputation or death from peripheral vascular disease [37]. During the same period, a reduction in the incidence of macrovascular complications, including stroke, myocardial infarction, heart failure and cataracts, was not as pronounced, ranging from 12% to 19% [37].

The UKPDS findings expand on the data from the DCCT, which showed a hyperbolic risk progression for microvascular complications as HbA1c increased in patients with type 1 diabetes [121, 122]. Patients in the intensive therapy group achieved a median HbA1c of 7.2%, compared with 9.1% in the conventional therapy group over a mean follow-up of 6.5 years. Intensive therapy reduced the adjusted mean risk for retinopathy 76% in the primary prevention cohort and reduced the occurrence of microalbuminuria 39% and of clinical neuropathy 60% in the combined primary and secondary intervention cohorts. In addition, UKPDS showed that the adjusted rate of microvascular events was ~14% in patients with type 2 diabetes who had HbA1c between 7% and 8% at study end [37].

Hyperglycemia, as measured by HbA1c, is a predictor of coronary heart disease (CHD) risk. In a Finnish study that followed elderly men and women (of whom ~16% and ~19% had type 2 diabetes, respectively at baseline) for up to 3.5 years, HbA1c >7.9% were associated with a 21% incidence of CHD-related events and a 12% incidence of CHD mortality [123]. In the Norfolk cohort of the European Prospective Investigation of Cancer and Nutrition (EPIC-Norfolk), 82% of the excess mortality associated with HbA1c ≥5% was accounted for by the 70% of the population whose HbA1c was between 5% and 6.9% [124]. It is not clear from these findings at which HbA1c percentage the transition from disease risk to accelerated event causation occurs.

The relation between glucose tolerance and the development of CVD has been investigated in several studies [125-128]. The Paris Prospective Study showed a 2-fold increase in CHD mortality in patients with IGT and a 2.5-fold increase in patients with known diabetes [125, 126, 128]. The Finnish study showed elevated fasting and postprandial insulin concentration to be strongly predictive of the development of coronary disease at 5 years, independent of other risk factors, including glucose concentrations [127, 128]. A meta-regression analysis of several longitudinal studies suggests a linear relation between both fasting and prandial glucose and CVD, with such risk extending into the nondiabetes range. This risk is somewhat stronger for prandial than for fasting glucose [129].

Data from the Nurses' Health Study showed that many individuals are at increased CV risk before the diagnosis of type 2 diabetes is made. In this analysis, the women who entered and remained nondiabetic throughout the study were assigned a baseline risk of 1. For women diagnosed with type 2 diabetes during the trial, there was a 2.82-fold increase in relative CV risk before their diagnosis and a 3.71-fold increased risk after their diagnosis. Women who had been diagnosed with type 2 diabetes before study entry had a 5-fold increased risk of CV events [130].

Despite mechanistic differences, standard treatment of patients with hyperglycemia has been shown to reduce the incidence of CV events. A meta-analysis involving 14 diabetes studies (including 8 in type 1 diabetes, involving 1,800 patients and 6 in type 2 diabetes, involving 4,472 patients) demonstrated that improved glycemic control, achieved through a reduction of HbA1c, reduced the incidence of macrovascular events in the evaluated trials for patients with diabetes [131]. Moreover, in another study, the control of postprandial plasma glucose was shown to lead to a regression of carotid atherosclerosis [132].

Several large studies provide evidence regarding the impact of intensive glycemic control on CV complications, including the Action to Control Cardiovascular Risk in Diabetes (ACCORD) study [133], the Diabetes and Vascular Disease: Preterax and Diamicron Modified Release Controlled Evaluation (ADVANCE) study [134], and the Veterans Affairs Diabetes Trial (VADT) [135]. None of these studies found a significant benefit for aggressive glucose lowering on CV events, although there was a reduction in microvascular complications, primarily through a decrease in the risk of nephropathy [134].

One controversial finding in the ACCORD study associated intensive antidiabetes management with increased mortality. This was not supported by the ADVANCE trial. Notably, patients in the ACCORD study had known heart disease or additional CV risk factors at baseline, a mean HbA1c of 8.3% and a 10-year duration of diabetes. Moreover, given the atherosclerotic profile of these patients, it is unclear whether the aggressive glycemic lowering actually may have led to greater plaque instability.

In the VADT, during a median 5.6-year follow up, no significant difference was seen between the intensive and standard therapy groups in any component of the primary outcome, which was time to occurrence of a major CV event that was a composite of MI, stroke, CV death, congestive heart failure, surgery for vascular disease, inoperable coronary disease and amputation for ischemic gangrene or in all-cause mortality between the 2 groups.

Post hoc analyses of these type 2 diabetes studies suggested that patients with a disease duration of <12 years may have benefited from intensive treatment [136]. Moreover, in a subset of patients who underwent coronary or aortic computed tomography calcium scoring at baseline, a lower coronary artery calcium score at baseline was associated with better outcomes with intensive therapy than was a higher calcium burden at baseline [136].

Similarly, the UKPDS study evaluated long term glucose control on atherosclerotic risk factors or events such as microvascular complications and MI. This included surviving patients from the original UKPDS cohort who underwent post-trial monitoring for up to 10 years post-intervention [137]. Patients in the treatment phase, which included conventional therapy (i.e. diet) or intensive therapy (i.e. sulfonylurea, metformin, insulin), reduced microvascular risk and emergent risk factors for MI and death from any cause. This was sustained over 10 years of follow-up.

Almost 50% of patients with type 2 diabetes have HbA1c above the generally recommended goal of <7%. However, microvascular complications may occur in many patients whose HbA1c is below the current target.

Macrovascular complications may represent the greatest cause of morbidity in patients with type 2 diabetes. Recent large studies, such as ACCORD and VADT, suggest that late adoption of intensive glycemic treatment may be detrimental to CV outcomes. Underlying atherosclerosis develops early in the course of the disease, when intensive glycemic control appears to be more advantageous. There is a growing need for improved biomarkers in order to identify and treat more aggressively patients at higher risk for microvascular and macrovascular complications.

Management of Hypertension

The more we appreciate the links between the increasing incidence of hypertension, type 2 diabetes and obesity throughout the years the more we understand the additional facets of the problem and therefore we can better understand the resistant nature of hypertension in many of these patients with such clustering of pathologies and therby attempt to address more and more of the individual components.

The current goal set forth for the treatment of hypertension in diabetic patients is to achieve a blood pressure less than 130/80 mm Hg. The intention of treating hypertension to a target range is to slow the progression of target organ damage or ideally to prevent it entirely. This is crucial because hypertension and type 2 diabetes act synergistically through endothelial damage. The pathologies to be delayed or prevented are coronary artery disease, left ventricular hypertrophy, renal disease and stroke.

Angiotensin-Converting Enzyme Inhibitors

Numerous large trials have demonstrated benefits attributed to angiotensin-converting enzyme (ACE) inhibitor therapy that addresses almost every site of target organ damage. In addition to the effective reduction of blood pressure, various studies have shown that ACE inhibitors reduce rates of death, myocardial infarction, stroke, diabetic retinopathy progression, microalbuminuria and congestive heart failure. Among other outcomes the HOPE trial has yielded data showing ramipril has beneficial effects on left ventricular structure and function [138] and prevented or delayed progression of microalbuminuria [139]. The EUCLID trial demonstrated a dramatic 50% reduction in retinopathy progression associated with the use of lisinopril in type 1 diabetic patients [140]. More recent trials such as the ONTARGET have not used a placebo arm but have only compared other agents with ACE inhibitors. Several studies suggest that ACE inhibitor use decreases the incidence of new-onset type 2 diabetes. These include the HOPE trial [141], the CAPP [142], ALLHAT [143] and ANBP-2 [143].

ACE inhibitors overall are quite well tolerated. Adverse drug reactions typically include dry cough and sometimes hyperkalemia. With all demonstrated benefits of ACE inhibitor therapy in the treatment of hypertension in patients with type 2 diabetes along with a relative low side-effect profile, this class of drugs is considered a first line choice for this indication.

Angiotensin Receptor Blockers

The angiotensin receptor blockers (ARBs) exert their effects in a very similar pharmacologic fashion to ACE inhibitors and numerous studies have demonstrated similar benefit derived between these two drug classes. Much data has come from the ONTARGET which compared the use of telmisartan with ramipril, each alone and also in combination. This trial reports noninferiority of the ARB telmisartan with the ACE inhibitor ramipril. The telmisartan group did have slightly greater reduction in blood pressure but had statistically equivalent rates of reduction in death from cardiovascular causes, myocardial infarction, stroke and hospitalization for heart failure. Additionally, the telmisartan group had a reduced incidence of cough and angioedema. However, corresponding to the greater reduction in blood pressure, there was an increased incidence of hypotension-related symptoms [144]. These results of class comparison are quite similar to those found previously in the VALIANT [145]. A noteworth aspect of ONTARGET and possibly the most important question that is answered is in regard to renal protection. Telmisartan therapy was found to reduce proteinuria and provide statistically equivalent nephroprotective benefit to ramipril. However, the combination of these two medications was inferior to either drug alone in preventing or slowing renal dysfunction and in fact increased its incidence [146]. Although hyperkalemia remains a potential adverse drug reaction associated with ARBs, the risk of cough associated with ACE inhibitors is eliminated. The risk of hyperkalemia may be lessened when combining the ARB with a thiazide or thiazide –type diuretic. The ARBs are also a first line choice in the treatment of hypertension and prevention of renal complications in diabetic patients.

Diuretics

Diuretics, specifically thiazide and thiazide-type diuretics have been in common use for the treatment of hypertension for many years as monotherapy and as frequent add-on agents. Numerous studies have shown their benefit in reducing blood pressure and target organ damage. The NORDIL study found diuretics to be equal in efficacy to β blockers and diltiazem in reducing the risk of myocardial infarction, cardiovascular death and stroke [147]. There is also evidence that thiazide diuretics provide benefit to elderly patients. This was demonstrated for elderly diabetic patients in the STOP Hypertension-2, in which a combination of hydrochlorothiazide and amiloride was found to be statistically equal in efficacy to β blockers, ACE inhibitors and calcium channel blockers in reducing cardiovascular death [148]. Although not specific to diabetic patients, further evidence in favor of diuretic use in elderly hypertensive patients was provided more recently by HYVET, which found significant benefit with indapamide with or without the addition of the ACE inhibitor perindopril [149].

Adrenergic Receptor Antagonists

The adrenergic receptor agents mostly fall into one of four categories: the 'traditional' β blockers, the α blockers (α1), combined α and β blockers and centrally acting α2 agonists. B blockers have been used for many years in the treatment of hypertension. The more β1-selective agents (eg atenolol, metoprolol and bisoprolol) have taken the forefront because of their cleaner mechanism of action and lower side-effect profile. Numerous trials have shown that β blockers improve nearly all parameters over placebo but the comparative evidence against other hypertensive agents seems conflicting. In a long term follow up study, atenolol has shown to provide comparable reduction in end points to captopril [150]. However, a more recent trial demonstrated the inferiority of atenolol to losartan [151].

Pure α1 receptor agonists have generally played little role in the treatment of hypertension in the diabetic population. Combined α and β blockers and chiefly carvedilol are widely used for patients with congestive heart failure. Centrally acting α2 agonists, specifically clonidine, remain a potent antihypertensive agent for patients with resistant hypertension.

Finally, the newest adrenergic receptor agent, nebivolol, is the most β1-selective agent and has also nitric oxide-dependent vasodilating properties. In a recent study, this property resulted in decreased endothelial cell stiffness as well as growth [152]. Clinical trials have demonstrated nebivolol to have statistically similar effects to atenolol on blood pressure reduction and aortic stiffness [153].

Calcium Channel Blockers

There is a sharp distinction in calcium channel blockers between the dihydropyridine and nondihydropyridine agents. Although the nondihydropiridines treat hypertension, they are more typically used in the setting of cardiac arrythmias. However, these agents are notable for reducing proteinuria to a similar extent as ACE inhibitors [154]. The dihydropyridines, such as amlodipine and felodipine, find more use in the treatment of hypertension in type 2 diabetic patients and obesity. One of the most noteworthy trials was the ACCOMPLISH trial, which compared the combination of benazepril and amlodipine with the combination of benazepril and hydrochlorothiazide. The amlodipine group was found to have fewer cardiovascular events in individuals who were at high risk for such events, such as diabetic patients [155]. These findings have led to an increase in the use of these agents as second or third line choice for patients at high risk for cardiac events.

Aldosterone Antagonists

The role of aldosterone and aldosterone antagonists, namely spironolactone and eplerenone, has been recognized for several years in advanced heart failure. More recent research has demonstrated that aldosterone plays a significant role in the development of insulin resistance and pancreatic β cell function [156]. Spironolactone has been demonstrated to be beneficial as an add-on agent for reducing blood pressure in patients with resistant hypertension, a problem encountered frequently in this population [157].

Renin Inhibitors

Aliskiren, a direct renin inhibitor, is one of the newer antihypertensive agents. Several studies have demonstrated the positive effects of aliskiren on reduction of blood pressure and target organ damage. It has been shown to be superior to hydrochlorothiazide in obese patients regarding blood pressure reduction and with fewer adverse drug reactions [158-159]. Aliskiren was proven to be as effective as an ARB in reduction of left ventricular mass in patients with hypertension and left ventricular hypertrophy [160]. Additionally, the combination of aliskiren and an ARB may have a synergistic effect on reduction of cardiovascular and renal injury [161]. Although this agent's precise place in clinical practice remains to be determined, it appears to be quite promising.

Management of Dyslipidemia

Advances in the treatment of lipid disorders during the last two decades have resulted in the ability to conduct clinical trials that have clearly demonstrated the benefits of management of dyslipidemia for the prevention of cardiovascular disease. People with type 2 diabetes derive particular benefit from the lowering of LDL cholesterol with HMG-CoA reductase inhibitors (statins), as recent clinical trials have shown. Other agents can also contribute to the management of diabetic dyslipidemia and therefore to the cardiovascular risk prevention.

Statins

HMG-CoA reductase inhibitors or statins are the most important advance in the treatment of lipid disorders since their introduction in 1987. Statins lower LDL cholesterol levels primarily via inhibition of hepatic cholesterol synthesis and up-regulation of LDL receptors. This increases the liver's receptor-mediated clearance of LDL and VLDL remnants. In mixed dyslipidemia (insulin resistance, type 2 diabetes), high dose statins also decrease production of apo B lipoproteins from the liver, which further lowers both VLDL and LDL levels [162]. Statins therefore are excellent for removal of atherogenic lipoproteins.

In the Scandinavian Simvastatin Survival Study, there was a 42% reduction in major coronary events in the simvastatin treated diabetics and a 48% reduction in coronary revascularization [163-164].

The largest study to date of cholesterol lowering in people with diabetes is the Heart Protection Study [165]. 20536 high risk subjects aged 40-80 years with coronary heart disease, peripheral vascular disease, diabetes or hypertension were randomized to simvastatin 40 mg or placebo, resulting in an average difference in LDL cholesterol of 39 mg/dl between the two groups. After 5 years of treatment, there was a 13% decrease in all cause mortality primarily due to a reduction in coronary death rate. They also observed a 27% decrease in major coronary events, 25% decrease in stroke and 25% decrease in revascularizations. There was a 22% decrease in major coronary events, strokes or revascularizations in the diabetic group compared to 24% for the overall population. The greatest risk reduction (33%) was in those without previous vascular disease. The risk reduction was independent of the baseline LDL cholesterol, glycemic control, duration or type of diabetes, age or presence of hypertension. The authors concluded that statin therapy was beneficial in patients with diabetes and should be considered routinely for all diabetic patients at high risk of major vascular events, independently of their initial cholesterol concentrations.

The Collaborative Atorvastatin Diabetes Study (CARDS) was a primary prevention trial that examined the effectiveness of LDL cholesterol lowering on major CV events in patients with type 2 diabetes and without elevated LDL cholesterol [166]. Median duration of follow-up was 3.9 years. Average treatment effect across the study was: total cholesterol -26%, LDL-C -40%, HDL-C +1%, TG -19%. These changes resulted in a 37% reduction in major cardiovascular events with atorvastatin. When the components of the primary endpoint were assessed separately, acute CHD events were reduced by 36%, coronary revascularizations by 31% and stroke by 48%. There was also a 27% reduction in death rate in the atorvastatin group. There was no evidence of a threshold level of baseline LDL-C for determining the benefit of statin therapy, and the authors suggested that all patients with diabetes would benefit from statin therapy, independent of baseline LDL-C. Although these results from CARDS were impressive, another study of similar design (ASPEN), also with atorvastatin, did not reach statistical significance [167].

The TNT study investigated whether intensive lipid lowering with high dose statin (atorvastatin 80 mg/day) provided significant clinical benefit compared to starting dose statin (atorvastatin 10 mg/dl) in patients with stable CHD. A post hoc subset analysis of the diabetic patients in the TNT study included 1501 of 10,001 patients with diabetes and CHD [168]. In order to qualify for the study, LDL-C levels were required to be < 130 mg/dl on atorvastatin 10 mg/dl. Subjects were randomized to either atorvastatin 10 mg or 80 mg daily, and followed for a median 4.9 years. Primary end-point was time to first major CV event (death from CHD, nonfatal MI, resuscitate cardiac arrest, or fatal/nonfatal stroke). End of study lipids were similar in the diabetic sub-group as the group overall (atorvastatin 10 vs 80 mg): LDL-C 99 vs 77 mg/dl; total cholesterol 178 vs 151 mg/dl; triglycerides 178 vs 145 mg/dl; HDL-C 44.0 vs 44.9 mg/dl. This difference in lipids resulted in a 25% reduction in risk of major CV events. There were also trends toward benefit with atorvastatin 80 mg for several primary endpoint components (non-procedure-related MI, fatal/nonfatal stroke and CHD death). Secondary outcomes showed significant benefit with atorvastatin 80 mg for cerebrovascular events and CV events. As in other studies, there was a higher incidence of events in subjects with diabetes than in the overall group. The authors concluded that the benefits of intensive cholesterol lowering with high dose statin were similar in subjects with and without diabetes and clinically evident CHD. They suggested that these results support the use of high-dose statins to achieve an LDL-C < 70 mg/dl as an appropriate therapeutic option in diabetic patients with CVD.

The Cholesterol Treatment Trialist Collaborators (CTTC) [169] performed a meta-analysis of 14 randomized trials of statin therapy in people with diabetes. They analyzed data from 18686 individuals. They found a 9% reduction in all-cause mortality per mmol/L reduction in LDL-C due to a significant reduction in vascular mortality. There was also a 21% reduction in major vascular events per mmol/L reduction in LDL-C due to a reduction in MI or coronary death, coronary revascularization and stroke. These results in individuals with diabetes were similar to those without diabetes (9% vs 13% reduction in all-cause mortality). The relative risk reduction was similar irrespective of previous history of vascular disease, baseline characteristics, lipid profile or type of diabetes.

Fibrates

Fibrates are most useful in patients with hypertriglyceridemia and low HDL-C. Fibrates activate peroxisome proliferator-activated receptor-alpha (PPARalpha), which is a member of the steroid hormone nuclear receptor superfamily, and modulates several aspects of lipid metabolism. Fibrates decrease triglycerides and VLDL levels by increasing VLDL catabolism and triglyceride clearance. This is achieved through an increase in lipoprotein lipase (LPL) activity, and a decrease in ApoC-III production (an inhibitor of LPL). Fibrates also initiate a shift from small, dense, atherogenic LDL particles to large, less atherogenic LDL particles. Fibrates increase HDL production by increasing ApoAI and ApoAII synthesis, and stimulate reverse cholesterol transport by increasing synthesis of the ATP binding cassette A1 (ABCA1) transporter [170].

The Helsinki heart study (HHS) was a primary prevention trial with gemfibrozil in middle-aged men with high non-HDL-C (> 200 mg/dL) [171]. 135 of 4081 subjects enrolled in the HHS had known T2DM [172]. The incidence of MI and cardiac death was higher in the subjects with T2DM than non-diabetic subjects (7.4% vs 3.3%). Changes in lipid and lipoprotein levels in the gemfibrozil treated diabetic subjects were similar to those in non-diabetic subjects

The Veterans affairs HDL-C intervention trial (VA-HIT) was also a secondary prevention trial with gemfibrozil in 2531 men with known CHD [173]. This population was different from HHS in that the VA-HIT subjects were selected for low HDL-C (< 40 mg/dl) and "normal" LDL-C (< 140 mg/dl). Primary outcome was nonfatal myocardial infarction (MI) or coronary death. During the trial, the effect on lipids at 1 year was: HDL-C 6% higher, TG 31% lower, total cholesterol 4% lower and LDL-C was not different in the gemfibrozil compared to the placebo group. The trial reported a 22% reduction in nonfatal MI or CHD death, and a 24% reduction in the combined endpoint of CHD death, nonfatal MI and stroke. Of the lipid changes reported in the study, only the increase in HDL-C significantly predicted a lower risk of CHD [174]. 30% of subjects in VA-HIT had known (n=627) or undiagnosed (n=142) diabetes [175]. As expected, the event rates for major CV events in the placebo group with known (36.5%) and undiagnosed (34.3%) diabetes was higher than in non-diabetic group with normal fasting glucose (21%). Gemfibrozil treatment was associated with a risk reduction for the combined end point of 32% for subjects with diabetes compared to 18% for those without diabetes. Both groups had comparable 22–21% reduction in nonfatal MI. The group with diabetes had 41% reduction in CHD death and 40% reduction in stroke compared to a non-significant reduction in the non-diabetic group of 3% and 10%, respectively. The rate of new CV events and reduction of events with gemfibrozil was greatest in subjects with insulin resistance (as estimated by HOMA-IR) than without [176]. The benefit of fibrate therapy was less dependent on levels of HDL-C or TG than on presence or absence of insulin resistance.

The Fenofibrate intervention and event lowering in diabetes (FIELD) study [177] was a cardiovascular outcome study with another fibrate (fenofibrate) in individuals with Type 2 DM aged 50–75 years not taking statin at study entry. 2131 (21%) of the subjects had known CVD and 7664 were without CVD at study entry. Lipids to qualify for the study were: cholesterol 116–251 mg/dl and chol/HDL>4.0 or TG 89–444 mg/dl. Subjects were randomized to fenofibrate 200 mg/day or placebo and followed for an average of 5 years. Primary study outcome was coronary events (CHD death or non-fatal MI). Outcome for pre-specified subgroup analyses was: total CV events (composite of CV death, MI, stroke, coronary and carotid revascularization). The effect of fenofibrate on lipids at the end of study (fenofibrate vs placebo) was: total cholesterol reduced 7.2%, LDL-C reduced 6.5%, TG reduced 21%, HDL-C increased < 1%. There was no difference in coronary events between the two groups (5.9% placebo vs 5.2% fenofibrate). The relative reduction of 11% consisted of a 24% reduction in non-fatal MI but a nonsignificant increase in CHD mortality. Total CV events were reduced significantly by 11%, primarily due to a 21% reduction in coronary revascularization. The authors' concluded that fenofibrate did not significantly reduce risk of coronary events (primary outcome). Fenofibrate did reduce total CV events, mainly due to fewer non-fatal MI and revascularizations. However, the higher rate of starting statin therapy in the placebo group compared to the fenofibrate group made it difficult to determine the benefit of fenofibrate treatment. The authors speculated that the use of fenofibrate should be considered in the context of the well established benefits of statin therapy, and that its main use will probably be in combination with a statin. Although the addition of fenofibrate to a statin can be effective for the treatment of mixed dyslipidemia [178], the additional benefit in terms of CV outcomes is unknown [179].

The ACCORD trial addressed the question of the potential benefit of adding fenofibrate to statin therapy for prevention of CVD in patients with type 2 diabetes mellitus who were at high risk for cardiovascular disease. The combination of fenofibrate and simvastatin did not reduce the rate of fatal cardiovascular events, nonfatal myocardial infarction, or nonfatal stroke, as compared with simvastatin alone [180].

Niacin

Nicotinic acid is the most effective agent available for raising HDL-C and lowering triglycerides. However, the only cardiovascular outcome study to date with niacin is the Coronary Drug Project. This study reported a modest benefit in decreasing myocardial infarctions after 15 years of follow-up [181]. A small angiographic study (HATS) did show improvement in coronary stenosis and clinical benefits with 3 years treatment with simvastatin and niacin [182]. A recent study also reported a significant regression of carotid intima-media thickness and major cardiovascular events with niacin in combination with statin [183].

Nicotinic acid should be used with caution in patients with diabetes, as it may worsen plasma glucose levels [184, 185]. This effect appears to be modest and reversible, especially if low doses are used [186]. The adverse effect of niacin on glucose metabolism appears to be secondary to worsening insulin resistance [187].

Ezetimibe

The cholesterol absorption inhibitor ezetimibe can lower LDL-C by about 15–20% [188]. This agent is most useful in combination with statins. A cardiovascular outcome study comparing ezetimibe plus simvastatin versus simvastatin alone is currently on-going [189]. A study in type 2 diabetes on carotid atherosclerosis showed that equivalent LDL-C reductions with a statin plus ezetimibe vs a statin alone resulted in similar regression of common carotid artery intima-media thickness [190, 191].

Conclusion

Patients with type 2 diabetes mellitus display a high risk for cardiovascular disease, with these two conditions sharing a common pathogenesis. Diabetes leads to the appearance of cardiovascular complications via several mechanisms, such as hyperglycemia, inflammation, oxidation and insulin resistance. Concomitant metabolic perturbations including obesity and hypertension frequently coexist and aggravate the effect of impaired glucose metabolism on cardiovascular function. The management of cardiovascular risk ought to be multifactorial in order to confront all the aspects of the problem via lifestyle changes (dietary intervention, exercise) as well as using appropriate medications in order to improve glycemic control, hypertension and lipid metabolism.

References

[1]   West KM. *Epidemiology of diabetes and its vascular lesions*. New York, Elsevier, 1978.

[2]   Vasan RS, Pencina MJ, Cobain M et al. Estimated risks for developing obesity in the Framingham Heart Study. *Ann Intern Med* 2005;143:473-80.

[3]   Fox CS, Pencina MJ, Meigs JB et al. Trends in the incidence of type 2 diabetes mellitus from the 1970s to the 1990s: the Framingham Heart Study. *Circulation* 2006;113:2914-8.

[4]   Fox CS, Coady S, Sorlie PD et al. Trends in cardiovascular complications of diabetes. *JAMA* 2004;292:2495-9.

[5]   Fox CS, Coady S, Sorlie PD et al. Increasing cardiovascular disease burden due to diabetes mellitus: the Framingham Heart Study. *Circulation* 2007;115:1544-50.

[6]   Levitzky YS, Pencina MJ, D'Agostino RB et al. Impact of impaired fasting glucose on cardiovascular disease: the Framingham Heart Study. *J Am Coll Cardiol* 2008;51:264-70.

[7]   Wilson PW, Kannel WB, Silbershatz H, D'Agostino RB. Clustering of metabolic factors and coronary heart disease. *Arch Intern Med* 1999;159:1104-9.

[8]   Meigs JB, D'Agostino RB Sr, Wilson PW et al. Risk variable clustering in the insulin resistance syndrome. The Framingham Offspring Study. *Diabetes* 1997;46:1594-600.

[9]   Meigs JB. Metabolic syndrome and risk for type 2 diabetes. *Expert Rev Endocrin Metab* 2006;1:57-66.

[10] Wilson PW, D'Agostino RB, Parise H et al. Metabolic syndrome as a precursor of cardiovascular disease and type 2 diabetes mellitus. *Circulation* 2005;112:3066-72.

[11] Meigs JB, Wilson PW, Fox CS et al. Body mass index, metabolic syndrome, and risk of type 2 diabetes or cardiovascular disease. *J Clin Endocrinol Metab* 2006;91:2906-12.

[12] Yudkin JS, Eringa E, Stehouwer CD. "Vasocrine" signalling from perivascular fat: a mechanism linking insulin resistance to vascular disease. *Lancet* 2005;365:1817-20.

[13] Hivert MF, Sullivan LM, Fox CS et al. Associations of adiponectin, resistin, and tumor necrosis factor-alpha with insulin resistance. *J Clin Endocrinol Metab*;93:3165-72.

[14] Prokopenko I, Langenberg C, Florez JC et al. Variants in MTNR1B influence fasting glucose levels. *Nat Genet* 2009;41:77-81.

[15] Dupuis J, Langenberg C, Prokopenko I et al. New genetic loci implicated in fasting glucose homeostasis and their impact on type 2 diabetes risk. *Nat Genet* 2010;42:105-16.

[16] Saxena R, Hivert MF, Langenberg C et al,. Genetic variation in GIPR influences the glucose and insulin responses to an oral glucose challenge. *Nat Genet* 2010;42:142-8.

[17] Meigs JB, Shrader P, Sullivan LM et al. Genotype score in addition to common risk factors for prediction of type 2 diabetes. *N Engl J Med* 2008;359:2208-19.

[18] Stamler J, Vaccaro O, Neaton JD, Wentworth D. Diabetes, other risk factors, and 12-yr cardiovascular mortality for men screened in the Multiple Risk Factor Intervention Trial. *Diabetes Care* 1993;16:434-44.

[19] Mazzone T, Chait A, Plutzky J. Cardiovascular disease risk in type 2 diabetes mellitus: insights from mechanistic studies. *Lancet* 2008;371:1800-9.

[20] Sniderman AD, Scantlebury T, Cianflone K. Hypertriglyceridemic hyperapob: the unappreciated atherogenic dyslipoproteinemia in type 2 diabetes mellitus. *Ann Intern Med* 2001;135:447-59.

[21] Steinberg HO, Tarshoby M, Monestel R et al. Elevated circulating free fatty acid levels impair endothelium-dependent vasodilation. *J Clin Invest* 1997;100:1230-9.

[22] Moore RE, Navab M, Millar JS et al. Increased atherosclerosis in mice lacking apolipoprotein A-I attributable to both impaired reverse cholesterol transport and increased inflammation. *Circ Res* 2005;97:763-71.

[23] De Caterina R. Endothelial dysfunctions: common denominators in vascular disease. *Curr Opin Lipidol* 2000;11:9-23.

[24] Stehouwer CD, Lambert J, Donker AJ, van Hinsbergh VW. Endothelial dysfunction and pathogenesis of diabetic angiopathy. *Cardiovasc Res* 1997;34:55-68.

[25] Schalkwijk CG, Stehouwer CD. Vascular complications in diabetes mellitus: the role of endothelial dysfunction. *Clin Sci (Lond)* 2005;109:143-59.

[26] Cubbon RM, Rajwani A, Wheatcroft SB. The impact of insulin resistance on endothelial function, progenitor cells and repair. Diab Vasc Dis Res 2007;4:103-11.

[27] Hadi HA, Suwaidi JA. Endothelial dysfunction in diabetes mellitus. *Vasc Health Risk Manag* 2007;3(6):853-76.

[28] Libby P. Inflammation in atherosclerosis. *Nature* 2002;420:868-74.

[29] Quyyumi AA. Endothelial function in health and disease: new insights into the genesis of cardiovascular disease. *Am J Med* 1998;105:32S-39S.

[30] Tan KC, Chow WS, Ai VH, Lam KS. Effects of angiotensin II receptor antagonist on endothelial vasomotor function and urinary albumin excretion in type 2 diabetic patients with microalbuminuria. *Diabetes Metab Res Rev* 2002;18:71-6.

[31] Verma S, Anderson TJ. Fundamentals of endothelial function for the clinical cardiologist. *Circulation* 2002;105:546-9.

[32] Calles-Escandon J, Cipolla M. Diabetes and endothelial dysfunction: a clinical perspective. *Endocr Rev* 2001;22:36-52.

[33] Lehto S, Rönnemaa T, Haffner SM et al. Dyslipidemia and hyperglycemia predict coronary heart disease events in middle-aged patients with NIDDM. *Diabetes* 1997;46:1354-9.

[34] Kuusisto J, Mykkänen L, Pyörälä K, Laakso M. NIDDM and its metabolic control predict coronary heart disease in elderly subjects. *Diabetes* 1994;43:960-7.

[35] Kuusisto J, Mykkänen L, Pyörälä K, Laakso M. Non-insulin-dependent diabetes and its metabolic control are important predictors of stroke in elderly subjects. *Stroke* 1994;25:1157-64.

[36] Turner RC, Millns H, Neil HA et al. Risk factors for coronary artery disease in non-insulin dependent diabetes mellitus: United Kingdom Prospective Diabetes Study (UKPDS: 23). *BMJ* 1998;316:823-8.

[37] Stratton IM, Adler AI, Neil HA et al. Association of glycaemia with macrovascular and microvascular complications of type 2 diabetes (UKPDS 35): prospective observational study. *BMJ* 2000;321:405-12.

[38] UK Prospective Diabetes Study (UKPDS) Group. Intensive blood-glucose control with sulphonylureas or insulin compared with conventional treatment and risk of complications in patients with type 2 diabetes (UKPDS 33). *Lancet* 1998;352:837-53.

[39] Holman RR, Paul SK, Bethel MA et al. 10-year follow-up of intensive glucose control in type 2 diabetes. *N Engl J Med* 2008;359:1577-89.

[40] Nathan DM, Cleary PA, Backlund JY et al; Diabetes Control and Complications Trial/Epidemiology of Diabetes Interventions and Complications (DCCT/EDIC) Study Research Group. Intensive diabetes treatment and cardiovascular disease in patients with type 1 diabetes. *N Engl J Med* 2005;353:2643-53.

[41] Thomas GN, Chook P, Qiao M et al. Deleterious impact of "high normal" glucose levels and other metabolic syndrome components on arterial endothelial function and intima-media thickness in apparently healthy Chinese subjects: the CATHAY study. *Arterioscler Thromb Vasc Biol* 2004;24:739-43.

[42] Fadini GP, Pucci L, Vanacore R et al. Glucose tolerance is negatively associated with circulating progenitor cell levels. *Diabetologia* 2007;50:2156-63.

[43] Nacci C, Tarquinio M, Montagnani M. Molecular and clinical aspects of endothelial dysfunction in diabetes. *Intern Emerg Med* 2009;4:107-16.

[44] Cosentino F, Hishikawa K, Katusic ZS, Lüscher TF. High glucose increases nitric oxide synthase expression and superoxide anion generation in human aortic endothelial cells. *Circulation* 1997;96:25-8.

[45] Gutierrez J, Ballinger SW, Darley-Usmar VM, Landar A. Free radicals, mitochondria, and oxidized lipids: the emerging role in signal transduction in vascular cells. *Circ Res* 2006;99:924-32.

[46] Yan SF, Ramasamy R, Naka Y, Schmidt AM. Glycation, inflammation, and RAGE: a scaffold for the macrovascular complications of diabetes and beyond. *Circ Res* 2003;93:1159-69.

[47] Cai W, He JC, Zhu L et al. High levels of dietary advanced glycation end products transform low-density lipoprotein into a potent redox-sensitive mitogen-activated protein kinase stimulant in diabetic patients. *Circulation* 2004;110:285-91.

[48] Young LH, Renfu Y, Russell R et al. Low-flow ischemia leads to translocation of canine heart GLUT-4 and GLUT-1 glucose transporters to the sarcolemma in vivo. *Circulation* 1997;95:415-22.

[49] Oliver MF, Yates PA. Induction of ventricular arrhythmias by elevation of arterial free fatty acids in experimental myocardial infarction. *Cardiology* 1971;56:359-64.

[50] Kurien VA, Yates PA, Oliver MF. The role of free fatty acids in the production of ventricular arrhythmias after acute coronary artery occlusion. Eur J Clin Invest 1971;1:225-41.

[51] Ouchi N, Kihara S, Arita Y et al. Adipocyte-derived plasma protein, adiponectin, suppresses lipid accumulation and class A scavenger receptor expression in human monocyte-derived macrophages. *Circulation* 2001;103:1057-63.

[52] Desideri G, Ferri C, Bellini C et al. Effects of ACE inhibition on spontaneous and insulin-stimulated endothelin-1 secretion: in vitro and in vivo studies. *Diabetes* 1997;46:81-6.

[53] Lempiäinen P, Mykkänen L, Pyörälä K et al. Insulin resistance syndrome predicts coronary heart disease events in elderly nondiabetic men. *Circulation* 1999;100:123-8.

[54] Lehto S, Rönnemaa T, Pyörälä K, Laakso M. Cardiovascular risk factors clustering with endogenous hyperinsulinaemia predict death from coronary heart disease in patients with Type II diabetes. *Diabetologia* 2000;43:148-55.

[55] Laakso M. Insulin resistance and coronary heart disease. *Curr Opin Lipidol* 1996;7:217-26.

[56] Ruige JB, Assendelft WJ, Dekker JM et al. Insulin and risk of cardiovascular disease: a meta-analysis. *Circulation* 1998;97:996-1001.

[57] Laakso M. Cardiovascular disease in type 2 diabetes: challenge for treatment and prevention. *J Intern Med* 2001;249:225-35.

[58] Taskinen MR. Type 2 diabetes as a lipid disorder. *Curr Mol Med* 2005;5:297-308.

[59] Kim JA, Montagnani M, Koh KK, Quon MJ. Reciprocal relationships between insulin resistance and endothelial dysfunction: molecular and pathophysiological mechanisms. *Circulation* 2006;113:1888-904.

[60] Jiang ZY, Zhou QL, Chatterjee A et al. Endothelin-1 modulates insulin signaling through phosphatidylinositol 3-kinase pathway in vascular smooth muscle cells. *Diabetes* 1999;48:1120-30.

[61] Strawbridge AB, Elmendorf JS. Endothelin-1 impairs glucose transporter trafficking via a membrane-based mechanism. *J Cell Biochem* 2006;97:849-56.

[62] Folsom AR, Rosamond WD, Shahar E et al. Prospective study of markers of hemostatic function with risk of ischemic stroke. The Atherosclerosis Risk in Communities (ARIC) Study Investigators. *Circulation* 1999;100:736-42.

[63] Grau AJ, Buggle F, Becher H et al. The association of leukocyte count, fibrinogen and C-reactive protein with vascular risk factors and ischemic vascular diseases. *Thromb Res* 1996;82:245-55.

[64] Shurtz-Swirski R, Sela S, Herskovits AT et al. Involvement of peripheral polymorphonuclear leukocytes in oxidative stress and inflammation in type 2 diabetic patients. *Diabetes Care* 2001;24:104-10.

[65] Venugopal SK, Devaraj S, Yuhanna I et al. Demonstration that C-reactive protein decreases eNOS expression and bioactivity in human aortic endothelial cells. *Circulation* 2002;106:1439-41.

[66] Pasceri V, Willerson JT, Yeh ET. Direct proinflammatory effect of C-reactive protein on human endothelial cells. *Circulation* 2000;102:2165-8.

[67] Venugopal SK, Devaraj S, Jialal I. Effect of C-reactive protein on vascular cells: evidence for a proinflammatory, proatherogenic role. *Curr Opin Nephrol Hypertens* 2005;14:33-7.

[68] Narayan KM, Boyle JP, Thompson TJ et al. Effect of BMI on lifetime risk for diabetes in the U.S. *Diabetes Care* 2007;30:1562-6.

[69] Maggio CA, Pi-Sunyer FX. The prevention and treatment of obesity. Application to type 2 diabetes. *Diabetes Care* 1997;20:1744-66.

[70] Jonsson S, Hedblad B, Engström G et al. Influence of obesity on cardiovascular risk. Twenty-three-year follow-up of 22,025 men from an urban Swedish population. *Int J Obes Relat Metab Disord* 2002;26:1046-53.

[71] Goldstein DJ. Beneficial health effects of modest weight loss. *Int J Obes Relat Metab Disord* 1992;16:397-415.

[72] Williamson DF, Thompson TJ, Thun M et al. Intentional weight loss and mortality among overweight individuals with diabetes. *Diabetes Care* 2000;23:1499-504.

[73] Ridderstråle M, Gudbjörnsdottir S, Eliasson B et al; Steering Committee of the Swedish National Diabetes Register (NDR). Obesity and cardiovascular risk factors in type 2 diabetes: results from the Swedish National Diabetes Register. *J Intern Med* 2006;259:314-22.

[74] Look AHEAD Research Group, Pi-Sunyer X, Blackburn G, Brancati FL et al. Reduction in weight and cardiovascular disease risk factors in individuals with type 2 diabetes: one-year results of the look AHEAD trial. *Diabetes Care* 2007;30:1374-83.

[75] Ratner R, Goldberg R, Haffner S et al; Diabetes Prevention Program Research Group. Impact of intensive lifestyle and metformin therapy on cardiovascular disease risk factors in the diabetes prevention program. *Diabetes Care* 2005;28:888-94.

[76] Kern PA, Ranganathan S, Li C et al. Adipose tissue tumor necrosis factor and interleukin-6 expression in human obesity and insulin resistance. *Am J Physiol Endocrinol Metab* 2001;280:E745-51.

[77] Mohamed-Ali V, Goodrick S, Rawesh A et al. Subcutaneous adipose tissue releases interleukin-6, but not tumor necrosis factor-alpha, in vivo. J Clin Endocrinol Metab 1997;82:4196-200.

[78] Xu H, Uysal KT, Becherer JD et al. Altered tumor necrosis factor-alpha (TNF-alpha) processing in adipocytes and increased expression of transmembrane TNF-alpha in obesity. *Diabetes* 2002;51:1876-83.

[79] Sopasakis VR, Sandqvist M, Gustafson B et al. High local concentrations and effects on differentiation implicate interleukin-6 as a paracrine regulator. *Obes Res* 2004;12:454-60.

[80] Hotamisligil GS, Arner P, Caro JF et al. Increased adipose tissue expression of tumor necrosis factor-alpha in human obesity and insulin resistance. *J Clin Invest* 1995;95:2409-15.

[81] Gustafson B, Smith U. Cytokines promote Wnt signaling and inflammation and impair the normal differentiation and lipid accumulation in 3T3-L1 preadipocytes. *J Biol Chem* 2006;281:9507-16.

[82] Klover PJ, Clementi AH, Mooney RA. Interleukin-6 depletion selectively improves hepatic insulin action in obesity. *Endocrinology* 2005;146:3417-27.

[83] Rotter V, Nagaev I, Smith U. Interleukin-6 (IL-6) induces insulin resistance in 3T3-L1 adipocytes and is, like IL-8 and tumor necrosis factor-alpha, overexpressed in human fat cells from insulin-resistant subjects. *J Biol Chem* 2003;278:45777-84.

[84] Weyer C, Foley JE, Bogardus C et al. Enlarged subcutaneous abdominal adipocyte size, but not obesity itself, predicts type II diabetes independent of insulin resistance. *Diabetologia* 2000;43:1498-506.

[85] Hotamisligil GS. Inflammation and metabolic disorders. *Nature* 2006;444:860-7.

[86] Kim JA, Montagnani M, Koh KK, Quon MJ. Reciprocal relationships between insulin resistance and endothelial dysfunction: molecular and pathophysiological mechanisms. *Circulation* 2006;113:1888-904.

[87] Kim JA, Koh KK, Quon MJ. The union of vascular and metabolic actions of insulin in sickness and in health. *Arterioscler Thromb Vasc Biol* 2005;25:889-91.

[88] Potenza MA, Marasciulo FL, Chieppa DM et al. Insulin resistance in spontaneously hypertensive rats is associated with endothelial dysfunction characterized by imbalance between NO and ET-1 production. *Am J Physiol Heart Circ Physiol* 2005;289:H813-22.

[89] Eringa EC, Stehouwer CD, Merlijn T et al. Physiological concentrations of insulin induce endothelin-mediated vasoconstriction during inhibition of NOS or PI3-kinase in skeletal muscle arterioles. *Cardiovasc Res* 2002;56:464-71.

[90] Carey RM, Siragy HM. Newly recognized components of the renin-angiotensin system: potential roles in cardiovascular and renal regulation. *Endocr Rev* 2003;24:261-71.

[91] Paul M, Poyan Mehr A, Kreutz R. Physiology of local renin-angiotensin systems. *Physiol Rev* 2006;86:747-803.

[92] Carey RM. Cardiovascular and renal regulation by the angiotensin type 2 receptor: the AT2 receptor comes of age. *Hypertension* 2005;45:840-4.

[93] Liu Z. The renin-angiotensin system and insulin resistance. *Curr Diab Rep* 2007;7:34-42.

[94] Lim HS, MacFadyen RJ, Lip GY. Diabetes mellitus, the renin-angiotensin-aldosterone system, and the heart. *Arch Intern Med* 2004;164:1737-48.

[95] Goldberg IJ. Clinical review 124: Diabetic dyslipidemia: causes and consequences. *J Clin Endocrinol Metab* 2001;86:965-71.

[96] Garvey WT, Kwon S, Zheng D et al. Effects of insulin resistance and type 2 diabetes on lipoprotein subclass particle size and concentration determined by nuclear magnetic resonance. *Diabetes* 2003;52:453-62.

[97] Krauss RM. Lipids and lipoproteins in patients with type 2 diabetes. *Diabetes Care* 2004;27:1496-504.

[98] Boden G, Laakso M. Lipids and glucose in type 2 diabetes: what is the cause and effect? *Diabetes Care* 2004;27:2253-9.

[99] Ginsberg HN, Zhang YL, Hernandez-Ono A. Regulation of plasma triglycerides in insulin resistance and diabetes. *Arch Med Res* 2005;36:232-40.

[100] Stamler J, Wentworth D, Neaton JD. Is relationship between serum cholesterol and risk of premature death from coronary heart disease continuous and graded? Findings in 356,222 primary screenees of the Multiple Risk Factor Intervention Trial (MRFIT). *JAMA* 1986;256:2823-8.

[101] Randomised trial of cholesterol lowering in 4444 patients with coronary heart disease: the Scandinavian Simvastatin Survival Study (4S). *Lancet* 1994;344:1383-9.

[102] Prevention of cardiovascular events and death with pravastatin in patients with coronary heart disease and a broad range of initial cholesterol levels. The Long-Term Intervention with Pravastatin in Ischaemic Disease (LIPID) Study Group. *N Engl J Med* 1998;339:1349-57.

[103] Heart Protection Study Collaborative Group. MRC/BHF Heart Protection Study of cholesterol lowering with simvastatin in 20,536 high-risk individuals: a randomised placebo-controlled trial. *Lancet* 2002;360:7-22.

[104] Downs JR, Clearfield M, Weis S et al. Primary prevention of acute coronary events with lovastatin in men and women with average cholesterol levels: results of AFCAPS/TexCAPS. Air Force/Texas Coronary Atherosclerosis Prevention Study. *JAMA* 1998;279:1615-22.

[105] Sacks FM, Pfeffer MA, Moye LA et al. The effect of pravastatin on coronary events after myocardial infarction in patients with average cholesterol levels. *Cholesterol and Recurrent Events* Trial investigators. *N Engl J Med* 1996;335:1001-9.

[106] Shepherd J, Cobbe SM, Ford I et al. Prevention of coronary heart disease with pravastatin in men with hypercholesterolemia. West of Scotland Coronary Prevention Study Group. *N Engl J Med* 1995;333:1301-7.

[107] Ridker PM, Danielson E, Fonseca FA ct al; JUPITER Study Group. Rosuvastatin to prevent vascular events in men and women with elevated C-reactive protein. *N Engl J Med* 2008;359:2195-207.

[108] Pasanisi F, Contaldo F, de Simone G, Mancini M. Benefits of sustained moderate weight loss in obesity. *Nutr Metab Cardiovasc Dis* 2001;11:401-6.

[109] Ilanne-Parikka P, Eriksson JG, Lindström J et al; Finnish Diabetes Prevention Study Group. Prevalence of the metabolic syndrome and its components: findings from a Finnish general population sample and the Diabetes Prevention Study cohort. *Diabetes Care* 2004;27:2135-40.

[110] Knowler WC, Barrett-Connor E, Fowler SE et al; Diabetes Prevention Program Research Group. Reduction in the incidence of type 2 diabetes with lifestyle intervention or metformin. *N Engl J Med* 2002;346:393-403.

[111] U.S. Department of Agriculture, U.S. Department of Health and Human Services. *Dietary Guidelines for Americans* 2010. http://www.cnpp.usda.gov/dietary guidelines. htm

[112] Sacks FM, Svetkey LP, Vollmer WM et al; DASH-Sodium Collaborative Research Group. Effects on blood pressure of reduced dietary sodium and the Dietary Approaches to Stop Hypertension (DASH) diet. DASH-Sodium Collaborative Research Group. *N Engl J Med* 2001;344:3-10.

[113] Ohkawara K, Tanaka S, Miyachi M et al. A dose-response relation between aerobic exercise and visceral fat reduction: systematic review of clinical trials. *Int J Obes (Lond)* 2007;31:1786-97.

[114] Centers for Disease Control and Prevention. Centers for Disease Control National Diabetes Fact Sheet. *General information and national estimates on diabetes in the United States*. Atlanta, GA: *Centers for Disease Control and Prevention,* US Dept of Health and Human Services, 2007.

[115] Cowie CC, Rust KF, Byrd-Holt DD et al. Prevalence of diabetes and impaired fasting glucose in adults in the U.S. population: National Health And Nutrition Examination Survey 1999-2002. *Diabetes Care* 2006;29:1263-8.

[116] Executive summary: standards of medical care in diabetes--2009. *Diabetes Care* 2009;32 Suppl 1:S6-12.

[117] Rodbard HW, Blonde L, Braithwaite SS et al; AACE Diabetes Mellitus Clinical Practice Guidelines Task Force. American Association of Clinical Endocrinologists medical guidelines for clinical practice for the management of diabetes mellitus. *Endocr Pract* 2007;13 Suppl 1:1-68.

[118] Koro CE, Bowlin SJ, Bourgeois N, Fedder DO. Glycemic control from 1988 to 2000 among U.S. adults diagnosed with type 2 diabetes: a preliminary report. *Diabetes Care* 2004;27:17-20.

[119] Ong KL, Cheung BM, Wong LY et al. Prevalence, treatment, and control of diagnosed diabetes in the U.S. National Health and Nutrition Examination Survey 1999-2004. *Ann Epidemiol* 2008;18:222-9.

[120] Pirart J. Diabetes mellitus and its degenerative complications: a prospective study of 4,400 patients observed between 1947 and 1973. *Diabetes Care*. 1978;1:168-188.

[121] The effect of intensive treatment of diabetes on the development and progression of long-term complications in insulin-dependent diabetes mellitus. The Diabetes Control and Complications Trial Research Group. *N Engl J Med* 1993;329:977-86.

[122] Skyler JS. Diabetic complications. The importance of glucose control. *Endocrinol Metab Clin North Am* 1996;25:243-54.

[123] Kuusisto J, Mykkänen L, Pyörälä K, Laakso M. NIDDM and its metabolic control predict coronary heart disease in elderly subjects. *Diabetes* 1994;43:960-7.

[124] Khaw KT, Wareham N, Luben R et al. Glycated haemoglobin, diabetes, and mortality in men in Norfolk cohort of european prospective investigation of cancer and nutrition (EPIC-Norfolk). *BMJ* 2001;322:15-8.

[125] Ducimetiere P, Eschwege E, Papoz L et al. Relationship of plasma insulin levels to the incidence of myocardial infarction and coronary heart disease mortality in a middle-aged population. *Diabetologia* 1980;19:205-10.

[126] Eschwege E, Richard JL, Thibult N et al. Coronary heart disease mortality in relation with diabetes, blood glucose and plasma insulin levels. The Paris Prospective Study, ten years later. *Horm Metab Res Suppl* 1985;15:41-6.

[127] Pyörälä K. Relationship of glucose tolerance and plasma insulin to the incidence of coronary heart disease: results from two population studies in Finland. *Diabetes Care* 1979;2:131-41.

[128] Stolar MW. Atherosclerosis in diabetes: the role of hyperinsulinemia. *Metabolism* 1988;37:1-9.

[129] Coutinho M, Gerstein HC, Wang Y, Yusuf S. The relationship between glucose and incident cardiovascular events. A metaregression analysis of published data from 20 studies of 95,783 individuals followed for 12.4 years. *Diabetes Care* 1999;22:233-40.

[130] Hu FB, Stampfer MJ, Haffner SM et al. Elevated risk of cardiovascular disease prior to clinical diagnosis of type 2 diabetes. *Diabetes Care* 2002;25:1129-34.

[131] Stettler C, Allemann S, Jüni P et al. Glycemic control and macrovascular disease in types 1 and 2 diabetes mellitus: Meta-analysis of randomized trials. *Am Heart J* 2006;152:27-38.

[132] Esposito K, Giugliano D, Nappo F, Marfella R; Campanian Postprandial Hyperglycemia Study Group. Regression of carotid atherosclerosis by control of postprandial hyperglycemia in type 2 diabetes mellitus. *Circulation* 2004;110:214-9.

[133] Action to Control Cardiovascular Risk in Diabetes Study Group, Gerstein HC, Miller ME, Byington RP et al. Effects of intensive glucose lowering in type 2 diabetes. *N Engl J Med* 2008;358:2545-59.

[134] ADVANCE Collaborative Group, Patel A, MacMahon S, Chalmers J et al. Intensive blood glucose control and vascular outcomes in patients with type 2 diabetes. *N Engl J Med* 2008;358:2560-72.

[135] Duckworth W, Abraira C, Moritz T et al; VADT Investigators. Glucose control and vascular complications in veterans with type 2 diabetes. *N Engl J Med* 2009;360:129-39.

[136] Skyler JS, Bergenstal R, Bonow RO et al; American Diabetes Association; American College of Cardiology Foundation; American Heart Association. Intensive glycemic control and the prevention of cardiovascular events: implications of the ACCORD, ADVANCE, and VA Diabetes Trials: a position statement of the American Diabetes Association and a Scientific Statement of the American College of Cardiology Foundation and the American Heart Association. *J Am Coll Cardiol.* 2009;53:298-304.

[137] Holman RR, Paul SK, Bethel MA et al. 10-year follow-up of intensive glucose control in type 2 diabetes. N Engl J Med 2008;359:1577-89.

[138] Mathew J, Sleight P, Lonn E et al; Heart Outcomes Prevention Evaluation (HOPE) Investigators. Reduction of cardiovascular risk by regression of electrocardiographic markers of left ventricular hypertrophy by the angiotensin-converting enzyme inhibitor ramipril. *Circulation* 2001;104:1615-21.

[139] Bakris GL, Sowers JR; American Society of Hypertension Writing Group. ASH position paper: treatment of hypertension in patients with diabetes-an update. *J Clin Hypertens (Greenwich)* 2008;10:707-13; discussion 714-5.

[140] Chaturvedi N, Sjolie AK, Stephenson JM et al. Effect of lisinopril on progression of retinopathy in normotensive people with type 1 diabetes. The EUCLID Study Group. EURODIAB Controlled Trial of Lisinopril in Insulin-Dependent Diabetes Mellitus. *Lancet* 1998;351:28-31.

[141] Yusuf S, Gerstein H, Hoogwerf B et al; HOPE Study Investigators. Ramipril and the development of diabetes. *JAMA* 2001;286:1882-5.

[142] Hansson L, Lindholm LH, Niskanen L et al. Effect of angiotensin-converting-enzyme inhibition compared with conventional therapy on cardiovascular morbidity and mortality in hypertension: the Captopril Prevention Project (CAPPP) randomised trial. *Lancet* 1999;353:611-6.

[143] Barzilay JI, Davis BR, Cutler JA et al; ALLHAT Collaborative Research Group. Fasting glucose levels and incident diabetes mellitus in older nondiabetic adults randomized to receive 3 different classes of antihypertensive treatment: a report from

the Antihypertensive and Lipid-Lowering Treatment to Prevent Heart Attack Trial (ALLHAT). *Arch Intern Med* 2006;166:2191-201.

[144] Wing LM, Reid CM, Ryan P et al; Second Australian National Blood Pressure Study Group. A comparison of outcomes with angiotensin-converting--enzyme inhibitors and diuretics for hypertension in the elderly. *N Engl J Med* 2003;348:583-92.

[145] ONTARGET Investigators, Yusuf S, Teo KK, Pogue J et al. Telmisartan, ramipril, or both in patients at high risk for vascular events. *N Engl J Med* 2008;358:1547-59.

[146] Pfeffer MA, McMurray JJ, Velazquez EJ et al; Valsartan in Acute Myocardial Infarction Trial Investigators. Valsartan, captopril, or both in myocardial infarction complicated by heart failure, left ventricular dysfunction, or both. *N Engl J Med* 2003;349:1893-906.

[147] Hansson L, Hedner T, Lund-Johansen P et al. Randomised trial of effects of calcium antagonists compared with diuretics and beta-blockers on cardiovascular morbidity and mortality in hypertension: the Nordic Diltiazem (NORDIL) study. *Lancet* 2000;356:359-65.

[148] Lindholm LH, Hansson L, Ekbom T et al. Comparison of antihypertensive treatments in preventing cardiovascular events in elderly diabetic patients: results from the Swedish Trial in Old Patients with Hypertension-2. STOP Hypertension-2 Study Group. *J Hypertens.* 2000 Nov;18(11):1671-5.

[149] Beckett NS, Peters R, Fletcher AE et al; HYVET Study Group. Treatment of hypertension in patients 80 years of age or older. *N Engl J Med* 2008;358:1887-98.

[150] UK Prospective Diabetes Study Group. Efficacy of atenolol and captopril in reducing risk of macrovascular and microvascular complications in type 2 diabetes: UKPDS 39. *BMJ* 1998;317:713-20.

[151] Lindholm LH, Ibsen H, Dahlöf B et al; LIFE Study Group. Cardiovascular morbidity and mortality in patients with diabetes in the Losartan Intervention For Endpoint reduction in hypertension study (LIFE): a randomised trial against atenolol. *Lancet* 2002;359:1004-10.

[152] Hillebrand U, Lang D, Telgmann RG et al. Nebivolol decreases endothelial cell stiffness via the estrogen receptor beta: a nano-imaging study. *J Hypertens* 2009;27:517-26.

[153] Dhakam Z, Yasmin, McEniery CM et al. A comparison of atenolol and nebivolol in isolated systolic hypertension. *J Hypertens* 2008;26:351-6.

[154] Bakris GL, Copley JB, Vicknair N et al. Calcium channel blockers versus other antihypertensive therapies on progression of NIDDM associated nephropathy. *Kidney Int* 1996;50:1641-50.

[155] Jamerson K, Weber MA, Bakris GL et al; ACCOMPLISH Trial Investigators. Benazepril plus amlodipine or hydrochlorothiazide for hypertension in high-risk patients. *N Engl J Med* 2008;359:2417-28.

[156] Sowers JR, Whaley-Connell A, Epstein M. Narrative review: the emerging clinical implications of the role of aldosterone in the metabolic syndrome and resistant hypertension. *Ann Intern Med* 2009;150:776-83.

[157] Lane DA, Shah S, Beevers DG. Low-dose spironolactone in the management of resistant hypertension: a surveillance study. *J Hypertens* 2007;25:891-4.

[158] Schmieder RE, Philipp T, Guerediaga J et al. Aliskiren-based therapy lowers blood pressure more effectively than hydrochlorothiazide-based therapy in obese patients with

hypertension: sub-analysis of a 52-week, randomized, double-blind trial. *J Hypertens* 2009;27:1493-501.

[159] Schmieder RE, Philipp T, Guerediaga J et al. Long-term antihypertensive efficacy and safety of the oral direct renin inhibitor aliskiren: a 12-month randomized, double-blind comparator trial with hydrochlorothiazide. *Circulation* 2009;119:417-25.

[160] Solomon SD, Appelbaum E, Manning WJ et al; Aliskiren in Left Ventricular Hypertrophy (ALLAY) Trial Investigators. Effect of the direct Renin inhibitor aliskiren, the Angiotensin receptor blocker losartan, or both on left ventricular mass in patients with hypertension and left ventricular hypertrophy. *Circulation* 2009;119:530-7.

[161] Yamamoto E, Kataoka K, Dong YF et al. Aliskiren enhances the protective effects of valsartan against cardiovascular and renal injury in endothelial nitric oxide synthase-deficient mice. *Hypertension* 2009;54:633-8.

[162] Myerson M, Ngai C, Jones J et al. Treatment with high-dose simvastatin reduces secretion of apolipoprotein B-lipoproteins in patients with diabetic dyslipidemia. *J Lipid Res* 2005;46:2735-44.

[163] Pyörälä K, Pedersen TR, Kjekshus J et al. Cholesterol lowering with simvastatin improves prognosis of diabetic patients with coronary heart disease. A subgroup analysis of the Scandinavian Simvastatin Survival Study (4S). *Diabetes Care* 1997;20:614-20.

[164] Haffner SM, Alexander CM, Cook TJ et al. Reduced coronary events in simvastatin-treated patients with coronary heart disease and diabetes or impaired fasting glucose levels: subgroup analyses in the Scandinavian Simvastatin Survival Study. *Arch Intern Med* 1999;159:2661-7.

[165] Heart Protection Study Collaborative Group. MRC/BHF Heart Protection Study of cholesterol lowering with simvastatin in 20,536 high-risk individuals: a randomised placebo-controlled trial. *Lancet* 2002;360:7-22.

[166] Colhoun HM, Betteridge DJ, Durrington PN et al; CARDS investigators. Primary prevention of cardiovascular disease with atorvastatin in type 2 diabetes in the Collaborative Atorvastatin Diabetes Study (CARDS): multicentre randomised placebo-controlled trial. *Lancet* 2004;364:685-96.

[167] Knopp RH, d'Emden M, Smilde JG, Pocock SJ. Efficacy and safety of atorvastatin in the prevention of cardiovascular end points in subjects with type 2 diabetes: the Atorvastatin Study for Prevention of Coronary Heart Disease Endpoints in non-insulin-dependent diabetes mellitus (ASPEN). *Diabetes Care* 2006;29:1478-85.

[168] Shepherd J, Barter P, Carmena R et al. Effect of lowering LDL cholesterol substantially below currently recommended levels in patients with coronary heart disease and diabetes: the Treating to New Targets (TNT) study. *Diabetes Care* 2006;29:1220-6.

[169] Cholesterol Treatment Trialists' (CTT) Collaborators, Kearney PM, Blackwell L, Collins R et al. Efficacy of cholesterol-lowering therapy in 18,686 people with diabetes in 14 randomised trials of statins: a meta-analysis. *Lancet* 2008;371:117-25.

[170] Lefebvre P, Chinetti G, Fruchart JC, Staels B. Sorting out the roles of PPAR alpha in energy metabolism and vascular homeostasis. *J Clin Invest* 2006;116:571-80.

[171] Frick MH, Elo O, Haapa K et al. Helsinki Heart Study: primary-prevention trial with gemfibrozil in middle-aged men with dyslipidemia. Safety of treatment, changes in risk factors, and incidence of coronary heart disease. *N Engl J Med* 1987;317:1237-45.

[172] Koskinen P, Mänttäri M, Manninen V et al. Coronary heart disease incidence in NIDDM patients in the Helsinki Heart Study. *Diabetes Care* 1992;15:820-5.

[173] Rubins HB, Robins SJ, Collins D et al. Gemfibrozil for the secondary prevention of coronary heart disease in men with low levels of high-density lipoprotein cholesterol. Veterans Affairs High-Density Lipoprotein Cholesterol Intervention Trial Study Group. *N Engl J Med* 1999;341:410-8.

[174] Robins SJ, Collins D, Wittes JT et al; VA-HIT Study Group. Veterans Affairs High-Density Lipoprotein Intervention Trial. Relation of gemfibrozil treatment and lipid levels with major coronary events: VA-HIT: a randomized controlled trial. *JAMA* 2001;285:1585-91.

[175] Rubins HB, Robins SJ, Collins D et al. Diabetes, plasma insulin, and cardiovascular disease: subgroup analysis from the Department of Veterans Affairs high-density lipoprotein intervention trial (VA-HIT). *Arch Intern Med* 2002;162:2597-604.

[176] Robins SJ, Rubins HB, Faas FH et al; Veterans Affairs HDL Intervention Trial (VA-HIT). Insulin resistance and cardiovascular events with low HDL cholesterol: the Veterans Affairs HDL Intervention Trial (VA-HIT). *Diabetes Care* 2003;26:1513-7.

[177] Keech A, Simes RJ, Barter P et al; FIELD study investigators. Effects of long-term fenofibrate therapy on cardiovascular events in 9795 people with type 2 diabetes mellitus (the FIELD study): randomised controlled trial. *Lancet* 2005;366:1849-61.

[178] Grundy SM, Vega GL, Yuan Z et al. Effectiveness and tolerability of simvastatin plus fenofibrate for combined hyperlipidemia (the SAFARI trial). *Am J Cardiol* 2005;95:462-8.

[179] Abourbih S, Filion KB, Joseph L et al. Effect of fibrates on lipid profiles and cardiovascular outcomes: a systematic review. *Am J Med* 2009;122:962.e1-8.

[180] ACCORD Study Group, Ginsberg HN, Elam MB, Lovato LC et al. Effects of combination lipid therapy in type 2 diabetes mellitus. *N Engl J Med* 2010;362:1563-74.

[181] Canner PL, Berge KG, Wenger NK et al. Fifteen year mortality in Coronary Drug Project patients: long-term benefit with niacin. *J Am Coll Cardiol* 1986;8:1245-55.

[182] Brown BG, Zhao XQ, Chait A et al. Simvastatin and niacin, antioxidant vitamins, or the combination for the prevention of coronary disease. *N Engl J Med* 2001;345:1583-92.

[183] Taylor AJ, Villines TC, Stanek EJ et al. Extended-release niacin or ezetimibe and carotid intima-media thickness. *N Engl J Med* 2009;361:2113-22.

[184] Garg A, Grundy SM. Nicotinic acid as therapy for dyslipidemia in non-insulin-dependent diabetes mellitus. *JAMA* 1990;264:723-6.

[185] Grundy SM, Vega GL, McGovern ME et al; Diabetes Multicenter Research Group. Efficacy, safety, and tolerability of once-daily niacin for the treatment of dyslipidemia associated with type 2 diabetes: results of the assessment of diabetes control and evaluation of the efficacy of niaspan trial. *Arch Intern Med* 2002;162:1568-76.

[186] Goldberg RB, Jacobson TA. Effects of niacin on glucose control in patients with dyslipidemia. *Mayo Clin Proc* 2008;83:470-8.

[187] Kahn SE, Beard JC, Schwartz MW et al. Increased beta-cell secretory capacity as mechanism for islet adaptation to nicotinic acid-induced insulin resistance. *Diabetes* 1989;38:562-8.

[188] Bays HE, Moore PB, Drehobl MA et al; Ezetimibe Study Group. Effectiveness and tolerability of ezetimibe in patients with primary hypercholesterolemia: pooled analysis of two phase II studies. *Clin Ther* 2001;23:1209-30.

[189] Cannon CP, Giugliano RP, Blazing MA et al; IMPROVE-IT Investigators. Rationale and design of IMPROVE-IT (IMProved Reduction of Outcomes: Vytorin Efficacy International Trial): comparison of ezetimbe/simvastatin versus simvastatin monotherapy on cardiovascular outcomes in patients with acute coronary syndromes. *Am Heart J* 2008;156:826-32.

[190] Howard BV, Roman MJ, Devereux RB et al. Effect of lower targets for blood pressure and LDL cholesterol on atherosclerosis in diabetes: the SANDS randomized trial. *JAMA* 2008;299:1678-89.

[191] Fleg JL, Mete M, Howard BV et al. Effect of statins alone versus statins plus ezetimibe on carotid atherosclerosis in type 2 diabetes: the SANDS (Stop Atherosclerosis in Native Diabetics Study) trial. *J Am Coll Cardiol* 2008;52:2198-205.

In: Current Advances in Cardiovascular Risk. Volume 2   ISBN: 978-1-62081-746-9
Editor: Sandeep Ajoy Saha   © 2012 Nova Science Publishers, Inc.

Chapter XV

Cardiovascular Risk in Patients with Chronic Kidney Disease

Radica Z. Alicic[1] and Katherine R. Tuttle[1,2]
[1]Providence Medical Research Center,
Sacred Heart Medical Center, Spokane, WA, US
[2]Division of Nephrology, Department of Medicine,
University of Washington School of Medicine,
Spokane and Seattle, WA, US

Abstract

The prevalence of chronic kidney disease (CKD) in the United States' population 20 years of age and older is about 11% in men and 15% in women. In 2008 it was estimated that more than 28 million people had CKD. This population is considered to be the "highest risk group" for subsequent cardiovascular disease (CVD) events. The cardiovascular morbidity and mortality rates sharply rise with a drop in kidney function and are particularly high in dialysis patients. Etiology of the increased risk is not completely understood and possible explanations include the high prevalence of traditional risk factors, as well as the so-called non-traditional risk factors specific for the CKD population. In the setting of decreased kidney function, the cardiovascular system is exposed to a number of unique abnormalities leading to unique differences in the presentation, diagnosis and management of CVD in the CKD population. Faced with the escalating numbers of CKD patients worldwide, it is of paramount importance to improve the understanding, early recognition, and development of new treatment strategies for CVD in the CKD population.

Abbreviations

ACCORD	Action to Control Cardiovascular Risk in Diabetes
ADVANCE	Action in Diabetes and Cardiovascular Disease: Preterax and Diamicron Modified Release Controlled Evaluation

DCCT/EDIC   Diabetes Control and Complications Trial/Epidemiology of Diabetes
              Interventions and Complications
UKPDS   United Kingdom Prospective Diabetes Study
RENAAL   Reduction of Endpoints in NIDDM with the Angiotensin II Antagonist
              Losartan
CREATE   The Cardiovascular risk Reduction by Early Anemia Treatment with
              Epoetin Beta
CHOIR   Correction of anemia with epoetin alpha in chronic kidney disease.
TREAT   Trial to Reduce Cardiovascular Events with Aranesp Therapy
MRFIT   The multiple Risk Factor Intervention Trial
GUSTO IV   Global Utilization of Strategies To open Occluded arteries-IV
4D   Deutsche Diabetes Dialyze Studie
AURORA   A Study to Evaluate the Use of Rosuvastatin in Subjects on Regular
              Hemodialysis: An Assessment of Survival and Cardiovascular Events
WOSCOP   Pravastatin Pooling Project, West of Scotland Coronary Prevention Study
CARE   Cholesterol and Recurrent Events
SHARP   Study of Heart and Renal Protection
CTT   Cholesterol Treatment Trialists
JUPITER   Justification for the Use of Statins in Prevention: an Intervention Trial
              Evaluating Rosuvastatin
SEARCH   The Study of the Effectiveness of Additional Reductions in Cholesterol
              and Homocysteine
HOT   Hypertension Optimal Treatment Study.

Introduction

The interaction between the kidneys and the heart is one of close cooperation in maintaining blood volume, vascular tone and hemodynamic stability. The dysfunction of one organ initiates and perpetuates the dysfunction of the other. The following chapter will discuss the epidemiology, risk factors, pathophysiology, clinical presentation and updates in the treatment of cardiovascular disease (CVD) in patients with chronic kidney disease (CKD).

As per the National Health and Nutrition Examination Survey (NHANES), in the period between 1999 and 2004 the prevalence of CKD in the population 20 years of age and older was 11.1% in men and 15% in women. This translates to more than 28 million people (estimated in the year 2008) [1]. The prevalence of CVD in CKD steeply rises with a drop in kidney function, and is up to 63% in the population with severe CKD. In comparison, the prevalence of CVD in the population without CKD is 5.8% [1]. Although the most recognizable outcome of CKD is end-stage renal disease (ESRD), only 2% of all patients with CKD will progress to this stage. [1,2]. If kidney function is mildly or moderately decreased, patients are 20 times more likely to die before ever needing kidney replacement therapy in the form of dialysis or transplantation. Even if kidney function is severely decreased the prospect of death is approximately 2-fold greater than the likelihood of starting renal replacement therapy [3]. Once patients are on dialysis, they are 10 to 30 times more likely to die from CVD than the general population. [4]. The 10-year mortality rate in pooled individuals from two large population-based cohort studies with estimated glomerular filtration rate (eGFR) 15–60 ml/ min /1.73 m^2 exceeded 35% in men and 20% in women [5]. After only 16 months of follow-up, the population with combined CKD and CVD had a 3-fold increased risk of death with a documented steep gradient between eGFR and CVD mortality [6] In 1998, the National Kidney Foundation Task Force on Cardiovascular Disease in Chronic Renal Disease recommended that CKD patients should be considered the "highest risk group" for subsequent CVD events [4].

Similarly to the mortality data, there is a graded association between a decreased eGFR and the risk of cardiovascular events and hospitalizations. The adjusted risk of any cardiovascular event ranges from a 43% increased risk with an eGFR of 45-59 ml/min 1.73 m^2 to a 343% increased risk with an eGFR of less than 15 ml/min /1.73 m^2 compared to population with eGFR bigger than 60 ml/min /1.73 m^2. [7]. The adjusted risk for hospitalization ranges from a 14 % increase with an eGFR of 45-59 ml/min 1.73 m^2. / to an increase of 315 % with an eGFR of less 15 ml/min/1.73 m^2. [7] Likewise, the latest data from United States Renal Data System (USRDS) shows an advancing graded impact of CKD on adjusted rates for hospitalization. Rates of hospitalization are 38% higher in Medicare patients with CKD than in patients without the disease, 19 % greater in patients in stage 3-5 than those with CKD 1-2, and 20 % higher in CKD 1-2 patients than in non-CKD patients. Follow-up studies confirmed graded associations between all stages of CKD and CVD morbidity and mortality [7-10]. Renal function is considered to be one of the most important independent risk factors for poor outcomes and all-cause mortality in patients with heart failure (HF) [11,12] At the same time, the merged data from 2 large, community-based longitudinal studies demonstrated that CVD *per se* is independently associated with the development of kidney disease [13,14]. This bidirectional interaction through common hemodynamic, neurohormonal, and immunological and biochemical pathways is now recognized as the 'cardiorenal syndrome' [11].

Definition of Chronic Kidney Disease

As per the 2002 The National Kidney Foundation Kidney Disease Outcome Quality Initiative (NKF-KDOQI) clinical practice guidelines, CKD is defined as either [1] kidney damage for ≥3 months, as confirmed by kidney biopsy or markers of kidney damage, such as proteinuria, abnormal urinary sediment or abnormal kidney imaging, with or without a decrease in eGFR, or [2] eGFR ≤60 ml/min / 1.73 m² for ≥3 months. The cutoff value of 60 ml/min/ 1.73 m² is selected because it represents a loss of approximately half of the normal GFR and is associated with the onset of laboratory abnormalities and complications characteristic of kidney failure. Based on eGFR, there are 5 stages of CKD (Table 1). eGFR ≤ 15 ml/min/1.73 m² is defined as kidney failure typically requiring treatment by dialysis or transplant [15]. In clinical practice, eGFR is most commonly calculated by the Modification of Diet in Renal Disease (MDRD) equation based on serum creatinine, age, sex, and race (black or non-black).

Table 1. Stages of chronic kidney disease, prevalence (%) of different stages of chronic kidney disease in US population per NHANES 1999-2006, and prevalence (%) of cardiovascular disease in different stages of CKD per NHANES 1999-2006

CKD Stage	Description of CKD stage	eGFR	Prevalence (%) of CKD by stages	Prevalence (%) of CVD in different stages of CKD
		≥90	3.2	7.7.
		60-89	4.1	18.4
3	Moderately decreased GFR	30-59	7.8	31.4
4	Severely decreased GFR	15-29	0.5	62.8
5	Kidney failure	≤15		

eGFR – estimated glomerular filtration rate in ml/min/1.73 m² (MDRD).
CKD – chronic kidney disease.
CVD – cardiovascular disease.
(Modified from U.S. Renal Data System, Annual Data Report: Disease. National Institutes of Health, National Institute of Diabetes and Digestive and Kidney Diseases, Bethesda, MD, 2010).

Spectrum and Pathophysiology of Cardiovascular Disease in Patients with Chronic Kidney Disease – How Is it Different from the General Population?

The milieu of decreased kidney function exposes the cardiovascular system to a number of unique abnormalities including: alterations in blood pressure and flow resulting in increased arterial tensile and shear stress; inflammation, malnutrition; anemia, dyslipidemia; sub-diabetic disturbances in glucose metabolism, hyperhomocysteinemia; bone and mineral metabolism disorders; renin-angiotensin-aldosteron system activation; and dysregulation of hemostasis.

As in the general population, arterial vessels in patients with decreased kidney function undergo at least two pathogenic processes: atherosclerosis and arteriosclerosis. These processes frequently co-exist and share common risk factors. Moreover, they contribute to each other through several proposed mechanisms including endothelial dysfunction, biomechanical stress to endothelial cells, elastic fiber fragmentation [16 -19]. In 1974, Lindner at al demonstrated the presence of greatly accelerated atherosclerosis in chronic dialysis patients receiving chronic dialysis treatment [20] In addition to a pre-existing disease related to CKD, it is possible that hemodialysis itself may aggravate CVD [21].

*Atherosclerosi*s is primarily an intimal process, usually focal and involving preferentially carotid bifurcation, coronary, renal, femoral arteries [22].There is a higher prevalence and severity of atherosclerotic changes in patients with CKD [23, 24]. Atherosclerotic plaque is most pronounced in arteries where shear stress is high (e.g. bifurcations) and in the upper body arteries where blood pressure tends to be higher. A post-mortem study of hemodialysis patients with CVD showed significantly more severe changes of the ascending aorta when compared to patients with normal kidney function who had CVD [25]. Patients with CKD have a higher degree of arterial calcifications and lower collagenous fibers content than compared to people with normal kidney function. [26-28]. The frequency of advanced atherosclerotic lesions in carotid arteries as types IV-VI by the American Heart Association (AHA) [29] increases gradually from 34% to 53% with the decreasing eGFR. A similar gradual increase in the frequency of calcified lesions was observed in coronary arteries. (30 Figure 1). Another morphological study of coronary arteries of uremic patients showed considerably reduced lumen with thickening of the media [31]. *Surrogates* of atherosclerosis include intima–media thickness of the carotid artery detected by ultrasound, inducible ischemia detected by stress test, ischemic ECG changes reflecting coronary atherosclerotic lesions, and electron-beam computed tomography detecting vascular calcifications. Clinical presentations of atherosclerosis include ischemic heart disease (angina, myocardial infarction and sudden death), cerebrovascular disease, peripheral vascular disease and heart failure [4].

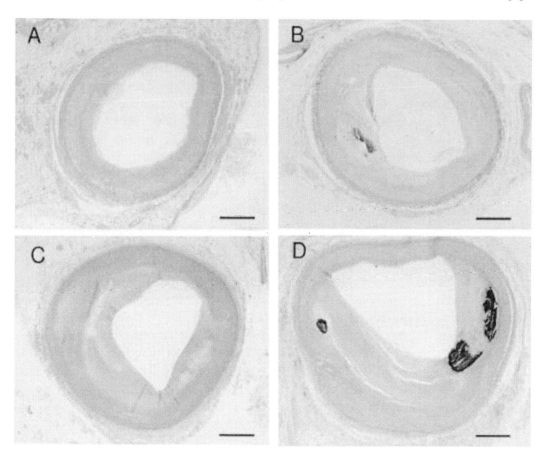

Figure 1. Typical arteries for each classification by glomerular filtration rate (GFR). (A-D) Typical light microscopic views of coronary arteries from respective cases with estimated GFR(A) ≥60, (B) 45-59, (C) 30-44, and (D) <30 mL/min/1.73 m². Stenosis rates of respective arteries were (A) 36.8%, (B) 42.3%, (C) 54.2%, and (D) 58.9%. All sections were stained with hematoxylin and eosin. Scale bars = 1.0 mm.
Permission obtained from Elsevier Copyright Clearance Center, Nakano, T, and et al. Am J Kidney Dis 2010 55, 21-30.

Arteriosclerosis in ESRD patients is characterized by structural remodeling similar to changes seen with aging and consists of diffuse dilation, hypertrophy, and stiffening of the aorta and major arteries [32]. However, in comparison with nonuremic patients the intima-media thickness is increased in ESRD. Some features of arterial remodeling such as fibroblastic intimal thickening, calcification of vascular smooth muscle cells (VSMCs), and ground substance depositions are specific for kidney patients [31-33]. As a consequence of arterial wall hypertrophy and calcifications of VSMCs there is a decrease in arterial distensibility resulting in increased pulse wave velocity (PWV) - a measure of arterial stiffening, and early return of wave reflection [33-36]. Systolic blood pressure and eGFR appear to be major determinants of arterial stiffness independent of conventional risk factors [37]. Both decreased aortic compliance and increased pulse pressure have been found to be independent risk factors for CVD in CKD in dialysis patients [38] with a stepwise increase of PWV [36-38]. Surrogates of arteriosclerosis are increased aortic pulse velocity, altered coronary perfusion, calcification of aorta, left ventricular hypertrophy and increased pulse pressure. These abnormalities typically result in clinical presentations of ischemic heart disease and congestive heart failure.

The heart muscle is one of the major targets of atherosclerosis, arteriosclerosis, and associated hemodynamic disturbances resulting in left ventricular hypertrophy (LVH). LVH is directly proportional to the decrease in aortic distensibility [39]. Two major consequences of LVH are reduction of coronary reserve and compromised coronary perfusion with decreased subendocardial blood flow [40]. In addition, alteration of left ventricular myoperfusion is a result of abnormalities in the intramyocardial microvasculature. Amen et al have shown a "myocyte/capillary mismatch" in patients with uremia. This mismatch is a result of lower capillary length and their diminished density on one side, and increased myocyte diameter and volume density of myocardial interstitial tissue on the other. [41]. Pressure overload as a result of hypertension and arteriosclerosis leads to more prevalent *concentric* hypertrophy (increased wall–to–lumen ratio), whereas volume overload as a result of anemia, fluid excess, and arteriovenous fistulas results in *eccentric* hypertrophy with left ventricular dilation (a proportional increase in left ventricular mass and diameter) [4,42]. Heart failure, ischemic heart disease, and decreased peripheral perfusion are clinical presentations of LVH. Diastolic dysfunction occurs early in the course of CKD [42] even before morphological changes are evident. LVH is evident in 27% of patients with eGFR >50 ml/min/ 1.73 m^2. [4], and up to 75% of patients with ESRD who are starting dialysis treatment [43]. In a retrospective study of 980 patients with CKD, the frequency of low left ventricular ejection fraction (LVEF) increased with declining GFR and was independently associated with all-cause mortality regardless of the presence of angiographic coronary artery disease (CAD) or other risk factors including anemia, hypertension, male sex, and age [44]. LVH is shown to be a strong predictor of the risk of worsening of kidney function and progression to dialysis [45], and a predictor of survival in dialysis patients [46] and in CKD patients with heart failure [47].

Risk Factors for Cardiovascular Disease in Chronic Kidney Disease

Between 1980 and 2000, the death rate from CVD in the general population fell by more than 40%. Half of this decline has been attributed to the reduction of major risk factors and the other half to specific therapeutic interventions for acute events. Unfortunately, this improving trend did not carry over to patients with CKD [48].

Traditional CVD risk factors, as defined by the Framingham Heart Study, are highly prevalent in CKD populations and include age, gender, family history, hypertension, hypercholesterolemia, diabetes, and smoking [4, 49]. Hypertriglyceridemia, obesity and inadequate exercise, as surrogates of metabolic syndrome, are considered additional components of the Framingham paradigm. Even after adjustment for a high burden of traditional CVD risk factors, CKD patients have excess CVD risk that is not fully explained. Therefore, this excess CVD risk is attributed to a host of candidate non-traditional risk factors (table 2).

Table 2. Traditional and Nontraditional Cardiovascular Risk Factors in Patients with CKD

Traditional Risk Factors	Nontraditional Factors
Age	Anemia
Gender	Abnormal mineral metabolism
Hypertension	Volume overload
Dyslipidemia	Albuminuria
Diabetes	Homocysteine
Smoking	Oxidative stress/inflammation
Family history	Thrombogenic factors
Physical inactivity	Altered nitric oxide/endothelin balance
	Malnutrition

Traditional Risk Factors in CKD Population

The evaluation of the Framingham equation on a pool of participants of two large community based studies with eGFR 15-60 ml/min/1.73 m^2 (mean 53 ml/min/1.73 m^2.) led to two conclusions: first, the overall accuracy of the Framingham instrument in predicting the primary cardiovascular events in patients with CKD is poor [50-52], and second that the conventional risk factors differ in magnitude of importance [50] from populations with normal renal function. For instance, importance of diabetes increases while hypertension and elevated cholesterol do not carry the same risk seen in the population without CKD. Well-known associations between hypertension, hypercholesterolemia and obesity and adverse cardiovascular outcomes are not noted in dialysis patients. On the contrary, there is a strong correlation between low body mass, low blood pressure and low cholesterol and increased morbidity and mortality. This paradoxical relationship is frequently referred as "reverse epidemiology" or "reverse causality" [53- 56].

Blood pressure is high in most patients with CKD; by the later stages 90% of patients carry a diagnosis of hypertension. [1]. This is a dynamic and self-perpetuating relationship. Uncontrolled hypertension accelerates the progression of CKD, and kidney dysfunction further elevates blood pressure. In CKD stages 2 and 3, hypertension is associated with increased risk of new or recurrent CVD events. Among renal transplant recipients, hypertension is associated with increased risk of congestive heart failure and coronary heart disease [57]. In diabetic patients with hypertension, there is an almost linear relationship between an increase in mean arterial blood pressure and yearly decrease in GFR [58]. In dialysis patients the expected linear correlation between the blood pressure and adverse CVD events is lost. The correlation assumes a J-shape - indicating a higher incidence of cardiovascular mortality and morbidity with low blood pressure - and is referred to as a "reverse epidemiology" [55] (Figure 2). It appears that the concept of the J-curve is not limited to dialysis patients only, but it is also noticed in the subset of high-risk hypertensive patients such as those with multiple risk factors, diabetes, CKD or previous history of CAD. Recent analysis of several international randomized trials showed an increased risk of CAD, mostly myocardial infarction, in patients who achieved the lowest blood pressure [58a] (Figure 3).

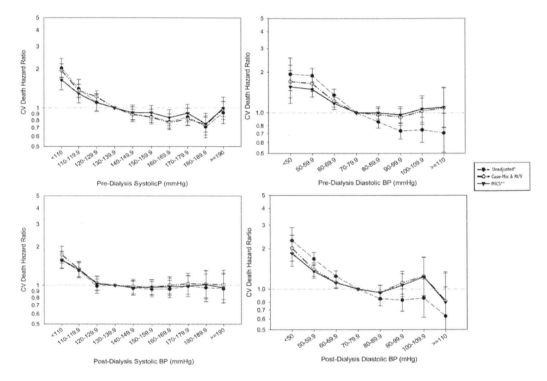

Figure 2. Association between BP and 15-month CV death in 40 933 MHD patients [95% confidence interval bars are depicted). Note that the unadjusted models also include entry quarter. **MICS-adjusted models also include all covariates in the previous models. Reproduced with permission from ref. no. 55.

Dyslipidemia in patents with CKD depends on stage and presence of nephrotic syndrome (table 3). Patients with mild to moderate CKD often display hypercholesterolemia and elevated low-density lipoprotein (LDL) levels [59]. However, in later stages of CKD and ESRD, total cholesterol and LDL tend to be normal or even reduced. In contrast, elevation of triglycerides is an early feature of CKD especially in patients with diabetes. Hypertriglyceridemia reflects increased synthesis by the liver and impaired clearance of very low-density lipoproteins and chylomicrons by the muscle and adipose tissue and their atherogenic remnants by the liver. Decreased catabolism also leads to the accumulation of small dense LDL particles. The other major CKD–associated lipid abnormalities include a reduction in levels of apoA-1 and high–density lipoprotein (HDL) cholesterol concentration.

Maturation of HDL is impaired, and its anti-inflammatory, antioxidant and reverse transport properties are defective. In addition, LDL cholesterol and lipoprotein remnants undergo oxidative modifications. As a result of lipid metabolism abnormalities, uptake of oxidized LDL by artery wall macrophages is increased, leading to the intensification of oxidative stress and inflammation and heightened injurious effects [60, 61]. The ability of VLDL and chylomicrons to deliver lipid fuel to muscle and adipose tissue is impaired contributing to muscle weakness and cachexia in ESRD. In CKD dyslipidemia ranks high among probable causes of premature atherosclerosis leading to cardiovascular morbidity and mortality. [62, 63] However, in the ESRD population there is evidence of a" reverse causality" relationship between cholesterol levels and CVD mortality with a "J" shaped curve demonstrating excess CVD events with lower cholesterol levels [64, 65].

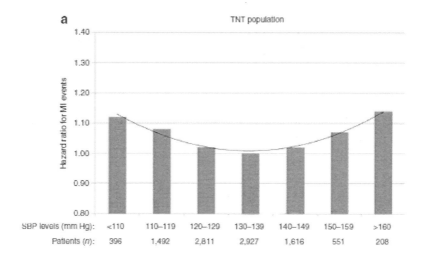

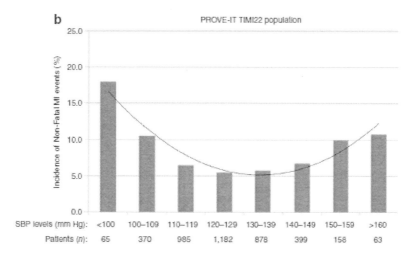

Figure 3. Incidence of myocardial infarction in the very high risk population enrolled in the (a) TNT and in (b) the PROVE IT-TIMI 22 trial, respectively. For each group the systolic blood pressure range and the population sample are reported.
[MI, myocardial infarction; SBP, systolic blood pressure].
Reproduced with permission from ref. no. 58a.

Diabetes is responsible for approximately 50% of CKD. Among the diabetic population, kidney disease is one of the most common microvascular complications occurring in 30-40 % cases [1]. In spite of diabetes being independent risk factor for ischemic heart disease, heart failure, and all cause-mortality few studies documented direct associations between glycemic control and cardiovascular outcomes. In 2008 two landmark studies involving diabetic patients at high CVD risk were released: ACCORD and ADVANCE [66, 67]. Both studies enrolled predominantly older diabetic patients (mean age of 60 years) at high CVD risk and both studies failed to demonstrate improved CVD outcomes with strict glycemic control (near normal hemoglobin A1C of 6.5). ACCORD was suspended 17 months earlier due to increased risk of death from all causes and CVD in the group randomized to intensive glycemic control, while intensive glycemic control was found to be risk –neutral in ADVANCE. The benefit-to risk ratio of intensive glycemic control is even more uncertain in the CKD population because ACCORD excluded patients with elevated creatinine.

Likewise, initial results from two other trials, DCCT/EDIC and UKPDS, did not demonstrate a positive effect of glycemic control on CVD [68, 69]. Both studies enrolled populations with no previous history of CV events. However, post-trial follow ups (> 10 years) of UKPDS patients in strict glycemic control group showed a significant reduction in all–cause mortality by 13%, and a 15% reduction in myocardial infarctions (MI) (p= 0.01) This extended benefit of intensive glucose control is a so-called legacy effect. [70] Similarly, by the end of the 11 year long observational follow-up of DCCT-EDIC participants the risk of any cardiovascular disease event was reduced by 42% in the intensive glycemic control group After 6 years, the intensive control group had decreased progression of carotid intima-media thickening [71].

Table 3. Lipid abnormalities in the chronic kidney disease

	CKD	CKD
	Stage 1-4	Stage 5
Total cholesterol	normal	normal
Triglyceride	normal or ↑	↑
LDL-cholesterol	normal or ↑	normal or ↓
HDL-cholesterol	↓ or normal	↓
Small dense LDL	↑	↑
Lipoprotein a	↑	↑
Hepatic lipase activity	↓	↓

CKD – chronic kidney disease.
LDL cholesterol – low-density cholesterol.
HDL –cholesterol – high-density cholesterol.
Modified from Yamamoto et al., Curr Opin Nephrol Hypertens, 2009 18, 181-188.

Non-Traditional Risk Factors for Cardiovascular Disease in Chronic Kidney Disease

Inflammation is present in all stages of CKD especially in dialysis patients [72, 73]. Increased prevalence of inflammation is probably the result of multiple parallel processes: reduced renal clearance of inflammatory substances, increased production of inflammatory mediators and reactive oxygen species, complications of dialyses treatment, and occult infections. Low grade inflammation as measured by high sensitivity C-reactive protein can predict all-cause mortality in non-dialysis-dependent CKD patients independent of age, estimated GFR, left ventricular mass index and vascular disease [74, 75]. Other studies showed association of inflammatory biomarkers and all-cause and cardiovascular mortality in dialysis and patients with CKD 2-4 [76, 77]. The highest tertile of high sensitivity C-reactive protein and interleukin (IL)-6 were each associated with doubling in the risk of sudden cardiac death [78]. Compared with the lowest tertile, the impact of circulating markers of inflammation was independent of traditional CVD risk factors [79, 80].

CKD is considered as a state of high *oxidative stress* with decreased production of nitric oxide as a result of substrate limitation (L-arginine). At the same time, levels of asymmetric dimethylarginine (ADMA), an endogenous inhibitor of nitric oxide, are increased. ADMA levels trend upward with loss of kidney function and are associated with increased CVD risk and all-cause mortality [73, 81].

Low eGFR, anemia, and microalbuminuria were each independently associated with CVD in a cohort of 37,153 patients screened for the National Kidney Foundation's Kidney Early Evaluation Program (KEEP), with a 3-fold increase in CVD mortality in the population with all 3 conditions [6].

Anemia typically develops once GFR is 20-40 ml/min/1.73m2, except in diabetic nephropathy where it is often seen with eGFR <60 ml/min/1.73m2. It is present in 43% patients with CKD 1-2, and nearly 57% of those with CKD 3-5. [1] Chronic anemia stresses the heart by increasing cardiac output, volume overload, pulse rate, and ultimately, LVH and diastolic dysfunction. As such anemia is a recognized risk factor for new-onset CHF [82]. In the RENAAL study, reduced hemoglobin, even within range considered "normal" was associated with an increased risk of ESRD and death [83]. However, CREATE, CHOIR and TREAT- 3 large randomized studies- failed to show that correction of anemia with the use of erythropoiesis – stimulating agents (ESA) has a beneficial effect on CVD outcomes or CVD death. The TREAT trial evaluated the effects of ESA (darbepoetin alfa) on cardiovascular and renal events in population with CKD, diabetes type II and anemia. There were no differences between groups in any of primary CV or renal end- points including all-cause death, CV death, non-fatal myocardial infarction (MI), heart failure, hospitalization for MI, or death from ESRD. However, risk of fatal and non-fatal stroke doubled over the course of the study (median 29.1 months) in those treated with darbepoetin (5.0% versus 2.6%; hazard ratio 1.92; 95% confidence interval, 1.38–2.68; p < 0.001), as well as risk of cancer deaths in those with pre-existing malignancies and thromboembolism (venous and arterial) [84-86].

Albuminuria emerged as a strong predictor of progression of CKD and an important risk factor for atherosclerotic CVD [87-89]. Ample data support the importance of albuminuria as a risk factor for increased mortality and morbidity. Documented presence of overt proteinuria is an independent predictor of death, cardiovascular events, and hospitalizations [7]. The risk of all-cause mortality, MI, and progression to kidney failure were increased in patients with higher levels of proteinuria in 920, 985 adults in Canadian study [90]. A meta-analysis derived from 14 studies (105,872 subjects) with available ACR measurements and 7 studies (1,128,310 subjects) with urine dipstick determination of proteinuria and eGFR <60 ml/min/1.73 m^2 showed graded association between proteinuria and cardiovascular and all-cause mortality [91].

Albuminuria is thought to be a biomarker of endothelial dysfunction. [92] as well as abnormalities of fibrinolytic and coagulation pathways, and ongoing inflammation [93] that signifies greater severity of target-organ damage.

Bone and mineral metabolism disorders are common complications of advancing CKD. Elevated phosphate and/or calcium trigger calcium precipitates in VSMCs. Arterial calcification is similar to bone formation, involving differentiation of VSMCs into phenotypically distinct osteoblast-like cells [33]. Serum phosphorus levels have been associated with death and myocardial infarction in patients with stages 3-4 CKD [94]. In the recent study each 1-mg/dl increase in phosphorus level imparted odds risks comparable to traditional CVD risk factors [95].These data imply a role for phosphorus in mechanisms of CVD, for example coronary artery calcification, even when kidney function is mot measurable decreased.

Increased extracellular volume is present in most patients with CKD, especially at advanced stages. Sodium and water overload cause volume expansion leading to heart muscle strain and LVH (as discussed above).

Clinical Presentations of Cardiovascular Disease in Chronic Kidney Disease

Ischemic heart disease (IHD) is prevalent in all stages of CKD. An estimated 40% of incident dialysis patients have coronary heart disease. [73]. In the MRFIT study even a mild increase in serum creatinine was an independent risk factor for coronary artery disease (CAD) [96]. Coronary angiograms of 264 patients with CKD showed more significant CAD and increased lesion complexity with decreased renal function. [97]. At the same time, IHD can be present in the absence of large-vessel disease with negative angiography in patients with CKD [98]. Typical chest pain is a poor predictor of presence of IHD, and absence of symptoms is not a safe criterion for the identification of disease-free patients. In ESRD patients, only 17%-20% had either stable or unstable angina symptoms. [99]. However, as seen in a study of 558 pre-kidney transplant patients, 23% of asymptomatic patients had evidence of inducible ischemia on nuclear stress test, while 14 % had apparent CAD by angiogram. [98]

The prevalence of CKD among patients with ST elevation myocardial infarction (STEMI) is ~30% and is >40% in patients with non-ST elevation myocardial infarction (NSTEMI).After reviewing national registry of 50,000 cases of STMI and NSTMI Fox and colleagues, demonstrated a graded relationship of CKD stage and short-term mortality which was twofold increased even in the patients with CKD stage 3. [100] One year mortality for patients aged 65 years and older who have CKD and myocardial infarction is 51% compared to 36% for non-CKD patients. This group is also at increased risk for hospital readmission and readmission resulting in death [1].

Troponin C. The GUSTO IV trial demonstrated that elevated troponin C (cTns) levels are strong predictors of reduced short-term survival in symptomatic patients with acute coronary syndrome (ACS) regardless of kidney function, and that predictive importance was even greater in patients with mild to moderate CKD [101]. At the same time, cTns are elevated in the absence of ACS in up to 30-75% of ESRD patients. [102] Accumulating data suggest that prevalence of elevated levels of cTns correlate with increased risk of CVD, and may predicate death [103]. Pathophysiology of the random elevation of cTns in CKD and ESRD is not clear, but it is unlikely to be result of decreased clearance [104, 105] It is proposed that the elevation may reflect ongoing myocardial damage in cardiomyopathy, microvascular disease, or LVH [106].

Heart failure and CKD commonly occur together. In the Acute Decompensated Heart Failure National Registry (ADHERE), 30% of patients hospitalized with heart failure had a history of CKD with serum creatinine >2 mg/dl. The meta-analysis of 16 studies involving over 80,000 patients with heart failure showed that 63% patients had mild and 20% had moderate to severely decreased kidney function. There was a consistent risk relationship of a 7% increase in mortality for every 10 ml/min decrease in eGFR. ADHERE date showed that admission levels of serum creatinine and blood urea nitrogen were among the strongest independent risk predictors for in–hospital mortality. [107]. Similarly, Japanese Cardiac Registry of Heart failure in Cardiology (JCARE-CARD) demonstrated increased risk of all-cause death and hospital readmissions with reduced eGFR. Prevalence of CKD in this study was 70%. [108] Per USRDS data on Medicare patients, one-year mortality for non-CKD patients with heart failure is 21% compared with 27% for patients with CKD stages 3-5. In the same population, one year probability for hospital readmission and readmission resulting in death is 68% and 73% respectively [1].

Diagnosis of heart failure is challenging in dialysis patients as salt and water retention are treated by ultrafiltration leaving only hypotension, fatigue and anorexia as clinical clues. Role of biomarkers used for diagnosis of heart failure in non-CKD population is unclear as CKD patients were excluded from early studies. Recently, Niizuma and al. showed that left ventricular end-diastolic wall stress (LVEDWS) was a strong determinant of brain natriuretic peptide (BNP) levels in the CKD population. Anemia, obesity and heart failure type (systolic versus diastolic) should also be considered in interpreting the BNP in CKD population. The cut-point for detection of heart failure when the eGFR <60 ml/min may need to be higher. In ESRD patients, the correlation between LVEDWS and BNP concentration was only modest. Currently, the clinical utility of BNP in CKD and ESRD populations is limited [109]. Several small studies indicate that combination measurements of BNP and Troponin C (cTns) in patients with heart failure might be effective for risk stratification. Unfortunately, studies were small and excluded patients with severe CKD, so the practical significance of this finding is not clear [110,111].

Arrhythmias are common in advanced CKD and ESRD. Sudden cardiac death (SCD) is the single largest cause of death for ESRD patients [1]. It accounts for 26% of all deaths and is attributed to arrhythmias [1]. A study of Japanese peritoneal dialysis patients reported very similar rate of sudden deaths of about 24%. The most powerful predictor of SCD in this study was LVEF: 1 – point drop equals 6% increase in SCD hazard. Cardiac troponin was predictive of SCD independent of echocardiographic findings. [112]. Atrial fibrillation is considered a predictor of very high cardiovascular morbidity and mortality. Comparing Medicare non-CKD patients with atrial fibrillation to stage 3-5 CKD patients, probabilities of hospital readmission within 6 months are 41 and 55%, respectively, with probabilities of readmission resulting in death of 43 and 63% [1].

Valvular heart disease is commonly caused by calcifications of the annulus and leaflets of aortic and mitral valves. Valvular disease evolves more rapidly in the setting of CKD leading to hemodynamicaly significant stenosis [113]. Incidence of valvular heart disease in

ESRD patients is 5 times greater than in general population [114]. Two–year mortality after valve replacement therapy is about 60% [115].

Treatment of Cardiovascular Disease in Patients with Chronic Kidney Disease

Management of chronic CVD. Review of available datasets including Medicare (population 65 years and older), Ingenix i3 (50-64 years old population), and MarketScan it appears that angiotensin- converting enzymes inhibitors(ACE) and angiotensin receptors blockers (ARB), beta blockers and statins are widely used in CKD patients. Over-all 56-57% of CKD patients receive treatment with ACEI/ARB, and this percent reaches 72-77 % in patients with concurrent diagnosis of diabetes and hypertension. In employer group health plans use of this group of medications is even higher: 74-83% of CKD patients with diagnosis of diabetes are on it Beta blockers are used in 67-80% of patients with CKD and congestive heart failure, and in 40-54% of those with diagnosis of CKD and hypertension with higher use in stages 3-5. [1] In spite of wide use of pharmacological agents only 20% of 1999-2006 NHANES participants age 20 years and older with CKD 3-4 were aware of diagnosis of hypertension and were adequately controlled [1].

Statins are used in 57-72% CKD patients with a diagnosis of diabetes or cardiovascular disease. [1]. The rate of usage drops in patients on hemodialysis to just over 30%. These data suggest that some dialysis patients may be taken off statins. This action may explained by results of two large-scale clinical trials of hemodialysis patients treated with atorvastatin and rosuvastatin (4D and AURORA) which showed significant reduction of LDL levels, yet no reduction in cardiovascular death or other CVD endpoints [116,117]. Until results of the SHARP trial were presented in abstract form in 2010, the major clinical trials providing evidence for use of statins in patients with non-dialysis-treated CKD, WOSCOP and CARE, were based on secondary, sub-group or *post-hoc* analyses [118-120] The SHARP trial studied over 9,000 patients with CKD defined as a creatinine equal or bigger than 1.7 mg/dl in men or equal or bigger than 1.3 mg/dl in women for longer than 2 months(mean eGFR of 26.5 ml/min/1.73m^2). One third of the SHARP participants were receiving treatment by hemodialysis or peritoneal dialysis. Patients younger than 40 years of age who had definitive diagnosis of MI or who underwent coronary revascularization procedure were excluded from study. The average LDL cholesterol at the beginning of study was 108 mg/dl. After a median of 4.9 years follow-up, use of simvostatin/ezetimibe (Vytorin®) combination resulted in significant reduction of the first major atherosclerotic event defined as non-fatal myocardial infarction or cardiac death, revascularization procedure, or stroke (15.2 % in Vytorin group vs. 17.9 % in placebo group, p=0.001) [121] This reduction of major vascular events is similar to the improvement in clinical outcomes predicted by meta-analysis of the large scale trials - CTT. [122]. Another sub-analysis of the JUPITER trial of subjects without hyperlipidemia (LDL cholesterol <130 mg/dl), but with elevated high-sensitivity CRP level (>2mg per liter) and GFR <60 ml/min/1.73m^2 also suggested that statins are effective for primary prevention of cardiovascular events and all-cause mortality in CKD [123].

Studies evaluating use of vitamin B12 and folic acid have been disappointing for CVD risk reduction in the CKD population, as has also been observed for the general population. In a study of folic acid, vitamin B12 and B6 supplementation in German hemodialysis patients, there was no significant difference in total mortality or CVD events versus placebo after 2 years of follow-up [124]. The SEARCH study involved >1200 survivors of MI in a randomized, double–blind comparison of folic acid and vitamin B12 versus placebo. In spite of a 28% reduction in the mean serum homocysteine level, there was no difference in the major coronary events, stroke or non-coronary revascularization. [125]

Management of acute CVD by evidence-based therapies is under-utilized in patients with CKD. In a study of acute myocardial infarction CKD patients were less likely to undergo early invasive therapies, and medical interventions were used to a lesser extent including aspirin (ASA), beta blockers, and statins. Discharge counseling was also documented less frequently in the CKD population [100]. Per 2007 data, use of ACE/ARB after acute myocardial infarction in the Medicare population with CKD was 40.7% compared with 50.3% in the non-CKD population [1]. Treatment of CKD patients with ACS is based on secondary or *post hoc* analyses of data accumulated in clinical trials of the general population with ACS and from the observational data. [126]. Data to support the use of ASA for primary prevention comes from secondary analysis of the HOT study. In subjects with a low eGFR of <45 ml/min/1.73m^2, treatment with 75 mg of ASA demonstrated a 65% reduced risk of the primary endpoints of myocardial infarction, stroke, or cardiovascular mortality. This analysis projected that for every 1000 patients with low eGFR treated for 3.8 years, 76 major cardiovascular events and 54 deaths could be prevented at a "cost" of 27 excess major bleeds [127].

Revascularization and surgery in patients with CKD using either percutaneous coronary interventions (PCI) or coronary artery bypass grafting (CABG) is associated with significantly more complications [128-130]. Restenosis of both drug-eluting (30%) and bare metal (40%) stents for HD patients is markedly higher than for non-dialysis patients [131]. In addition, the pattern of restenosis of drug eluted vs. bare metal stents was different in a study of patients receiving hemodialysis treatment in Japan. For example, focal restenosis occurred more frequently in drug eluted than bare metal stents, and diffuse restenosis occurred more frequently in bare metal stents. In the same study, there was no difference in 3-year mortality (22.5% for drug eluted and 22.2% for bare metal stents) [132]. CABG is associated with at least 3-fold higher rates of in-hospital and long-term mortality in patients on hemodialysis than in general population [131]. Outcomes of newer surgical approaches, such as "off-pump," demonstrated a modest reduction in mortality risk of 8% with no difference in survival rates as compared to traditional "on-pump" approaches. [133].

The use of tissue valves in ESRD populations was supported by a recent study of 1335 renal transplant patients undergoing left–sided valve replacement. The hazard ratio of death for tissue valves compared with non-tissue valves was 17 % lower. [134].

Conclusion

CVD is the most common chronic disease and accounts for 30% of all global deaths. [135]. Over the last decade, there is evidence of a decline in CV mortality in developed countries, but this decrease is not reported in developing countries, minority populations, or in people with CKD [136]. The presence of CKD is a strong risk factor for CVD independent of diabetes, hypertension or other conventional risk factors [6,137]. The etiology of this increased risk has not been fully elucidated. Kidney function has been suggested as a potential "test" for cardiovascular risk prediction, with recent studies demonstrating increased cardiovascular death with an eGFR of less than 92-95 mg/ml/ 1.73 m^2 [138,139]. With diabetes fuelling the CKD epidemic the close interaction between kidney disease and systemic CVD poses the clinically relevant and intriguing question of whether the interventions targeted towards prevention, early detection and slowing the progression of kidney disease can help reduce CVD risk. This question remains to be answered.

References

[1] U.S. Renal Data System, USRDS 2010 Annual Data Report: Disease. *National Institutes of Health, National Institute of Diabetes and Digestive and Kidney Diseases*, Bethesda, MD, 2010. Accessed on April 20, 2011.

[2] Castro, AF, Coresh, J. CKD surveillance Using Laboratory Date from the Population – Based National Health and Nutrition Examination Survey (NHANES). *Amer J Kidney Dis,* 2009 53, S46-55.

[3] Keith, DS, Nichols, GA. Longitudinal Follow-up and Outcomes Among a Population With Chronic Kidney Disease in a Large Managed Care Organization. *Arch Intern Med* 2004 164, 659-663.

[4] Sarnak, MJ, Levey, AS. Kidney Disease as a Risk Factor for Development of Cardiovascular Disease. A Statement from the American Heart Association Councils on Kidney in Cardiovascular Disease, High Blood Pressure Research, Clinical Cardiology, and Epidemiology and Prevention. *Circulation* 2003 108, 2154-2169.

[5] Weiner, DE, Tighiouart, H. Kidney Disease, Framingham Risk Score, and Cardiac and Mortality Outcomes. *Am J Med*, 2007 120, 552e1-e8.

[6] McCullough, PA, Jurkovitz, CT. Independent Components of Chronic Kidney Disease as a Cardiovascular Risk State. *Arch Intern Med,* 2007 167, 1122-1120. (KEEP)

[7] Go, AS, Chertow, GM. Chronic Kidney Disease and the Risks of Death, Cardiovascular Events, and Hospitalization. *N Engl J Med,* 2004 351, 1296-1305.

[8] Roderick, PJ, Atkins, RJ. CKD and Mortality Risk in Older People: A Community-Based Population Study in the United Kingdom. *Am J Kidney Dis,* 2009 53, 950-960.

[9] Henry, RMA, Kostense, PJ. Mild renal insufficiency is associated with increased cardiovascular mortality: The Hoorn Study. *Kidney International,* 2002 62, 1402-1407.

[10] Brantsma AH, Bakker, SJL for the PREVEND Study Group. Cardiovascular and renal outcome in subjects with K/DOQI stage 1–3 chronic kidney disease: the importance of urinary albumin excretion. *Nephrol Dial Transplant,* 2008 23, 3851–3858.

[11] Bock, JS, Gottlieb, SS. Cardiorenal Syndrome New Perspectives. *Circulation,* 2010 121, 2592-2600.

[12] Forman, DE, Butler, J. Incidence, predictors at admission, and impact of worsening renal function among patients hospitalized with heart failure. *J Am Coll Cardiol,* 2004 43, 61–67.

[13] The ARIC Investigators. The Atherosclerosis Risk in Communities (ARIC) study: design objectives. *Am J Epidemiol,* 1989 129,687–702.

[14] Fried, LP, Borhani, NO. The Cardiovascular Health Study: design and rationale. *Ann Epidemiol,* 1991 1, 263–76.

[15] National Kidney Foundation. K/DOQI clinical practice guidelines for chronic kidney disease: evaluation, classification and stratification. A J Kidney Dis, 2002 39, S1-S266.

[16] Guerin, AP, Pannier, B. Assessment and significance of arterial stiffness in patients with chronic kidney disease. *Curr Opin Nephrol Hypertens,* 2008 17, 635–641.

[17] García-Cardeña, G, Gimbrone, M A Jr. Biomechanical modulation of endothelial phenotype: implications for health and disease. *Handb Exp Pharmacol,* 2006 176, 79–95.

[18] Chung, AW. Upregulation of matrix metalloproteinase-2 in the arterial vasculature contributes to stiffening and vasomotor dysfunction in patients with chronic kidney disease. *Circulation,* 2009 120, 792–801.

[19] Van Herck, JL. Impaired fibrillin-1 function promotes features of plaque instability in apolipoprotein E-deficient mice. *Circulation,* 2009 120, 2478–2487.

[20] Lindner, A, Charra, B.Accelerated atherosclerosis in prolonged maintenance hemodialysis. *N Engl J Med*, 1974 290,697—701.

[21] Glagov, S, Zarins, C. Hemodynamics and atherosclerosis: Insights and perspectives gained from the studies of human arteries. *Arch Pathol Lab Med,* 1988 112, 1018—1031.

[22] Rostand, SG, Gretes, JC. Ischemic heart disease in patients with uremia undergoing maintenance hemodialysis. *Kidney Int*, 1979 16, 600–611.

[23] Weiner, DE, Tabatabai, H. Cardiovascular outcomes and all-cause mortality: exploring the interaction between CKD and cardiovascular disease. *Am J Kidney Dis*, 2006 48, 392–401.

[24] Anavekar, NS, McMurray, JJ Relation between renal dysfunction and cardiovascular outcomes after myocardial infarction. *N Engl J Med*, 2004 351, 1285–1295. (Valiant)

[25] Suzuki, C, Nakamura. S. Evidence for severe atherosclerotic changes in chronic hemodialysis patients: Comparative autopsy study against cardiovascular disease patients without chronic kidney disease. *Ther Apher Dial*, 2010 15, 51-57.

[26] Pelisek, J, Assadian, A. Carotid plaque composition in chronic kidney disease: A retrospective analysis of patients undergoing carotid endarterectomy. *Eur J Vasc Endovasc Surg,* 2010 39, 11-16.

[27] Gross, ML, Meyer HP. Calcification of coronary intima and media immunohistochemistry, backscatter imaging, and X-ray analysis in renal and nonrenal patients. *Clin J Am Soc Nephrol,* 2007 2, 121–134.

[28] Nakamura, S, Ishibashi-Ueda, H. Coronary calcification in patients with chronic kidney disease and coronary artery disease. *Clin J Am Soc Nephrol*, 2009 4, 1892–1900.

[29] Stary, HC, Chandler, AB. A definition of advanced types of atherosclerotic lesions and a histological classification of atherosclerosis. A report from the Committee on Vascular Lesions of the Council on Arteriosclerosis, American Heart Association. *Circulation,* 1995 92, 1355–1374.

[30] Nakano, T, Ninomiya, T. Association of kidney function with coronary atherosclerosis and calcification in autopsy samples from Japanese elders: the Hisayama study. *Am J Kidney Dis, 2010* 55, 21–30.

[31] Schwarz, U, Buzello, M. Morphology of coronary atherosclerotic lesions in patients with end-stage renal failure. *Nephrol Dial T ransplant,* 2000 15, 218–223.

[32] London, GM, Drueke, T. Atherosclerosis and arteriosclerosis in chronic renal failure. *Kidney Int*, 1997 51, 1678-1695.

[33] London GM, Marchais, SJ. Arteriosclerosis, vascular calcifications and cardiovascular disease in uremia. *Curr Opin Nephrol Hypertens*, 2005 6, 525-531.

[34] Cheu, CD, Townend, JN. Arterial stiffness in chronic kidney disease: causes and consequences. *Heart*, 2010 11: 817-823.

[35] Mitchell, GF, Izzo, JL. Omapatrilat reduces pulse pressure and proximal aortic stiffness in patients with systolic hypertension: results of the conduit hemodynamics of omapatrilat international research study. *Circulation*, 201 23, 2955-2961.

[36] Townsend, RR, Wimmer, NJ. Aortic PWV in chronic kidney disease: A CRIC Ancillary Study. *American Journal of Hypertension*, 2010 23, 282-289.

[37] Wang, MC, Tsai, WC. Stepwise Increase in arterial stiffness corresponding with the stages of chronic kidney disease. *Am J Kidney Dis*, 2005 45, 494-501.

[38] Guerin AP, Blacher J, Pannier B, et al. Impact of aortic stiffness attenuation on survival of patients in end-stage renal failure. *Circulation*, 2001 103: 987–992.

[39] O'Rourke, M. Mechanical principles in arterial disease. Hypertension, 1995 26, 2-9.

[40] London, GM, Guerin, AP. Cardiac and arterial interactions in end-stage renal disease. *Kidney Int,* 1996 50:600—608.

[41] Amann, K, Neusub, R. Changes of vascular architecture independent of blood pressure in experimental uremia. *Am J Hypertens*, 1995 8, 409-417.

[42] Otsuka, T, Suzuki, M. Left ventricular diastolic dysfunction in the early stage of chronic kidney disease. *Am J Cardiol*, 2009 54, 199-204.

[43] Tonelli, M, Pfeffer, MA. Kidney disease and cardiovascular risk. *Annu Rev Med,* 2007 58,123-139.

[44] Wu, IW, Hung, MJ. Ventricular function and all cause-mortality in chronic kidney disease patients with angiographic coronary artery disease. *J Nephrol,* 2010 23, 181-188.

[45] Paoletti, E, Bellino, D. Is left ventricular hypertrophy a powerful predictor of progression to dialysis in chronic kidney disease? *Nephrol Dial Transplant,* 2011 26, 670-677.

[46] Hage, FG, Smalheiser, S. Predictors of survival in patients with end-stage renal disease evaluated for kidney transplantation. *Am J Cardiol,* 2007 100, 1020-1025.

[47] Ahmed, A, Rich, MW. Chronic kidney disease associated mortality in diastolic versus systolic heart failure: a propensity matched study. *Am J Cardiol,* 2007 99,393-398.

[48] Ford, ES, Ajani, UA. Explaining the decrease in U.S. deaths from coronary disease, 1980-2000. N Engl J Med, 2007 356, 2388-2398.

[49] Wilson, PW, Castelli, WP. Coronary risk prediction in adults (the Framingham Heart Study). *Am J Cardiol* 1987 57, 91G-94G.

[50] Weiner, DE, Tighiouart, H. The Framingham Predictive Instrument in Chronic Kidney Disease. *J Am Coll Cardiol* 2007 50, 217–224.

[51] The ARIC Investigators. The Atherosclerosis Risk in Communities (ARIC) study: design and objectives. *Am J Epidemiol* 1989 129, 687–702.

[52] Fried, LP, Borhani, NO. The Cardiovascular Health Study: design and rationale. *Ann Epidemiol* 1991 1,263–76.

[53] Port, FK, Hulbert-Shearon, TE1999. Predialysis blood pressure and mortality risk in a national sample of maintenance hemodialysis patients. *Am J Kidney Dis,* 1999 33, 507–517

[54] Kalantar-Zadeh, K, Block, G. Reverse epidemiology of cardiovascular risk factors in maintenance dialysis patients. *Kidney Int,* 2003 63,793–808.

[55] Kalantar-Zadeh, K, Kilpatrick, RD. Reverse epidemiology of hypertension and cardiovascular death in the hemodialysis population: the 58th annual conference and scientific sessions. *Hypertension*, 2005 45, 811-817.

[56] Kopple, JD: Nutritional status as a predictor of morbidity and mortality in maintenance hemodialysis patients. *ASAIO J,* 1997 43, 246-250.

[57] Brenner, M.B. (2008) Approach to the patient with the kidney disease. In 8th Ed. *Brenner and Rector's The Kidney* (705-713). Philadelphia. Saunders Elsevier.

[58] Muntner P, He, J. Traditional and nontraditional risk factors predict coronary heart disease in chronic kidney disease: results form the Atherosclerosis Risk in Communities Study. *J Am Nephrol*, 2005 16, 529-538.

[59] [58a] Volpe M, Tocsin G. Redefining blood pressure targets in high-risk patients?: Lessons from coronary endpoints in recent randomized clinical trials. *Am J Hyper* 2011 advanced online publication June 16.

[60] Vaziri, ND: Dyslipidemia of chronic renal failure: The nature, mechanisms and potential consequences. *Am J Renal Physiol* 2006 290, 262–272.

[61] Vaziri, ND, Norris, K. Lipid Disorders and Their Relevance to Outcomes in Chronic Kidney Disease. *Blood Purif* 2011 31, 189–196.

[62] Yamamoto, S, Kon, V. Mechanisms for increased cardiovascular disease in chronic kidney dysfunction. *Curr Opin Nephrol Hypertens.* 2009 18, 181–188.

[63] Baigent,C, Burbury, K. Premature cardiovascular disease in chronic renal failure. *Lancet*, 2000 356, 147-152.

[64] Wanner, C, Krane, V. Atorvastatin in patients with type 2 Diabetes Mellitus undergoing hemodialysis. *New Engl J Med*, 2005 353, 238-248.

[65] Kilpatrick, RD, McAllister, CJ. Association between serum lipids and survival in hemodialysis patients and impact of race. *J Am Soc Nephrol* 2007 18, 293–303.

[66] Prichard, SS. Impact of dyslipidemia in end-stage renal disease, *J AM Soc Nephrol*, 2003 14, S315-S320.

[67] ACCORD Study Group: Effects of intensive glucose lowering in type 2 diabetes. *N Engl J Med,* 2008 358, 2545-2559.

[68] The ADVANCE Collaborative Group: Intensive blood glucose control and vascular outcomes in patients with type 2 diabetes. *N Engl J Med*, 2008 358, 2560-2572.

[69] Diabetes Control and Complications Trial Research Group: The effect of intensive treatment of diabetes on the development and progression of long-term complications in insulin-dependent diabetes mellitus. *N Engl J Med,* 1993, 329,977-986.

[70] UK Prospective Diabetes Study Group: Intensive blood glucose control with sulfonylureas or insulin compared with conventional treatment and risk of complications in patients with type 2 diabetes (UKPDS 33). *Lancet,* 1998 352,837-853.

[71] Holman, RR, Paul, SK. 10-year follow-up of intensive glucose control in type 2 diabetes. N Engl J Med, 2008 359, 1577-1589.

[72] Diabetes Control and Complications Trial/Epidemiology of Diabetes Interventions and Complications Study Research Group: Retinopathy and nephropathy in patients with

type 1 diabetes four years after a trial of intensive therapy. *N Engl J Med*, 2000 342, 981-989.

[73]   Stenvinkel, P, Alvestrand, A. Inflammation in end-stage renal disease: sources, consequences, and therapy. *Semin Dial*, 2002 15,329–37.

[74]   Shastri, S, Sarnak, S. Cardiovascular disease and CKD: Core Curriculum 2010. *Am J Kidney Dis,* 2010 56, 399-417.

[75]   Vickery, S, Webb, MC. Prognostic value of cardiac biomarkers for death in a nondialysis chronic kidney disease population. *Nephrol Dial Transplant,* 2008 23, 3546–3553.

[76]   Shlipak, MG, Fried, LF. Cardiovascular mortality risk in chronic kidney disease: comparison of traditional and novel risk factors. *JAMA,* 2005 293, 1737–1745.

[77]   Pecoits-Filho, R, Barany, P. Interleukin-6 is an independent predictor of mortality in patients starting dialysis treatment. Nephrol Dial Transplant 2002 17,1684–8.

[78]   Romao, JE, Haiashi, AR. Positive acute-phase inflammatory markers in different stages of chronic kidney disease. *Am J Nephrol*, 2006 26, 59-66.

[79]   Parekh, RS, Plantinga, LC. The association of sudden cardiac death with inflammation and other traditional risk factors. *Kidney Int*, 2008 74, 1335–1342.

[80]   Soriano, S, Gonzalez, L. C-reactive protein and low albumin are predictors of morbidity and cardiovascular events in chronic kidney disease (CKD) 3–5 patients. Clin Nephrol, 2007 67, 352–357.

[81]   Shah DS, Polkinhorne, KR. Are traditional risk factors valid for assessing cardiovascular risk in end-stage renal failure patients? *Nephrology* (Carlton), 2008 3, 667–671.

[82]   Ravani, P, Tripepi, G. Asymmetrical dimethylarginine predicts progression to dialysis and death in patients with chronic kidney disease: a competing risks modeling approach. *J Am Soc Nephrol*, 2005 16, 2449-2455.

[83]   Sandgren, PE, Murray, AM. Anemia and new-onset congestive heart failure in the general Medicare population. *J Card Fail*, 2005 11,99–105.

[84]   Keane, WF, Lyle, PA. Recent advances in management of type 2 diabetes and nephropathy: lessons from the RENAAL study. *Am J Kidney Dis*, 2003 41, S22–S25.

[85]   Drueke, TB, Locatelli, F for the CREATE Investigators. Normalization of hemoglobin level in patients with chronic kidney disease and anemia. *N Engl J Med,* 2009 355, 2071–2084.

[86]   Singh, AK, Szczech, L for the CHOIR Investigators: Correction of anemia with epoetin alpha in chronic kidney disease. *N Engl J Med,* 2006 355, 2085–2098.

[87]   Pfeffer, MA, Burdmann, EA for the TREAT Investigators: A trial of darbepoetin alfa in type 2 diabetes and chronic kidney disease. *N Engl J Med,* 2009 361, 2019–2032.

[88]   Hillege, HL, Fidler, V, for the Prevention of Renal and Vascular End Stage Disease (PREVEND) Study Group: Urinary albumin excretion predicts cardio vascular and noncardiovascular mortality in general population. *Circulation*, 2002 106, 1777–1782.

[89]   Astor, BC, Hallan, SI. Glomerular filtration rate, albuminuria, and risk of cardiovascular and all-cause mortality in the US population. *Am J Epidemiol*, 2008, 167, 1226–1234.

[90]   Arnlöv, J, Evans, JC. Low-grade albuminuria and incidence of cardiovascular disease events in nonhypertensive and nondiabetic individuals: the Framingham Heart Study. *Circulation,* 2005 112, 969–975.

[91] Hemmelgarn, B, Manns, B. Relation between kidney function, proteinuria, and adverse outcomes. *JAMA*, 2010 303,423-429.

[92] Matsushita, K, van der Velde, M. Association of estimated glomerular filtration rate and albuminuria with all-cause and cardiovascular mortality in general population cohorts: a collaborative meta-analysis. *Lancet,* 2010 375, 2073-2081.

[93] Pedrinelli, R, Dell'Omo, G. Non-diabetic microalbuminuria, endothelial dysfunction and cardiovascular disease. *Vasc Med,* 2001 6, 257-264.

[94] Paisley, KE, Beaman, M. Endothelial dysfunction and inflammation in asymptomatic proteinuria. *Kidney Int,* 2003 63, 624-633.

[95] Tonelli, M, Sacks, F. Relation between serum phosphate level and cardiovascular event rate in people with coronary disease. Circulation, 2005 112, 2627–33.

[96] Tuttle, KR, Short, RA. Longitudinal Relationships among coronary artery calcification, serum phosphorus, and kidney function. Clin J Am Soc Nephrol, 2009 4, 1968-1973.

[97] Flack, JM, Neaton, JD. Ethnicity and renal disease: lessons from Multiple Risk Factor intervention Trial and Treatment of Mild Hypertension (MRFIT). *Am J Kidney Dis*, 1993 21, 31-40.

[98] Kilickesmez, KO, Abaci, O. Chronic kidney disease as a predictor of coronary lesion morphology. *Angiology*, 2010 61, 344-349.

[99] Tamagnone, LG, Tognarelli, GM. Assessment of cardiovascular risk in waiting-listed renal transplant patients: a single center experience in 558 cases. *Clin Transplant*, 2009 23, 653-659.

[100] Stack, AG, Bloembergen, WE. Prevalence and clinical correlates of coronary artery disease among new dialysis patients in the United States: a cross-sectional study. *J Am Soc Nephrol*, 2001 12, 1516 – 1523.

[101] Fox, CS, Muntner, P. Use of evidence-based therapies in short-term outcomes of ST-segment elevation myocardial infarction in patients with chronic kidney disease: a report from the National Cardiovascular Data Acute Coronary Treatment and Intervention Outcomes Network registry. *Circulation*, 2010 121, 357-365.

[102] Aviles, RJ, Askari, AT. Troponin T levels in patients with acute coronary syndromes, with or without renal dysfunction. *N Engl J Med*, 2002 346, 2047-2052.

[103] Abbas, NA, John, RI. Cardiac troponins and renal function in nondialysis patients with chronic kidney disease. *Clin Chem*, 2005 51, 2059-2066.

[104] Khan, NA, Hemmelgarn, BR. Prognostic value of troponin T and I among asymptomatic patients with end-stage renal disease. *Circulation,* 2005 112, 3088-3096.

[105] Fredericks, S, Chang, R. Circulating cardiac troponin-T in patients before and after renal transplantation. *Clin Chim Acta,* 2001 310, 199-203.

[106] Ellis, K, Dreisbach, AW. Plasma elimination of cardiac troponin I in end-stage renal disease. *South Med J,* 2001 94, 993-996.

[107] Iwanaga, Y, Miyazaki, S. Heart failure, chronic kidney disease, and biomarkers. *Circ J,* 2010 74, 1274-1282.

[108] Adams, KF, Fonarow, GC, for the ADHERE Scientific Advisory Committee and Investigators. Characteristics and outcomes of patients hospitalized for heart failure in the United States: rationale, design, and preliminary observations from the first 100,000 cases in the Acute Decompensated Heart Failure National Registry (ADHERE). *Am Heart J,* 2005 149, 209–216.

[109] Hamaguchi, S, Tsuchihashi-Makaya, M. Chronic kidney disease as an independent risk for long-term adverse outcomes in patients hospitalized with heart failure in Japan. Report from Japanese Cardiac Registry of Heart Failure in Cardiology (JCARE-CARD). *Circ J*, 2009 73, 1442-1447.

[110] Niizuma, S, Iwanaga, Y. Impact of left ventricular end-diastolic wall stress on plasma B- natriuretic peptide in heart failure with chronic kidney disease and end-stage renal disease. *Clin Chem*, 2009 55, 1347-1353.

[111] Ishii, J, Cui, W. Prognostic value of combination of cardiac troponin T and B-type natriuretic peptide after initiation of treatment in patients with chronic heart failure. *Clin Chem*, 2003 49, 2020-2029.

[112] Taniguchi, R, Sato, Y. Combined measurements of cardiac troponin T and N-terminal pro-brain natriuretic peptide in patients with heart failure. *Circ J,* 2004 68, 1160-1164.

[113] Wang, AY, Lam, CW. Sudden cardiac death in end-stage renal disease patients: a 5-year prospective analysis. *Hypertension*, 2010 56, 210–216.

[114] Umana, E, Ahmed, W. Valvular and perivalvualr abnormalities in end-stage renal disease. *Am J Med Sci,* 2003 325, 237-242.

[115] Herzog, CA. Kidney disease in cardiology. *Nephrol Dial Transplant*, 2011 26, 46-50.

[116] Herzog, CA, Ma JZ. Long-term survival of dialysis patients in the United States with prosthetic heart valves: should ACC/AHA practice guidelines on valve selection be modified? *Circulation*, 2002 105, 1336-1341.

[117] Wanner, C, Krane, V for the German Diabetes and Dialysis Study Investigators. Atorvastatin in patients with type 2 diabetes mellitus undergoing hemodialysis. *New Engl J Med,* 2005 353, 238–248.

[118] Fellstrom, BC, Jardine, AG, for the AURORA Study Group: Rosuvastatin and cardiovascular events in patients undergoing hemodialysis. *New Engl J Med,* 2009 360, 1395–1407.

[119] Tonelli, M, Keech, A. Effect of pravastatin in people with diabetes and chronic renal hypercholesterolemia disease. *J Am Soc Nephrol*, 2005 16,3748–3754.

[120] Shepherd, J, Cobbe, SM, for the West of Scotland Coronary Prevention Study Group: Prevention of coronary heart disease with pravastatin in men with. *N Engl J Med* 1995 333, 1301–1307.

[121] Sacks, FM, Pfeffer, MA, for the Cholesterol and Recurrent Events Trial Investigators: The effect of pravastatin on coronary events after myocardial infarction in patients with average cholesterol levels. *N Engl J Med*, 1996 335, 1001–1009.

[122] Sharp Collaborative Group et al. Study of Heart and Renal Protection (SHARP): randomized trial to assess the effects of lowering low-density lipoprotein cholesterol among 9,438 patients with chronic kidney disease. *Am Heart J,* 2010 160, 785-794.

[123] Cholesterol Treatment Trialists (CTT) Collaboration, Baigent, C, Blackwell, L. Efficacy and safety of mote intensive lowering of LDL cholesterol: a meta-analysis of data from 170, 000 participants in 26 randomized trials. *Lancet,* 2010 376, 1670-1681.

[124] Ridker, PM, MacFadyen, J. Efficacy of rosuvastatin among men and women with moderate chronic kidney disease and elevated high-sensitivity C-reactive protein: a secondary analysis from the JUPITER (Justification for the Use of Statins in Prevention- an Intervention Trial Evaluating Rosuvastatin) trial. *J Am Coll Cardiol,* 2010 55, 1266–1273.

[125] Hein, J, Kropf, S. B vitamins and the risk of total mortality and cardiovascular disease in end-stage renal disease: results of a randomized controlled trial. *Circulation,* 2010 121, 1432–1438.

[126] SEARCH Collaborative Group. Effects of homocysteine-lowering with folic acid plus vitamin B12 vs. placebo on mortality and major morbidity in myocardial infarction survivors: a randomized trial. *JAMA*, 2010 303, 2486-2494.

[127] Smith, GL, Lichtman, JH. Renal impairment and outcomes in heart failure: Systemic review and meta-analysis. *J Am Coll Cardiol*, 2006 47, 1987-1996.

[128] Jardine, MJ, Ninomiya, T. Aspirin is beneficial in hypertensive patients with chronic kidney disease: a post-hoc subgroup analysis of a randomized controlled trial. *J Am Coll Cardiol,* 2010 56, 956–965.

[129] Koganei, H, Kasanuki, H. Association of glomerular filtration rate with unsuccessful primary percutaneous coronary intervention and subsequent mortality in patients with acute myocardial infarction: from the HIJAMI registry. *Circ J*, 2008 72, 179-185.

[130] Ix, JH, Mercado, N. Association of chronic kidney disease with clinical outcomes after coronary revascularization: the Arterial Revascularization Therapies Study (ARTS). *Am Heart J* 2005 149, 512-519.

[131] Blackman, DJ, Pinto, R. Impact of renal insufficiency on outcome after contemporary percutaneous coronary intervention. *Am Heart J* 2006 151, 146-152.

[132] Herzog, CA, Gilbertson, DT. Survival and repeat revascularization in US dialysis patients after surgical versus percutaneous coronary intervention. [Abstract]. *Circulation* 2009; 120: S941.

[133] Ichimoto E, Kobayashi Y. Long-term clinical outcomes after sirolimus-eluting stent implantation in dialysis patients. *Int Heart J*, 2010 51, 92–97.

[134] Shroff, GR, Li, S. Survival of patients on dialysis having off-pump versus on-pump coronary artery bypass surgery in the United States. *J Thorac Cardiovasc Surg*, 2010 139, 1333–1338.

[135] Sharma, A, Gilbertson, DT. Survival of kidney transplantation patients in the United States after cardiac valve replacement. *Circulation,* 2010 121, 2733–2739.

[136] World Health Organization. 2008-2013 action plan for global strategy for the prevention and control of noncommunicable diseases. Available online at http://whqlibdoc.who.int/ publications/2009/9789241597418_ eng.pdf. Accessed April 20, 2011.

[137] Narayan, KM, Ali, MK. Global noncommunicable diseases-where worlds meet. *N Engl J Med,* 2010 363, 1196-1198.

[138] Tonelli, M, Wiebe, N. Chronic kidney disease and mortality risk: a systemic review. *J Am Soc Nephrol*, 2006 17, 2034-2047.

[139] Soveri, I, Arnlov, J. Kidney function and discrimination of cardiovascular risk in middle-aged men. *J Intern Med,* 2009 266, 406-413.

[140] Foley, RN, Wang, C. Kidney function and risk triage in adults: threshold values and hierarchical importance. *Kidney Int*, 2011 79, 99-111.

In: Current Advances in Cardiovascular Risk. Volume 2   ISBN: 978-1-62081-746-9
Editor: Sandeep Ajoy Saha   © 2012 Nova Science Publishers, Inc.

Chapter XVI

Cardiovascular Risks in Patients with Polycystic Ovary Syndrome: An Update

Manfredi Rizzo[1] and Enrico Carmina[2,]*

[1] Department of Internal Medicine and Medical Specialties,
University of Palermo, Italy
[2] Department of Biological and Medical Sciences,
University of Palermo, Italy

Abstract

Cardiovascular diseases represent the major cause of death in most of developed countries and ultimately kill as many men as women. However, as shown in several prospective studies, it seems that the onset of cardiovascular diseases is somewhat delayed in women than in men. Men and women are exposed to the same risk factors but their rates of cardiovascular morbidity and mortality are very different until old age. Only at age 75 and above cardiovascular rates of women approximate those of men. It has been suggested that differences in hormonal status and mainly in androgen levels may explain the gender disparity.

Consistent with the hypothesis that high androgen levels play a main role in determining increased cardiovascular risk, it has been shown that women with polycystic ovary syndrome (PCOS) have elevated cardiovascular risk despite their young age. However, the risk is not the same in all PCOS women, and an individual risk profile should be assessed. The number of cardiovascular events is probably increased but longitudinal studies are needed.

The discrepancy between increased cardiovascular risk at young age and postmenopausal number of cardiovascular events may be dependent on changes in androgen ovarian function after the forties.

* Corresponding author. Prof. Enrico Carmina, MD. Department of Biological and Medical Sciences, University of Palermo, Via delle Croci 47, 90139 – Palermo – Italy. Fax: +39 (091) 328997; E-mail: enricocarmina@libero.it.

1. Introduction

Cardiovascular diseases represent the major cause of death in most of developed countries and ultimately kill as many men as women [1, 2]. However, as shown in several prospective studies, it seems that the onset of cardiovascular diseases (including coronary heart disease, cerebrovascular disease and peripheral vascular disease) is somewhat delayed in women than in men [3]. It has been calculated that such onset is delayed of about 10-15 years between the two genders and for this reason the National Cholesterol Education Program in the Adult Treatment Panel III [1] defined age as a risk factor in women at age 55, compared to age 45 for men.

Men and women are exposed to the same risk factors but their rates of cardiovascular morbidity and mortality are very different until old age. Only at age 75 and above cardiovascular rates of women approximate those of men [4]. The reasons for such disparity in ages of onset of cardiovascular diseases between women and men are still not fully understood, and it cannot be explained on the basis of the differences in major established risk factors only [5].

It has been suggested that differences in hormonal status and mainly in androgen levels may explain the gender disparity. Consistently with the hypothesis that high androgen levels play a main role in determining increased cardiovascular risk, it has been shown that women with polycystic ovary syndrome (PCOS) have elevated cardiovascular risk despite their young age [6]. However, PCOS is a complex, heterogeneous disorder, associated to many other alterations that are associated to CV risk like insulin resistance and abdominal obesity, and it is unclear which factors determine the increased CV risk in these patients.

2. Cardiovascular Risk in the General Population

The possibility that androgens may increase cardiovascular risks remains controversial. Hyperandrogenism, as isolated androgen excess, has not been clearly recognized so far as a risk factor for cardiovascular disease, even though many authors have tried to correlate it with the earlier onset of atherosclerosis in men than women. In fact, some authors measured circulating androgens in post-menopausal women and they found that those with clinical or subclinical atherosclerosis had lower SHBG levels [7] or increased free testosterone concentrations [8]. In addition, acne and hirsutism were common features in women undergoing coronary revascularizations, and these women were also found to have greater involvement of coronary vessels [9]. Finally, weak associations were found between the presence of androgenic alopecia and cardiovascular risk in both men and women [10]. However, prospective studies performed on pre- and post-menopausal women failed to show a clear association between androgen levels and future cardiovascular events [10-12]. In addition, exogenous administration of testosterone to women or to female-to-male transsexuals has not led to an increased risk of cardiovascular disease [13]. Thus, at the present time, there is no evidence that androgens constitute an important risk factor for cardiovascular diseases.

3. Cardiovascular Risk
in Women with PCOS

PCOS represents the most frequently encountered endocrinopathy in women, affecting up to 10% of those in reproductive age [14]. Despite their young age, women with PCOS have an increased cardiovascular risk and this finding has been consistently reported across several geographic areas and ethnic groups.

Women with PCOS are more likely than normally cycling women to have insulin resistance, central adiposity and hypertension [15]; in addition, several markers of clinical and subclinical atherosclerosis, including serum markers (such as C-reactive protein and homocysteine), carotid intima-media thickness, coronary artery calcium and echocardiographic patterns have been found to be altered too [16-21]. Dyslipidemia is very common in women with PCOS and generally presents with the characteristics of atherogenic dyslipidemia (low HDL-cholesterol levels, elevated triglyceride concentrations [14] and lower LDL particle size due to increased levels of small, dense subclasses [21]. Increased LDL and total cholesterol have been also found and may be present in up to 30% of the patients [19, 21]. Interestingly, differently on the lipid alterations of atherogenic dyslipidemia, in PCOS, LDL increase is not influenced by body weight and is present with similar prevalence in different ethnic groups [22].

Although cardiovascular risk factors are more prevalent in women with PCOS, the risk of premature cardiovascular diseases in PCOS is at present uncertain. In fact, long-term studies examining the prevalence of cardiovascular diseases among women with PCOS did not demonstrate an increased number of events of cardiovascular morbidity and mortality [23-27].

On the basis of the observed alterations in several markers of clinical and subclinical atherosclerosis these results were somehow unexpected. Yet, it is likely that the most important confounding factor that interfered in such studies was the definition of PCOS and this makes the interpretation of the results quite difficult. PCOS by definition is a syndrome made by signs or symptoms that occur together, e.g. a combination of different phenotypes. Even after the recent revised consensus on diagnostic criteria [28], the controversy regarding characteristics of PCOS still remains [29].

Lack of universally accepted diagnostic criteria for the syndrome makes comparison of studies assessing cardiovascular risk or metabolic abnormalities very problematic [30]. Therefore, we wait for new long-term outcome studies that should include well-defined PCOS populations, without heterogeneity in their diagnostic criteria.

Another confounding factor may be related to changes in ovarian androgen production that occur with increasing age. In fact, ovarian androgen secretion starts decreasing after the age of forties.

It probably reduces the risk linked to androgen excess and may partially explain the discrepancy between the cardiovascular risk at young age and the number of cardiovascular events. Interestingly, in the study of Shaw et al. [31], the cardiovascular mortality was related to postmenopausal androgen levels of women who had PCOS during their fertile age. It suggests that the patients who maintain the highest androgen levels may have a larger number of cardiovascular events.

4. Assessment of the Cardiovascular Risk in Women with PCOS

Because of the presence of insulin resistance, abdominal obesity and androgen excess, PCOS presents an increased lifetime risk of type-2 diabetes, cardiovascular diseases and endometrial cancer. This risk combines with that linked to environmental factors, including the quantity of food, the quality of food and the physical activity. There are also some genetic factors to consider, including gene polymorphisms associated to cardiovascular diseases, as well as genes related to type-2 diabetes.

Because of all these variables, metabolic and cardiovascular risk may be vary in different ethnic groups, different PCOS phenotypes inside the same ethnic group as well as in different patients inside the same phenotype. The difference in BMI among PCOS women from different countries is shown in Figure 1, while the differences in insulin levels are shown in Figure 2.

Further, PCOS is a heterogeneous disorder and several phenotypes can be distinguished (see Figure 3). For instance, regarding our population [32,33], in classic PCOS phenotype we found that: 1) Insulin resistance is very mild or absent in 30% of the patients; 2) Body weight is normal in 35% of the patients; 3) Abdominal obesity is absent in 30% of the patients; 4) Biochemical hyperandrogenism is very mild or absent in 30% of the patients. In Figures 4-6 are shown BMI, insulin levels and LDL subclasses in the different PCOS phenotypes in our population.

It should be highlighted that there are many important differences in cardiovascular risk between the different PCOS phenotypes. In fact, most studies have been performed in severe (classic) PCOS phenotype that are generally associated to insulin resistance and increased body weight. On the contrary, few studies have included patients with mild PCOS phenotypes (ovulatory PCOS and normo-androgenic PCOS) who often present normal insulin sensitivity and normal body weight [32]. While it indicates the need of an individual assessment of cardiovascular risk in PCOS women, the few available data also suggest that patients with mild PCOS phenotype present some increase of cardiovascular risk [33-35].

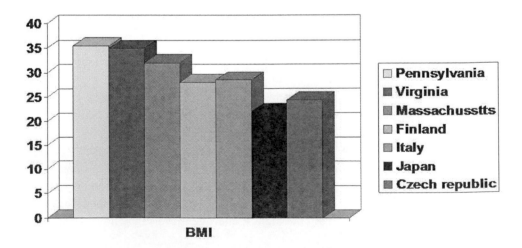

Figure 1. BMI in different PCOS populations.

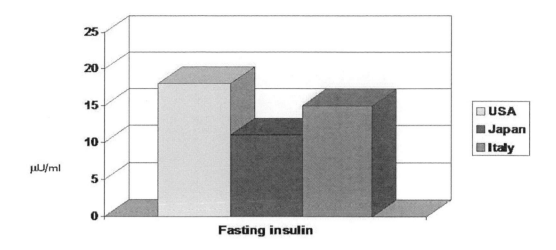

Carmina E et al. Am J Obstet Gynecol 1992; 167: 1807-12

Figure 2. Insulin levels in different PCOS populations.

5. Individual Cardiovascular Risk Profile in Women with PCOS

Because of all these variables, the risk is not the same in all PCOS patients and an individual risk profile should be assessed. In this view, the Androgen Excess & Polycystic Ovary Syndrome (AE-PCOS) Society has recently published a position statement on this topic [36].

	Androgen levels	LH/FSH	Insulin resistance	CV risk
Type I Classic PCOS	Increased	Increased	Increased	Increased
Type II Classic PCOS	Increased	Mild increase	Increased	Increased
Ovulatory PCOS	Increased	Normal	Mild increase	Mild increase
Normoandrogenic PCOS	Normal	Increased	Normal	Normal?

Figure 3. Characteristics of main PCOS phenotypes.

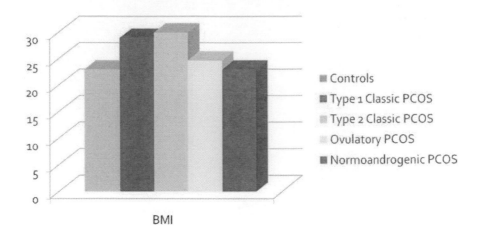

Guastella E et al. Fertil Steril 2010

Figure 4. BMI in different PCOS phenotypes [32].

According to these guidelines, the PCOS risk categories were distinguished in: 1) At regular risk; 2) At risk; 3) At high risk. PCOS patients at risk for metabolic and cardiovascular diseases were identified as all PCOS patients with Obesity, Cigarette smoking, Dyslipidemia, Complete atherogenic dyslipidemia, Increased LDL-C or non-HDL-C, Hypertension, Impaired glucose tolerance, Subclinical vascular disease. By contrast, PCOS patients probably at risk for metabolic and cardiovascular diseases were identified as all PCOS patients with mood disturbances, mostly severe depression and maybe also anxiety and reduced quality of life. Finally, PCOS patients at high risk for metabolic and cardiovascular diseases were identified as all PCOS patients with the metabolic syndrome, Type-2 diabetes or overt cardiovascular or renal disease.

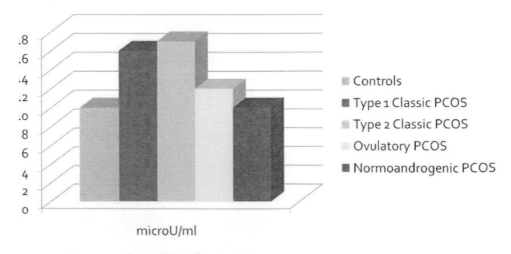

Guastella E et al. Fertil Steril 2010

Figure 5. Insulin levels in different PCOS phenotypes [32].

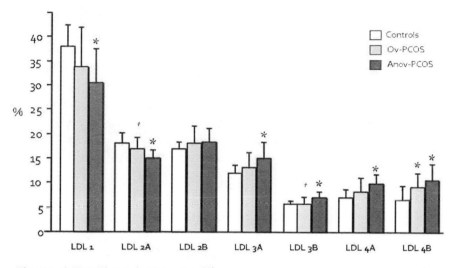

Rizzo et al. Hum Reprod 2009; 24: 2286-2292

Figure 6. LDL subclasses in different PCOS phenotypes [33].

For a correct assessment of metabolic and cardiovascular risk, the statement suggested that in all PCOS patients, the following parameters should be assessed: Family history, including type II diabetes and early cardiovascular diseases, Clinical history, including cigarette smoking, BMI, waist circumference, Blood pressure, Fasting glucose, complete lipid profile. Regarding treatment, PCOS patients at regular risk should not have any treatment related to metabolic and cardiovascular issues. Also, PCOS patients at risk or at high risk should be treated by lifestyle modification as first line therapy. PCOS patients who do not normalize their risk profile should be further treated with specific therapies according their risk factors.

	Risk	LDL cut-off values	Non-HDL cut-off values
PCOS patients at regular risk	Regular	130	160
PCOS patients at risk	Increased	130	160
PCOS patients at high risk	Severely increased	100	130

R Wild, E Carmina et al. J Clin Endocrinol Metab 2010

Figure 7. PCOS risk categories and lipid target values [36].

For instance, regarding dyslipidemia, lipid target values have been suggested (see Figure 7). For patients with atherogenic dyslipidemia, the statement suggested the following: 1) No treatment for isolated low HDL-C or high triglycerides; 2) Patients with atherogenic dyslipidemia may be treated by metformin; 3) In alternative, statins may be used; 4) The association metformin + statins does not get additional results. Further, for patients with increased LDL-cholesterol or non-HDL-cholesterol, the statement suggested the following: 1) Lipid goals depend on the degree of risk; 2) Statins should be used to reduce LDL- and non-HDL-C levels; 3) Metformin is not effective on LDL-C; 4) In particular conditions, fenofibrate, nicotinic acid or omega-3-fatty acids may be added to statins.

Conclusion

Women with PCOS have increased cardiovascular risk; however, the risk is not the same in all patients and an individual risk profile should be assessed. The number of cardiovascular events is probably increased but longitudinal studies are needed. The discrepancy between increased cardiovascular risk at young age and postmenopausal number of cardiovascular events may be depending on changes in androgen ovarian function after the forties.

Future Perspective

There is a need of future clinical studies to better clarify whether cardiovascular morbidity and mortality is increased in women with PCOS in the short-term and particularly in the long-term [37]; these studies would include observational and intervention studies, cohort studies, as well as randomized controlled studies. Indeed, evidence is accumulating that postmenopausal women with PCOS have an increased risk of cerebro-vascular events and cardiovascular morbidity; notably, these events are only in part related to persisting hyperandrogenism, but are mostly correlated with excessive body weight (mainly visceral obesity). Therefore, the best long-term strategy may be to inform women with PCOS on their high risk for metabolic and cardiovascular diseases.

References

[1]   National Cholesterol Education Program (NCEP). Expert Panel on Detection, Evaluation, and Treatment of High Blood Cholesterol in Adults (Adult Treatment Panel III). Third Report of the National Cholesterol Education Program (NCEP) Expert Panel on Detection, Evaluation, and Treatment of High Blood Cholesterol in Adults (Adult Treatment Panel III) final report. *Circulation* 2002; 106:3143-421. 23.

[2]   Am Heart Association. *Heart Disease and Stroke Statistics* - 2003 Update. http://www.americanheart.org/downloadable/heart/104039109 1015HDS_Stats_03.pdf.

[3]   Waldron, I. Trends in gender differences in mortality: relationships to changing gender differences in behaviour and other causal factors. 2000. in *Annandale and Hunt* (Eds.), Gender Inequalities in Health. Open University Press: London. p. 150-181.

[4]   Statistical Abstract of the United States. 1992, 112th Edition, *U.S. Department of Commerce, Economics and Statistics Administration,* Bureau of the Census.

[5]   Dauber TR, Meadows GF, Moore FE Jr. Epidemiological approaches to heart disease: the Framingham Study. *Am J Public Health* 1951; 41:279-81.

[6]   Guzick DS. Cardiovascular risk in PCOS. *J Clin Endocrinol Metab.* 2004; 89:3694-5.

[7]   Reinecke H, Bogdanski J, Woltering A, Breithardt Gu, Assmann G, Kerber S, von Eckardstein A. Relation of serum levels of sex hormone binding globulin to coronary heart disease in postmenopausal women. *Am J Cardiol* 2002; 90:364–368.

[8]   Phillips GB, Pinkernell TH, Jing TY. Relationship between serum sex hormones and coronary artery disease in postmenopausal women. *Arterioscler Thromb Vasc Biol* 1997; 17:695–70.

[9]   Wild RA, Grubb B, Hartz A, Van Nort JJ, Bachman W, Bartholomew M. Clinical signs of androgen excess as risk factors for coronary artery disease. *Fertil Steril* 1990; 54:255–259.

[10]   Rebora A Baldness and coronary artery disease: the dermatologic point of view of a controversial issue. *Arch Dermatol* 137:943–947.

[11]   Eckardestein A, Wu FCW. Testosterone and atherosclerosis. *Growth Hormone IGF Res* 2003; 13 (Suppl. 1): S72-S84.

[12]   Barrett-Connor E, Goodman-Gruen D. Prospective study of endogenous sex hormones and fatal cardiovascular disease in postmenopausal women. *BMJ* 1995; 17: 369-384.

[13]   Gorgels WJ, van der Graaf Y, Blankenstein MA, Collette HJ, Erkelens DW. Urinary sex hormone excretions in premenopausal women and coronary heart disease risk: a nested casereferent study in the DOM-cohort. *J Clin Epidemiol* 1997; 50:275–281.

[14]   Price JF, Lee AJ, Fowkes FG. Steroid sex hormones and peripheral arterial disease in the Edinburgh artery study. *Steroids* 1997; 62:789–794.

[15]   Lobo RA, Carmina E. The importance of diagnosing the polycystic ovary syndrome. *Ann Intern Med.* 2000; 132:989-93.

[16]   Talbott EO, Guzick DS, Sutton-Tyrrell K, McHugh-Pemu K, Zborowski J, Remsberg K, Kuller L. Evidence for association between polycystic ovary syndrome and premature carotid atherosclerosis in middle-aged women. *Arterioscler Thromb Vasc Biol* 2000; 20:2414–2421.

[17]   Christian RC, Dumesic DA, Behrenbeck T, Oberg A, Sheedy PF, Fitzpatrick L. Prevalence and predictors of coronary artery calcification in women with polycystic ovary syndrome. *J Clin Endocrinol Metab* 2003; 88:2562–2568.

[18]   Orio F, Palomba S, Spinellli L, Cascella T, Tauchmanova L, Zullo F, Lombardi G, Colao A. The cardiovascular risk of young women with polycystic ovary syndrome: an observational, analytical, prospective case-control study. *J Clin Endocrinol Metab* 2004; 89:3696–3701.

[19]   Carmina E, Chu MC, Longo RA, Rini GB, Lobo RA. Phenotypic variation in hyperandrogenic women influences the findings of abnormal metabolic and cardiovascular risk parameters. *J Clin Endocrinol Metab* 2005;90(5):2545-9.

[20]   Carmina E, Orio F, Palomba S, Longo RA, Cascella T, Colao A, Lombardi G, Rini GB, Lobo RA. Endothelial dysfunction in PCOS: role of obesity and adipose hormones. *Am J Med.* 2006;119(4):356.e1-6.

[21]   Berneis K, Rizzo M, Fruzzetti F, Lazzaroni V, Carmina E. Atherogenic lipoprotein phenotype and LDL size and subclasses in women with polycystic ovary syndrome. *J Clin Endocrinol Metab* 2007; 92:186-189.

[22]   Rizzo M, Longo RA, Guastella E, Rini GB, Carmina E. Assessing cardiovascular risk in mediterranean women with polycystic ovary syndrome. J *Endocrinol Invest* 2011; 34: 422-426

[23]   Dahlgren E, Janson PO, Johansson S, Lapidus L, Oden A. Polycystic ovary syndrome and risk for myocardial infarction. Evaluated from a risk factor model based on a prospective population study of women. *Acta Obstet Gynecol Scand* 1992; 71:599–604.

[24]   Pierpoint T, McKeigue PM, Isaacs AJ, et al. Mortality of woman with polycystic ovary syndrome at long term follow up. *J Clin Epidemiol* 1998;51:581-86.

[25]   Wild SH, Pierpoint T, Mckeigue PM, et al. Cardiovascular disease in women with polycystic ovary syndrome at long-term follow-up: a retrospective cohort study. *Clin Endocrinol* 2000;52:595-600.

[26]   Cibula D, Cifkova R, Fanta M, Poledne R, Zivny J, Skibova J. Increased risk of non-insulin dependent diabetes mellitus, arterial hypertension and coronary artery disease in perimenopausal women with a history of the polycystic ovary syndrome. 2000 *Hum Reprod* 15:785–789.

[27]   Talbott EO, Zborowski JV, Sutton-Tyrrell K, McHugh-Pemu KP, Guzick DS. Cardiovascular risk in women with polycystic ovary syndrome. *2001 Obstet Gynecol Clin North Am* 28:111–133.

[28]   The Rotterdam ESHRE/ASRM-sponsored PCOS consensus Workshop Group. Revised 2003 consensus on diagnostic criteria and long term health risks related to polycystic ovary syndrome. *Fertility Sterility* 2004; 81:19-25.

[29]   Azziz R. Diagnosis of polycystic ovary syndrome: the Rotterdam criteria are premature. *J Clin Endocrinol Metab* 2006; 91:781-85.

[30]   Dagre AG, Lekakis J. *Cardiovascular Disease in Polycystic Ovary Syndrome:* Questioning the Obvious. Published online. 2006. http://www.athero.org.

[31]   Shaw LJ, Merz CN, Azziz R, Stanczyk FZ, Sopko G, Braunstein GD, Kelsey SF, Kip KE, Cooper-Dehoff RM, Johnson BD, Vaccarino V, Reis SE, Bittner V, Hodgson TK, Rogers W, Pepine CJ. Post-Menopausal Women with a History of Irregular Menses and Elevated Androgen Measurements at High Risk for Worsening Cardiovascular Event-Free Survival: Results from the National Institutes of Health National Heart, Lung, and Blood Institute (NHLBI) Sponsored Women's Ischemia Syndrome Evaluation (WISE). *J Clin Endocrinol Metab.* 2008; 93:1276-84.

[32]   Guastella E, Longo RA, Carmina E. Clinical and endocrine characteristics of the main polycystic ovary syndrome phenotypes. *Fertil Steril* 2010;94:2197-201.

[33]   Rizzo M, Berneis K, Hersberger M, Pepe I, Di Fede G, Rini GB, Spinas GA, Carmina E. Milder forms of atherogenic dyslipidemia in ovulatory vs. anovulatory polycystic ovary syndrome phenotype. *Hum Reprod* 2009; 24: 2286-2292.

[34]   Carmina E, Napoli N, Longo RA, Rini GB, Lobo RA. Metabolic syndrome in polycystic ovary syndrome (PCOS): lower prevalence in southern Italy than in the USA and the influence of criteria for the diagnosis of PCOS. *Eur J Endocrinol* 2006; 154: 141-145.

[35] Berneis K, Rizzo M, Hersberger M, Rini GB, Di Fede G, Pepe I, Spinas GA, Carmina E. Atherogenic forms of dyslipidemia in women with polycystic ovary syndrome. *Int J Clin Pract* 2009; 63:56-62.

[36] R Wild, E Carmina, E Diamanti-Kandarakis, A Dokras, H Escobar-Morreale, W Futterweit, R Lobo, R Norman, E Talbott, D Dumesic. Assessment of cardiovascular risk and prevention of cardiovascular disease in women with the polycystic ovary syndrome: a position statement by the androgen excess & polycystic ovary syndrome (AE-PCOS) society. *J Clin Endocrinol Metab* 2010; 85:2038-49.

[37] Rizzo M, Berneis K, Spinas GA, Rini GB, Carmina E. Long-term consequences of polycystic ovary syndrome on cardiovascular risk. *Fertil Steril* 2009; 91(4 Suppl):1563-7.

In: Current Advances in Cardiovascular Risk. Volume 2   ISBN: 978-1-62081-746-9
Editor: Sandeep Ajoy Saha   © 2012 Nova Science Publishers, Inc.

Chapter XVII

Cardiovascular Risk in Patients with Obstructive Sleep Apnea: Pathophysiology, Epidemiology and Management

Miranda M. Lim[1],* and Indira Gurubhagavatula[1,2]
[1]Division of Sleep Medicine, University of Pennsylvania Medical Center,
Philadelphia, PA, US
[2]Pulmonary, Critical Care and Sleep Section,
Philadelphia VA Medical Center, Philadelphia, PA, US

Abstract

Despite rising awareness of its high prevalence, myriad of health consequences and responsiveness to treatment, obstructive sleep apnea (OSA) still remains under-recognized and therefore untreated. One consequence of untreated OSA is cardiovascular disease, which has been attributed to several purported mechanisms: increased sympathetic drive, oxidative stress, inflammation, vascular endothelial dysfunction, large intra-thoracic pressure fluctuations, mechanically-mediated vessel wall changes and metabolic dysregulation. These mechanisms may be the basis for why OSA is more common among patients with hypertension, coronary artery disease, arrhythmias and stroke. Indeed, epidemiologic studies have provided evidence that untreated severe OSA confers increased risk of cardiovascular events, but data are limited by small sample sizes and incomplete control for obesity (the major risk factor for OSA). Data from controlled trials is scarce, but suggests that hypertension may improve with treatment of OSA, particularly in those with severe disease. The first-line treatment for OSA, continuous positive airway pressure (CPAP), is safe and effective, and should be offered to patients with severe OSA to reduce cardiovascular risk, and patients with mild to moderate apnea and known cardiovascular disease. Data from randomized intervention studies is needed

* Corresponding Author Address: Miranda Lim, MD, PHD. Division of Sleep Medicine; 3624 Market Street, Suite 205; Philadelphia, PA 19104; Miranda.Lim@uphs.upenn.edu.

to establish whether treatment of mild to moderate OSA improves cardiovascular outcomes.

I. Introduction

Obstructive sleep apnea (OSA) is a common form of sleep-disordered breathing characterized by intermittent obstruction of the upper airway during sleep, which results in drops in blood oxygen saturation. These events are terminated by a surge in sympathetic activity and an arousal from sleep.

Occult symptoms may be present for years without identification, and many patients with OSA are unaware of their difficulty breathing, even upon awakening. Often it is the patient's bed partner who observes the patient snoring or experiencing apneas during sleep. OSA is also frequently suspected by primary care physicians or cardiologists because of signs/symptoms such as refractory hypertension, obesity, insulin resistance and other potential cardiovascular and metabolic sequelae.

The diagnosis of OSA relies on overnight polysomnography, which typically measures airflow, respiratory effort, oximetry and electroencephalography (EEG) during sleep. Obstructive apneas are defined by complete absence of inspiratory airflow lasting at least 10 seconds despite ongoing ventilatory effort.

Hypopneas are defined by reduction of inspiratory airflow lasting at least 10 seconds, accompanied by either oxyhemoglobin desaturation or an arousal on EEG. The Apnea-Hypopnea Index (AHI) is calculated by summing the number of apneas and hypopneas and dividing the sum by total sleep time. OSA within the "mild" range is defined as an AHI value between 5 and 15 events per hour, "moderate" as 15 to 30 events per hour and "severe" as ≥ 30 events per hour.

In this chapter, we will review the evidence supporting the association between OSA and cardiovascular disease, possible pathophysiological mechanisms and treatment benefits and suggest basic guidelines for managing OSA in the high-risk cardiovascular patient.

II. Pathophysiology

The repetitive oxyhemoglobin desaturation that occurs in association with apnea events, the swings in intra-thoracic pressure that occur when effort to breathe is made against a closed upper airway, and the arousal from sleep that terminates these events, presumably form the basis for a range of pathophysiologic disturbances in OSA. These include neurobiological, metabolic, vascular and inflammatory changes which may contribute to the development of cardiovascular disease.

Specifically, potential biological pathways include: sympathetic hyperactivity, oxidative stress leading to chronic inflammation, vascular endothelial dysfunction, intra-thoracic pressure changes leading to hemodynamic instability, mechanically-mediated carotid atherosclerosis from snoring and metabolic dysfunction leading to the so-called "metabolic syndrome".

(A) Sympathetic Hyperactivity

In healthy subjects, different stages of sleep confer distinct changes in cardiovascular regulation, with a progressive decrease in sympathetic nervous traffic to muscle with deepening stages of non-REM sleep. In contrast, rapid eye movement (REM) sleep is accompanied by increased sympathetic drive, with correspondingly more labile blood pressure and heart rate, mimicking the levels seen during wakefulness [1].

Obstructive apneas are often accompanied by a surge in sympathetic activity which terminates after the apnea ends with an arousal or awakening from sleep [2]. Patients with OSA show increased sympathetic activity even during wakefulness with normal oxyhemoglobin saturation, as evidenced by microneurography and elevated catecholamine levels in blood and urine [2, 3]. Heightened sympathetic activity in the peripheral circulation appears to be independent of age, sex and obesity.

Chronically sympathetic hyperactivity may explain why OSA patients have faster heart rates, decreased heart rate variability and increased blood pressure variability [4]. These abnormalities have been linked to increased risk of hypertension, congestive heart failure and related mortality [4-7].

(B) Inflammation/Oxidative Stress

Intermittent, recurrent hypoxic injury and reperfusion generate highly-reactive oxygen free radical species which have been linked to atherosclerosis in both animal and human studies [8, 9]. The potential mechanisms for this include activation of nuclear factor kappa B (NFKB) and other plasma cytokines and pro-inflammatory markers, such as C-reactive protein and serum amyloid-A [10, 11]. In addition, *in vitro* studies have shown that cell adhesion molecule upregulation can lead to increased leukocyte activation and vascular endothelial binding in patients with OSA [12, 13].

Treatment of OSA with CPAP reduces the production of the free radical superoxide and the proinflammatory cytokines NFKB and tumor necrosis factor (TNF)-alpha [14, 15]. Treatment of OSA with CPAP also attenuates the increased leukocyte binding activity to endothelial lining [12, 13]. Withdrawal of CPAP therapy for one week does not reinstate the pro-inflammatory state, suggesting perhaps there are long-lasting anti-inflammatory effects of CPAP [16]. These studies provide some evidence that OSA, like obesity, can lead to the so-called "inflammatory state" which predisposes patients to cardiovascular disease.

(C) Vascular Endothelial Dysfunction

Endothelial dysfunction is often seen in patients with hypertension, hyperlipidemia, diabetes and smoking and has been linked to increased risk of cardiovascular events [17]. The combination of hypoxia, hypercapnia and heart rate/blood pressure changes during obstructive events have been linked to impaired endothelial function. Release of vasoactive substances such as endothelin may contribute to a sustained vasoconstrictive state, resulting in increased blood pressure [18]. Recent data show that endothelial nitric oxide synthase (eNOS) and phosphorylation of eNOS is reduced in patients with OSA, which reverses after 4 weeks of treatment with CPAP [19].

In addition to impaired vascular endothelial dysfunction, patients with untreated OSA may also have an increased risk of clot formation. This may be in part mediated by increased hematocrit, increased levels of fibrinogen and increased blood viscosity [20-22]. Also, platelet aggregation increases in patients with OSA and is reversed by CPAP therapy [23-25]. These platelet effects may be in part due to elevated nocturnal catecholamine levels [24].

(D) Intrathoracic Pressure Changes

The mechanics of the obstructive apnea are characterized by recurrent inspiratory effort against a closed upper airway resulting in negative intrathoracic pressures. Such abrupt and repetitive intrathoracic pressure changes can consequently affect hemodynamics of cardiac filling and cardiac function by increasing transmural gradients across the atria, ventricles and aorta [26-28]. Changes in transmural pressures may increase afterload, impair left ventricular relaxation and reduce left ventricular preload filling, thereby decreasing stroke volume and cardiac output [28, 29]. These cardiac changes may contribute to the development of heart failure in patients with untreated OSA. Furthermore, one study suggests that patients with OSA may be at a higher risk of thoracic aortic dissection [30].

(E) Mechanically-mediated Atherosclerosis

One recent study showed an association between heavy snoring and atherosclerosis of the carotid artery [31]. The hypothesis is that vibration produced by snoring might directly damage the wall of the carotid artery, leading to increased atherosclerotic plaque deposition.

Mouse models of OSA using cyclic intermittent hypoxia have shown that atherosclerosis can be induced in the presence of a high-fat diet [32]. While these mice were not subject to the mechanical disruption seen with heavy snoring, this points to the fact that there are multiple parallel pathways engaged during OSA that can lead to atherosclerosis. Indeed, patients with OSA show early signs of atherosclerosis [33] and there is a strong positive correlation between OSA severity and atherosclerotic plaque volume [34].

(F) Metabolic Syndrome

Several lines of evidence hint that OSA is associated with metabolic dysregulation that leads to obesity, thus amplifying cardiovascular risk. Patients with OSA are predisposed to significant weight gain prior to the diagnosis of sleep apnea [35]. After controlling for obesity, patients with OSA show significantly higher levels of circulating leptin compared to non-OSA controls [35, 36]. This suggests that OSA confers resistance to leptin, which is a hormone that suppresses appetite by promoting satiety, thereby predisposing OSA patients to weight gain. Accordingly, treatment with CPAP reduces leptin levels and decreases visceral fat volume [37].

OSA may also contribute to cardiovascular risk via impaired glucose tolerance and insulin resistance. Patients with OSA have higher fasting blood glucose levels, insulin and hemoglobin A1c (HgA1c) values even after controlling for body mass index (BMI) [36]. The severity of OSA correlates with the degree of insulin resistance and severe OSA increases the risk of Type 2 Diabetes Mellitus by five-fold [38-40]. However, there are conflicting reports regarding whether treatment with CPAP can improve insulin sensitivity and these results may be confounded by the degree of obesity across subjects [41-44].

III. Epidemiology

(A) Prevalence and Risk Factors

One of the largest and most comprehensive studies on OSA, the Wisconsin Sleep Cohort study, estimates that approximately 20% of adults have at least mild OSA, while 7% of adults have at least moderate OSA (AHI > 15 events/hour) [45, 46]. This prevalence is expected to rise as the prevalence of obesity increases, because the strongest risk factor for OSA is obesity. Indeed, BMI, a proxy variable for obesity and enlarged neck circumference, an indicator of central obesity, have been used as screening tools for OSA. Other risk factors include advancing age, male gender, post-menopausal status and reduced upper airway caliber, and [47]. Other suspected risk factors for OSA include family history/genetics, smoking, use of alcohol, narcotics or benzodiazepines before sleep and nighttime nasal congestion [47]. It is important to note that most of these risk factors have also shown to be independent risk factors for the occurrence of cardiovascular disease.

Because of its high prevalence, obesity as a risk factor for OSA deserves particular attention. Obesity alone increases the risk of developing OSA [48] . Untreated OSA may contribute to weight gain through metabolic syndrome [35, 36]. The prevalence of OSA increases with several markers of obesity, including visceral adiposity [49]. Given the rapid rise in obesity rates in the United States, it is crucial from a public health standpoint to clearly understand what role OSA plays in obesity [50].

Obesity and OSA share the same biological pathways (oxidative stress, inflammation, vascular endothelial dysfunction, metabolic syndrome). If OSA indeed carries risk for cardiovascular disease that is independent of obesity, then we would expect that the combination of OSA and obesity would correlate with cardiovascular risk that exceeds the risk from either condition existing alone.

The challenge, however, has been to reliably and accurately segregate the cardiovascular risk attributable to these two conditions when they tend to share a tight epidemiological linkage to one another. There may be inherent differences in the biological state of the mildly obese subject compared to the severely obese subject and this might explain conflicting epidemiologic and treatment data [51].

The fact that there is a safe and highly effective treatment of OSA (nasal continuous positive airway pressure, or CPAP), whereas there is not such an effective treatment for obesity, gives hope that we may be able to mitigate the cardiovascular consequences of obesity through treatment of OSA.

(C) Evidence for the link between OSA and Cardiovascular Outcomes

While the pathophysiology of OSA provides biologically plausible links to cardiovascular disease, the direct evidence establishing a causal link is still lacking. Current studies have been limited by several barriers, including lack of randomized controlled trials, confounding coexisting disease conditions such as obesity, hypertension, diabetes and the significant expense associated with polysomnography as the diagnostic gold standard for OSA. In this section, we will review the epidemiology data showing that patients with OSA have an increased risk for hypertension, coronary artery disease, arrhythmia, stroke and possibly even acute myocardial infarction. While these studies strongly suggest a causal link between OSA and cardiovascular burden, one should keep in mind that most of these studies offer indirect evidence at best.

(1) Hypertension

The Joint National Committee on Prevention, Detection, Evaluation and Treatment of High Blood Pressure has listed OSA as first on the list of identifiable causes of hypertension [52]. This is because the strongest evidence linking OSA to cardiovascular disease exists when hypertension is used as the outcome measure.

Hypertension has been induced in rats subjected to cyclic intermittent hypoxia that is similar in magnitude and frequency to that seen in clinical OSA [53]. A canine model of OSA in which dogs were subjected to repetitive occlusion of the upper airway during sleep also produced elevated blood pressure in as little as two weeks, and reverses within four weeks after cessation of the occlusive events and restoration of a normal breathing pattern [54].

Human studies also support this association between sleep-disordered breathing and hypertension [55-58]. Prospective data from the large, community-based, Wisconsin Sleep Cohort Study showed that moderate to severe OSA (defined as an AHI $\geq$15 events/hour) is independently associated with a three-fold increased risk of developing hypertension after just four years [59]. The design included an initial cross-sectional component, with subjects being followed for many years thereafter and included participants between 30 and 60 years of age. Among the older cohort in the Sleep Heart Health Study, however, a similar association with hypertension was not found; nearly half of the subjects were greater than 65 years old [60], and this lack of association may be due to a survivor effect. This hypothesis was supported in a smaller study, which showed that the strength of the association between OSA and hypertension decreased with age [61]. Patients with OSA tend to be classified as "non-dippers," with respect to the observation that they do not show the typical decrease in blood pressure during sleep [62]. The "non-dipper" state has been shown to be an independent risk factor for cardiovascular morbidity [62].

Treatment of OSA with CPAP may in fact reverse hypertension [63]. Patients with OSA who start CPAP therapy may show significant lowering of daytime blood pressure, even if they have relatively refractory hypertension, defined as taking three or more antihypertensive medications at maximum doses [64]. This effect has also been shown in two separate randomized placebo-controlled trials with CPAP therapy reducing systolic blood pressure, between 1.3 and 5.3 mm Hg [65, 66]. While this degree of reduction may appear small, nevertheless, reductions of this magnitude are similar to those achieved by BP-lowering medication and have tremendous implications when we consider the global prevalence of OSA and hypertension. Therefore, convincing data exist implicating OSA in the development of hypertension, in both animal and human studies. Treatment of OSA with CPAP during sleep may lower blood pressure even in the daytime.

(2) Coronary Artery Disease (CAD)

OSA may contribute to the development of CAD through its effects on blood pressure, or by initiating vascular dysfunction via inflammation, oxidative stress and endothelial changes, as discussed earlier. Animal studies show that cyclic intermittent hypoxia can induce atherosclerosis in mice that are fed a high-fat diet [32].

While early, small-scale studies supported an association between OSA (or snoring) and CAD/myocardial infarction (MI) [67-70], it was not until 2001 that a large-scale, community-based, cross-sectional report of over 9,000 patients found that OSA was an independent risk factor for CAD [71].

More recent studies have shown a strong positive correlation between OSA severity and coronary atherosclerotic plaque volume, as measured by three-dimensional, intravascular ultrasound [34]. Furthermore, OSA may portend poorer survival in patients with CAD, as patients with OSA and established CAD have a significantly higher mortality (38%) than those without OSA and established CAD (9%)[72].

Treatment of OSA with CPAP appears to decrease the incidence of new cardiovascular events in patients with known CAD [73]. Another study reported that cardiovascular deaths were less common in CPAP-treated patients compared to CPAP-untreated patients, although this was based on retrospective data [74].

(3) Arrhythmias

A wide range of cardiac arrhythmias have been reported in patients with OSA and the frequency appears to increase with the severity of OSA [75-77]. The most common arrhythmias include sinus bradycardia, atrioventricular block and atrial fibrillation, although ventricular arrhythmias ranging from benign ectopy to fatal ventricular tachycardia have also been reported [75, 78-80].

Bradyarrhythmias are often temporally correlated to the occurrence of obstructive events and the following desaturation, due to the vagal response to apnea and hypoxia [81]. This may occur even in the absence of known conduction disease; thus, it is important to exclude OSA as a cause of sinus bradycardia prior to cardiac intervention such as placement of a permanent pacemaker. Use of a pacemaker rather than correction of hypoxia with appropriate CPAP therapy may put the patient at risk for demand ischemia, as pacing during apneic events would be expected to increase heart rate and oxygen demand during apneic events, a condition of relative hypoxia. Elimination of apnea and abolition of hypoxia with CPAP would be a more appropriate management approach.

Patients with OSA carry a greater risk for developing atrial fibrillation [82]. In addition, patients with untreated OSA that underwent cardioversion for atrial fibrillation had a two-fold increased likelihood of recurrence within one year, compared to patients with CPAP-treated OSA [83]. Potential mechanisms predisposing patients to atrial fibrillation include hypoxia, sympathetic surges, blood pressure fluctuations and transmural pressure changes during each obstructive event.

Ventricular arrhythmias vary widely. Benign premature ventricular contractions are seen in up to 60% of patients with OSA [75]. In contrast, even fatal ventricular tachycardia has been reported in patients with OSA [76]. A major epidemiologic study, Sleep Heart Health, reported a significant association between OSA and nocturnal ventricular ectopy [77].

Treatment of OSA with CPAP usually eliminates sinus bradycardia which occurs as a physiologic response to obstructive apneas [75, 78]. Removal of obstruction via CPAP or tracheostomy has also been reported to relieve atrioventricular nodal block and nocturnal ventricular arrhythmias [84-87].

(4) Stroke

The same hemodynamic, vascular, inflammatory and thrombotic disease mechanisms activated by OSA can contribute to the risk of stroke [88]. Obstructive respiratory events have been associated with reduced cerebral blood flow [89]. Even isolated snoring has been associated with an increased risk of stroke, independent of other cardiovascular risk factors [90, 91]. This finding may in part be related to the previously discussed finding that snoring is associated with increased carotid atherosclerosis [31].

The Sleep Heart Health data showed that men with moderate to severe OSA (AHI greater than 19) have a three-fold increased risk of stroke. In the mild to moderate range (AHI between 5-25), each unit increase in AHI was estimated to increase stroke risk by 6%. In women, stroke was not significantly associated with AHI, but increased risk was observed at an AHI greater than 25 [92].

In addition to the evidence that OSA confers a greater risk of stroke, OSA itself may be an important predictor of post-stroke outcome [71, 93, 94]. OSA is common post-stroke and increasing severity of OSA may confer worsening neuropsychological outcome and cognitive impairment, as well as risk of recurrent stroke and death [95]. Treatment of OSA post-stroke with CPAP has shown promising results, although studies have been limited by poor adherence [96, 97]. OSA may develop in the post-stroke patient for many reasons, including weight gain or injury to relevant regions of the brain.

(5) Acute cardiac Events

Patients with severe OSA experience recurrent, intermittent apneas with oxyhemoglobin desaturation, CO_2 retention and abnormal autonomic and hemodynamic profiles during sleep. Any of these and in particular oxyhemoglobin desaturation, could hypothetically precipitate acute cardiovascular ischemia. Nocturnal sympathetic excess may be one condition that fosters the development of acute ischemic cardiovascular events in the sleep apnea patient. Data for this hypothesis comes from an investigation of the time of occurrence of myocardial infarction (MI) in patients with OSA, compared to those without OSA [98]. In the general population, MI is most likely to occur during daytime morning hours (6:00 am to 2:00 pm); in this group, sleep is a condition that is typically characterized by high parasympathetic tone and is relatively cardioprotective. In contrast, over 40% of patients with OSA suffered MI's during nighttime sleep hours (10:00 pm to 6:00 am); in this group, sleep is a time of sympathetic, rather than parasympathetic excess. These results suggest that OSA may precipitate nocturnal MI and may even lead to increased risk of sudden cardiac death seen in patients with OSA [99]. In patients without clinically significant coronary artery disease, OSA may result in nocturnal angina and ST-segment depression on electrocardiogram (EKG) [100], though these remain rare occurrences in sleep laboratory subjects. ST depression is more frequent in patients with severe OSA [101], albeit the widespread use of beta blockers may have reduced this frequency. Moreover, CPAP treatment of OSA significantly decreases

ST depression [102]. In summary, while these studies suggest an association between OSA and cardiovascular outcomes, definitive evidence regarding a causal role for OSA is still lacking. Small sample sizes, inadequate control for confounding variables such as medical illnesses, medication use and age, lack of control groups and lack of randomized treatment trials continue to hamper our understanding of this relationship. Thus, existing data addressing cardiovascular outcomes associated with OSA should be interpreted with caution.

IV. Management

The primary therapy for OSA is positive airway pressure (PAP), which consists of delivery of pressurized air to the nose and/or mouth to maintain patency of the upper airway [103, 104]. PAP has been shown to be safe and effective for treating OSA. Second-line therapies include weight loss, position therapy (in those whose apnea is dependent on body position during sleep), oral appliances and upper airway surgery. Other alternatives such as plastic adhesive nasal strips to flare the nostrils and nasal micro-valve devices to create more positive end-expiratory pressure (PEEP) are untested but may improve snoring.

(A) Positive Airway Pressure (PAP)

PAP therapy has been shown to reduce the AHI to a normal range (less than 5 events per hour) in many patients with OSA. In patients with moderate to severe OSA, PAP improves daytime sleepiness and neurocognitive function [105, 106]. PAP therapy may also reduce cardiovascular risk in patients with OSA, including a modest reduction in blood pressure [2], myocardial infarction [73], ventricular arrhythmias [84, 107], cardiac death [108], and the need for coronary angioplasty or coronary artery bypass grafting [73]. The mechanisms by which PAP improves cardiovascular outcomes may be related to a reduction in adrenergic activity and inflammatory markers and improved vascular endothelial function. Unfortunately, evidence-based guidelines are still lacking, as essential randomized clinical trials remain in the early stages of planning. In the meantime, empiric evidence supports that patients with existing cardiovascular disease should be actively screened for OSA symptoms and referred to a Sleep Center if indicated. This includes patients with obesity, refractory hypertension, known coronary artery disease or arrhythmias, as well as a clinical history of snoring, witnessed apneas and daytime sleepiness. Given that PAP is effective and safe, the following patient populations should be offered treatment with PAP to reduce cardiovascular risk: 1) Patients with severe OSA, 2) Patients with high cardiovascular risk and 3) Patients with mild to moderate OSA with daytime sleepiness [51, 109, 110].

(B) Weight Loss

Despite the recommendation by most sleep specialists that weight management be an integral part of OSA management, the actual data for the beneficial effects of weight loss on OSA is sparse [59, 111]. In many cases, weight loss may not completely eliminate OSA;

however, a study with mildly overweight subjects showed that loss of as little as 10% weight was associated with a decrease in OSA severity [59]. Some have hypothesized that treatment with PAP may facilitate weight loss, via mechanisms including restoration of sensitivity to leptin and perhaps increased physical activity due to improvements in daytime alertness; however, others studies have not borne this out [112].

(C) Other Treatment Options

In those who cannot tolerate or refuse PAP therapy, alternative treatment options include positional therapy, use of an oral appliance or upper airway surgery. None of these treatments has been proven to reduce cardiovascular risk, and should be used only if PAP fails to improve the patient's OSA.

Positional therapy refers to sleeping in a certain position that may reduce the frequency of obstructive respiratory events. OSA is often worse in the supine position; therefore, forced sleeping in the lateral position or cervical extension may be helpful to improve patency of the upper airway [113, 114]. However, this therapy should be considered only after PAP has been attempted, especially in patients with severe OSA.

The most common oral appliance used in the treatment of OSA is the mandibular advancement device. Oral appliances are a reasonable alternative to PAP therapy in patients with mild to moderate OSA and only minimal sleepiness or cardiovascular risk. These devices act to gradually advance the mandible thereby increasing the antero-posterior diameter of the oropharynx. Small studies have shown improvement in the severity of OSA and snoring, but there is still not yet evidence of reduced cardiovascular risk after treatment with oral appliances [115, 116].

Different surgical options to increase airway size and reduce airway resistance exist as second or third-line therapies for patients with OSA. The most common surgery is the uvulopalatopharyngoplasty (UPPP), followed by maxillomandibular advancement surgery. Both surgeries are complex and not without risk, without guarantee of success. About 40% of patients experience 50% reductions in AHI; if their baseline disease severity was severe, therefore, there is still significant likelihood that they would require ongoing PAP therapy. Therefore every effort should be made for patients to clearly understand the risks and benefits prior to proceeding with surgery [117]. Tracheostomy can be considered in patients with life-threatening OSA who fail or are non-adherent to PAP therapy, as an alternative approach to bypass the upper airway obstruction.

Conclusion and Future Directions

We have described the evidence linking OSA to cardiovascular disease and reviewed the data regarding putative pathophysiological mechanisms. We note the difficulty in separating an independent risk due to OSA from that due to obesity. The current evidence is limited by small sample sizes, inability to adequately control for obesity, comorbid conditions and/or medication use, age and a paucity of randomized controlled clinical trials. The primary treatment for OSA, positive airway pressure, is safe and effective in reducing the frequency of sleep-disordered breathing events and in restoring oxygen saturation levels. Given existing data from randomized clinical trials that shows improvement in blood pressure with treatment of OSA with PAP, particularly in patients with severe disease, we propose that all patients with severe OSA should be treated with PAP. Interventions aimed at adherence to weight loss and PAP therapy are crucial aspects of the management of OSA.

Two large randomized trials are evaluating the efficacy of CPAP on neurocognitive function, mood, sleepiness and quality of life. The first, the Apnea Positive Pressure Long-term Efficacy Study (APPLES) [118] is a randomized, sham-controlled, double-blinded, 6-month, intention-to-treat trial of CPAP therapy of 1100 subjects in five clinical centers. Sham-CPAP has recently been validated as the placebo intervention in another major randomized controlled trial for CPAP in mild to moderate OSA, known as the CPAP Apnea Trial, North America Program (CATNAP) [119]. Like APPLES, CATNAP also measures daytime functioning. Data from these and other larger-scale randomized studies are required to establish whether early identification and treatment of mild to moderate OSA improves cardiovascular outcomes.

References

[1]   Somers VK, Dyken ME, Mark AL, Abboud FM. Sympathetic-nerve activity during sleep in normal subjects. *N Engl J Med.* 1993 Feb 4;328(5):303-7.

[2]   Somers VK, Dyken ME, Clary MP, Abboud FM. Sympathetic neural mechanisms in obstructive sleep apnea. *J Clin Invest.* 1995 Oct;96(4):1897-904.

[3]   Narkiewicz K, van de Borne PJ, Cooley RL, Dyken ME, Somers VK. Sympathetic activity in obese subjects with and without obstructive sleep apnea. *Circulation.* 1998 Aug 25;98(8):772-6.

[4]   Narkiewicz K, Montano N, Cogliati C, van de Borne PJ, Dyken ME, Somers VK. Altered cardiovascular variability in obstructive sleep apnea. *Circulation.* 1998 Sep 15;98(11):1071-7.

[5]   Frattola A, Parati G, Cuspidi C, Albini F, Mancia G. Prognostic value of 24-hour blood pressure variability. *J Hypertens.* 1993 Oct;11(10):1133-7.

[6]   Palatini P, Penzo M, Racioppa A, Zugno E, Guzzardi G, Anaclerio M, et al. Clinical relevance of nighttime blood pressure and of daytime blood pressure variability. *Arch Intern Med.* 1992 Sep;152(9):1855-60.

[7]   Singh JP, Larson MG, Tsuji H, Evans JC, O'Donnell CJ, Levy D. Reduced heart rate variability and new-onset hypertension: insights into pathogenesis of hypertension: the Framingham Heart Study. *Hypertension.* 1998 Aug;32(2):293-7.

[8]   Dean RT, Wilcox I. Possible atherogenic effects of hypoxia during obstructive sleep apnea. *Sleep.* 1993 Dec;16(8 Suppl):S15-21; discussion S-2.

[9]   Halliwell B. The role of oxygen radicals in human disease, with particular reference to the vascular system. *Haemostasis.* 1993 Mar;23 Suppl 1:118-26.

[10]   Punjabi NM, Beamer BA. C-reactive protein is associated with sleep disordered breathing independent of adiposity. *Sleep.* 2007 Jan 1;30(1):29-34.

[11]   Svatikova A, Wolk R, Shamsuzzaman AS, Kara T, Olson EJ, Somers VK. Serum amyloid a in obstructive sleep apnea. *Circulation.* 2003 Sep 23;108(12):1451-4.

[12]   Dyugovskaya L, Lavie P, Lavie L. Increased adhesion molecules expression and production of reactive oxygen species in leukocytes of sleep apnea patients. *Am J Respir Crit Care Med.* 2002 Apr 1;165(7):934-9.

[13] Dyugovskaya L, Lavie P, Lavie L. Lymphocyte activation as a possible measure of atherosclerotic risk in patients with sleep apnea. Ann N Y Acad Sci. 2005 Jun;1051:340-50.

[14] Ryan S, Taylor CT, McNicholas WT. Selective activation of inflammatory pathways by intermittent hypoxia in obstructive sleep apnea syndrome. *Circulation.* 2005 Oct 25;112(17):2660-7.

[15] Schulz R, Mahmoudi S, Hattar K, Sibelius U, Olschewski H, Mayer K, et al. Enhanced release of superoxide from polymorphonuclear neutrophils in obstructive sleep apnea. Impact of continuous positive airway pressure therapy. *Am J Respir Crit Care Med.* 2000 Aug;162(2 Pt 1):566-70.

[16] Phillips CL, Yang Q, Williams A, Roth M, Yee BJ, Hedner JA, et al. The effect of short-term withdrawal from continuous positive airway pressure therapy on sympathetic activity and markers of vascular inflammation in subjects with obstructive sleep apnoea. *J Sleep Res.* 2007 Jun;16(2):217-25.

[17] Bonetti PO, Lerman LO, Lerman A. Endothelial dysfunction: a marker of atherosclerotic risk. *Arterioscler Thromb Vasc Biol.* 2003 Feb 1;23(2):168-75.

[18] Phillips BG, Narkiewicz K, Pesek CA, Haynes WG, Dyken ME, Somers VK. Effects of obstructive sleep apnea on endothelin-1 and blood pressure. *J Hypertens.* 1999 Jan;17(1):61-6.

[19] Jelic S, Padeletti M, Kawut SM, Higgins C, Canfield SM, Onat D, et al. Inflammation, oxidative stress, and repair capacity of the vascular endothelium in obstructive sleep apnea. *Circulation.* 2008 Apr 29;117(17):2270-8.

[20] Chin K, Ohi M, Kita H, Noguchi T, Otsuka N, Tsuboi T, et al. Effects of NCPAP therapy on fibrinogen levels in obstructive sleep apnea syndrome. *Am J Respir Crit Care Med.* 1996 Jun;153(6 Pt 1):1972-6.

[21] Hoffstein V, Herridge M, Mateika S, Redline S, Strohl KP. Hematocrit levels in sleep apnea. *Chest.* 1994 Sep;106(3):787-91.

[22] Wessendorf TE, Thilmann AF, Wang YM, Schreiber A, Konietzko N, Teschler H. Fibrinogen levels and obstructive sleep apnea in ischemic stroke. *Am J Respir Crit Care Med.* 2000 Dec;162(6):2039-42.

[23] Bokinsky G, Miller M, Ault K, Husband P, Mitchell J. Spontaneous platelet activation and aggregation during obstructive sleep apnea and its response to therapy with nasal continuous positive airway pressure. A preliminary investigation. *Chest.* 1995 Sep;108(3):625-30.

[24] Eisensehr I, Ehrenberg BL, Noachtar S, Korbett K, Byrne A, McAuley A, et al. Platelet activation, epinephrine, and blood pressure in obstructive sleep apnea syndrome. *Neurology.* 1998 Jul;51(1):188-95.

[25] Sanner BM, Konermann M, Tepel M, Groetz J, Mummenhoff C, Zidek W. Platelet function in patients with obstructive sleep apnoea syndrome. *Eur Respir J.* 2000 Oct;16(4):648-52.

[26] Buda AJ, Pinsky MR, Ingels NB, Jr., Daughters GT, 2nd, Stinson EB, Alderman EL. Effect of intrathoracic pressure on left ventricular performance. *N Engl J Med.* 1979 Aug 30;301(9):453-9.

[27] Stoohs R, Guilleminault C. Cardiovascular changes associated with obstructive sleep apnea syndrome. *J Appl Physiol.* 1992 Feb;72(2):583-9.

[28] Virolainen J, Ventila M, Turto H, Kupari M. Effect of negative intrathoracic pressure on left ventricular pressure dynamics and relaxation. *J Appl Physiol.* 1995 Aug;79(2):455-60.

[29] Bradley TD. Right and left ventricular functional impairment and sleep apnea. *Clin Chest Med.* 1992 Sep;13(3):459-79.

[30] Sampol G, Romero O, Salas A, Tovar JL, Lloberes P, Sagales T, et al. Obstructive sleep apnea and thoracic aorta dissection. *Am J Respir Crit Care Med.* 2003 Dec 15;168(12):1528-31.

[31] Lee SA, Amis TC, Byth K, Larcos G, Kairaitis K, Robinson TD, et al. Heavy snoring as a cause of carotid artery atherosclerosis. *Sleep.* 2008 Sep 1;31(9):1207-13.

[32] Savransky V, Nanayakkara A, Li J, Bevans S, Smith PL, Rodriguez A, et al. Chronic intermittent hypoxia induces atherosclerosis. *Am J Respir Crit Care Med.* 2007 Jun 15;175(12):1290-7.

[33] Drager LF, Bortolotto LA, Lorenzi MC, Figueiredo AC, Krieger EM, Lorenzi-Filho G. Early signs of atherosclerosis in obstructive sleep apnea. *Am J Respir Crit Care Med.* 2005 Sep 1;172(5):613-8.

[34] Turmel J, Series F, Boulet LP, Poirier P, Tardif JC, Rodes-Cabeau J, et al. Relationship between atherosclerosis and the sleep apnea syndrome: an intravascular ultrasound study. *Int J Cardiol.* 2009 Feb 20;132(2):203-9.

[35] Phillips BG, Kato M, Narkiewicz K, Choe I, Somers VK. Increases in leptin levels, sympathetic drive, and weight gain in obstructive sleep apnea. *Am J Physiol Heart Circ Physiol.* 2000 Jul;279(1):H234-7.

[36] Vgontzas AN, Papanicolaou DA, Bixler EO, Hopper K, Lotsikas A, Lin HM, et al. Sleep apnea and daytime sleepiness and fatigue: relation to visceral obesity, insulin resistance, and hypercytokinemia. *J Clin Endocrinol Metab.* 2000 Mar;85(3):1151-8.

[37] Chin K, Shimizu K, Nakamura T, Narai N, Masuzaki H, Ogawa Y, et al. Changes in intra-abdominal visceral fat and serum leptin levels in patients with obstructive sleep apnea syndrome following nasal continuous positive airway pressure therapy. *Circulation.* 1999 Aug 17;100(7):706-12.

[38] Elmasry A, Lindberg E, Berne C, Janson C, Gislason T, Awad Tageldin M, et al. Sleep-disordered breathing and glucose metabolism in hypertensive men: a population-based study. *J Intern Med.* 2001 Feb;249(2):153-61.

[39] Ip MS, Lam B, Ng MM, Lam WK, Tsang KW, Lam KS. Obstructive sleep apnea is independently associated with insulin resistance. *Am J Respir Crit Care Med.* 2002 Mar 1;165(5):670-6.

[40] Punjabi NM, Sorkin JD, Katzel LI, Goldberg AP, Schwartz AR, Smith PL. Sleep-disordered breathing and insulin resistance in middle-aged and overweight men. *Am J Respir Crit Care Med.* 2002 Mar 1;165(5):677-82.

[41] Harsch IA, Schahin SP, Radespiel-Troger M, Weintz O, Jahreiss H, Fuchs FS, et al. Continuous positive airway pressure treatment rapidly improves insulin sensitivity in patients with obstructive sleep apnea syndrome. *Am J Respir Crit Care Med.* 2004 Jan 15;169(2):156-62.

[42] Smurra M, Philip P, Taillard J, Guilleminault C, Bioulac B, Gin H. CPAP treatment does not affect glucose-insulin metabolism in sleep apneic patients. *Sleep Med.* 2001 May;2(3):207-13.

[43] Babu AR, Herdegen J, Fogelfeld L, Shott S, Mazzone T. Type 2 diabetes, glycemic control, and continuous positive airway pressure in obstructive sleep apnea. *Arch Intern Med.* 2005 Feb 28;165(4):447-52.

[44] West SD, Nicoll DJ, Wallace TM, Matthews DR, Stradling JR. Effect of CPAP on insulin resistance and HbA1c in men with obstructive sleep apnoea and type 2 diabetes. *Thorax.* 2007 Nov;62(11):969-74.

[45] Young T, Peppard PE, Gottlieb DJ. Epidemiology of obstructive sleep apnea: a population health perspective. *Am J Respir Crit Care Med.* 2002 May 1;165(9):1217-39.

[46] Phillipson EA. Sleep apnea--a major public health problem. *N Engl J Med.* 1993 Apr 29;328(17):1271-3.

[47] Young T, Skatrud J, Peppard PE. Risk factors for obstructive sleep apnea in adults. *JAMA.* 2004 Apr 28;291(16):2013-6.

[48] Young T, Palta M, Dempsey J, Skatrud J, Weber S, Badr S. The occurrence of sleep-disordered breathing among middle-aged adults. *N Engl J Med.* 1993 Apr 29;328(17):1230-5.

[49] Shinohara E, Kihara S, Yamashita S, Yamane M, Nishida M, Arai T, et al. Visceral fat accumulation as an important risk factor for obstructive sleep apnoea syndrome in obese subjects. *J Intern Med.* 1997 Jan;241(1):11-8.

[50] Mokdad AH, Bowman BA, Ford ES, Vinicor F, Marks JS, Koplan JP. The continuing epidemics of obesity and diabetes in the United States. *JAMA.* 2001 Sep 12;286(10):1195-200.

[51] Pack AI, Gislason T. Obstructive sleep apnea and cardiovascular disease: a perspective and future directions. *Prog Cardiovasc Dis.* 2009 Mar-Apr;51(5):434-51.

[52] Chobanian AV, Bakris GL, Black HR, Cushman WC, Green LA, Izzo JL, Jr., et al. The Seventh Report of the Joint National Committee on Prevention, Detection, Evaluation, and Treatment of High Blood Pressure: the JNC 7 report. *JAMA.* 2003 May 21;289(19):2560-72.

[53] Fletcher EC, Lesske J, Qian W, Miller CC, 3rd, Unger T. Repetitive, episodic hypoxia causes diurnal elevation of blood pressure in rats. *Hypertension.* 1992 Jun;19(6 Pt 1):555-61.

[54] Brooks D, Horner RL, Kozar LF, Render-Teixeira CL, Phillipson EA. Obstructive sleep apnea as a cause of systemic hypertension. Evidence from a canine model. *J Clin Invest.* 1997 Jan 1;99(1):106-9.

[55] Silverberg DS, Oksenberg A, Iaina A. Sleep-related breathing disorders as a major cause of essential hypertension: fact or fiction? *Curr Opin Nephrol Hypertens.* 1998 Jul;7(4):353-7.

[56] Fletcher EC, DeBehnke RD, Lovoi MS, Gorin AB. Undiagnosed sleep apnea in patients with essential hypertension. *Ann Intern Med.* 1985 Aug;103(2):190-5.

[57] Kales A, Bixler EO, Cadieux RJ, Schneck DW, Shaw LC, 3rd, Locke TW, et al. Sleep apnoea in a hypertensive population. *Lancet.* 1984 Nov 3;2(8410):1005-8.

[58] Lavie P, Ben-Yosef R, Rubin AE. Prevalence of sleep apnea syndrome among patients with essential hypertension. *Am Heart J.* 1984 Aug;108(2):373-6.

[59] Peppard PE, Young T, Palta M, Dempsey J, Skatrud J. Longitudinal study of moderate weight change and sleep-disordered breathing. *JAMA.* 2000 Dec 20;284(23):3015-21.

[60] Nieto FJ, Young TB, Lind BK, Shahar E, Samet JM, Redline S, et al. Association of sleep-disordered breathing, sleep apnea, and hypertension in a large community-based study. Sleep Heart Health Study. *JAMA.* 2000 Apr 12;283(14):1829-36.

[61] Lavie P, Herer P, Hoffstein V. Obstructive sleep apnoea syndrome as a risk factor for hypertension: population study. *BMJ.* 2000 Feb 19;320(7233):479-82.

[62] Pankow W, Nabe B, Lies A, Becker H, Kohler U, Kohl FV, et al. Influence of sleep apnea on 24-hour blood pressure. *Chest.* 1997 Nov 5;112(5):1253-8.

[63] Hla KM, Skatrud JB, Finn L, Palta M, Young T. The effect of correction of sleep-disordered breathing on BP in untreated hypertension. *Chest.* 2002 Oct;122(4):1125-32.

[64] Logan AG, Tkacova R, Perlikowski SM, Leung RS, Tisler A, Floras JS, et al. Refractory hypertension and sleep apnoea: effect of CPAP on blood pressure and baroreflex. *Eur Respir J.* 2003 Feb;21(2):241-7.

[65] Pepperell JC, Ramdassingh-Dow S, Crosthwaite N, Mullins R, Jenkinson C, Stradling JR, et al. Ambulatory blood pressure after therapeutic and subtherapeutic nasal

continuous positive airway pressure for obstructive sleep apnoea: a randomised parallel trial. *Lancet.* 2002 Jan 19;359(9302):204-10.

[66] Becker HF, Jerrentrup A, Ploch T, Grote L, Penzel T, Sullivan CE, et al. Effect of nasal continuous positive airway pressure treatment on blood pressure in patients with obstructive sleep apnea. *Circulation.* 2003 Jan 7;107(1):68-73.

[67] D'Alessandro R, Magelli C, Gamberini G, Bacchelli S, Cristina E, Magnani B, et al. Snoring every night as a risk factor for myocardial infarction: a case-control study. *BMJ.* 1990 Jun 16;300(6739):1557-8.

[68] Mooe T, Rabben T, Wiklund U, Franklin KA, Eriksson P. Sleep-disordered breathing in men with coronary artery disease. *Chest.* 1996 Mar;109(3):659-63.

[69] Mooe T, Rabben T, Wiklund U, Franklin KA, Eriksson P. Sleep-disordered breathing in women: occurrence and association with coronary artery disease. *Am J Med.* 1996 Sep;101(3):251-6.

[70] Hung J, Whitford EG, Parsons RW, Hillman DR. Association of sleep apnoea with myocardial infarction in men. *Lancet.* 1990 Aug 4;336(8710):261-4.

[71] Shahar E, Whitney CW, Redline S, Lee ET, Newman AB, Javier Nieto F, et al. Sleep-disordered breathing and cardiovascular disease: cross-sectional results of the Sleep Heart Health Study. *Am J Respir Crit Care Med.* 2001 Jan;163(1):19-25.

[72] Peker Y, Hedner J, Kraiczi II, Loth S. Respiratory disturbance index: an independent predictor of mortality in coronary artery disease. *Am J* Respir Crit Care Med. 2000 Jul;162(1):81-6.

[73] Milleron O, Pilliere R, Foucher A, de Roquefeuil F, Aegerter P, Jondeau G, et al. Benefits of obstructive sleep apnoea treatment in coronary artery disease: a long-term follow-up study. *Eur Heart J.* 2004 May;25(9):728-34.

[74] Doherty LS, Kiely JL, Swan V, McNicholas WT. Long-term effects of nasal continuous positive airway pressure therapy on cardiovascular outcomes in sleep apnea syndrome. *Chest.* 2005 Jun;127(6):2076-84.

[75] Guilleminault C, Connolly SJ, Winkle RA. Cardiac arrhythmia and conduction disturbances during sleep in 400 patients with sleep apnea syndrome. *Am J Cardiol.* 1983 Sep 1;52(5):490-4.

[76] Hoffstein V, Mateika S. Cardiac arrhythmias, snoring, and sleep apnea. *Chest.* 1994 Aug;106(2):466-71.

[77] Mehra R, Benjamin EJ, Shahar E, Gottlieb DJ, Nawabit R, Kirchner HL, et al. Association of nocturnal arrhythmias with sleep-disordered breathing: The Sleep Heart Health Study. *Am J Respir Crit Care Med.* 2006 Apr 15;173(8):910-6.

[78] Koehler U, Fus E, Grimm W, Pankow W, Schafer H, Stammnitz A, et al. Heart block in patients with obstructive sleep apnoea: pathogenetic factors and effects of treatment. *Eur Respir J.* 1998 Feb;11(2):434-9.

[79] Mooe T, Gullsby S, Rabben T, Eriksson P. Sleep-disordered breathing: a novel predictor of atrial fibrillation after coronary artery bypass surgery. *Coron Artery Dis.* 1996 Jun;7(6):475-8.

[80] Shepard JW, Jr., Garrison MW, Grither DA, Dolan GF. Relationship of ventricular ectopy to oxyhemoglobin desaturation in patients with obstructive sleep apnea. *Chest.* 1985 Sep;88(3):335-40.

[81] Zwillich C, Devlin T, White D, Douglas N, Weil J, Martin R. Bradycardia during sleep apnea. Characteristics and mechanism. *J Clin Invest.* 1982 Jun;69(6):1286-92.

[82] Gami AS, Hodge DO, Herges RM, Olson EJ, Nykodym J, Kara T, et al. Obstructive sleep apnea, obesity, and the risk of incident atrial fibrillation. *J Am Coll Cardiol.* 2007 Feb 6;49(5):565-71.

[83] Kanagala R, Murali NS, Friedman PA, Ammash NM, Gersh BJ, Ballman KV, et al. Obstructive sleep apnea and the recurrence of atrial fibrillation. *Circulation*. 2003 May 27;107(20):2589-94.

[84] Harbison J, O'Reilly P, McNicholas WT. Cardiac rhythm disturbances in the obstructive sleep apnea syndrome: effects of nasal continuous positive airway pressure therapy. *Chest*. 2000 Sep;118(3):591-5.

[85] Grimm W, Hoffmann J, Menz V, Kohler U, Heitmann J, Peter JH, et al. Electrophysiologic evaluation of sinus node function and atrioventricular conduction in patients with prolonged ventricular asystole during obstructive sleep apnea. *Am J Cardiol*. 1996 Jun 15;77(15):1310-4.

[86] Becker H, Brandenburg U, Peter JH, Von Wichert P. Reversal of sinus arrest and atrioventricular conduction block in patients with sleep apnea during nasal continuous positive airway pressure. *Am J Respir Crit Care Med*. 1995 Jan;151(1):215-8.

[87] Tilkian AG, Guilleminault C, Schroeder JS, Lehrman KL, Simmons FB, Dement WC. Sleep-induced apnea syndrome. Prevalence of cardiac arrhythmias and their reversal after tracheostomy. *Am J Med*. 1977 Sep;63(3):348-58.

[88] Somers VK, White DP, Amin R, Abraham WT, Costa F, Culebras A, et al. Sleep Apnea and Cardiovascular Disease. An American Heart Association/American College of Cardiology Foundation Scientific Statement From the American Heart Association Council for High Blood Pressure Research Professional Education Committee, Council on Clinical Cardiology, Stroke Council, and Council on Cardiovascular Nursing Council. *Circulation*. 2008 Jul 28.

[89] Netzer N, Werner P, Jochums I, Lehmann M, Strohl KP. Blood flow of the middle cerebral artery with sleep-disordered breathing: correlation with obstructive hypopneas. *Stroke*. 1998 Jan;29(1):87-93.

[90] Dyken ME, Somers VK, Yamada T, Ren ZY, Zimmerman MB. Investigating the relationship between stroke and obstructive sleep apnea. *Stroke*. 1996 Mar;27(3):401-7.

[91] Partinen M. Ischaemic stroke, snoring and obstructive sleep apnoea. *J Sleep Res*. 1995 Jun;4(S1):156-9.

[92] Redline S, Yenokyan G, Gottlieb DJ, Shahar E, O'Connor GT, Resnick HE, et al. Obstructive sleep apnea-hypopnea and incident stroke: the sleep heart health study. *Am J Respir Crit Care Med*. 2010 Jul 15;182(2):269-77.

[93] Good DC, Henkle JQ, Gelber D, Welsh J, Verhulst S. Sleep-disordered breathing and poor functional outcome after stroke. *Stroke*. 1996 Feb;27(2):252-9.

[94] Wessendorf TE, Dahm C, Teschler H. Prevalence and clinical importance of sleep apnea in the first night after cerebral infarction. *Neurology*. 2003 Mar 25;60(6):1053; author reply

[95] Yaggi H, Mohsenin V. Obstructive sleep apnoea and stroke. *Lancet Neurol*. 2004 Jun;3(6):333-42.

[96] Bassetti CL, Milanova M, Gugger M. Sleep-disordered breathing and acute ischemic stroke: diagnosis, risk factors, treatment, evolution, and long-term clinical outcome. *Stroke*. 2006 Apr;37(4):967-72.

[97] Wessendorf TE, Wang YM, Thilmann AF, Sorgenfrei U, Konietzko N, Teschler H. Treatment of obstructive sleep apnoea with nasal continuous positive airway pressure in stroke. *Eur Respir J*. 2001 Oct;18(4):623-9.

[98] Kuniyoshi FH, Garcia-Touchard A, Gami AS, Romero-Corral A, van der Walt C, Pusalavidyasagar S, et al. Day-night variation of acute myocardial infarction in obstructive sleep apnea. *J Am Coll Cardiol*. 2008 Jul 29;52(5):343-6.

[99] Gami AS, Howard DE, Olson EJ, Somers VK. Day-night pattern of sudden death in obstructive sleep apnea. *N Engl J Med*. 2005 Mar 24;352(12):1206-14.

[100] Hanly P, Sasson Z, Zuberi N, Lunn K. ST-segment depression during sleep in obstructive sleep apnea. *Am J Cardiol.* 1993 Jun 1;71(15):1341-5.

[101] Philip P, Guilleminault C. ST segment abnormality, angina during sleep and obstructive sleep apnea. *Sleep.* 1993 Sep;16(6):558-9.

[102] Peled N, Abinader EG, Pillar G, Sharif D, Lavie P. Nocturnal ischemic events in patients with obstructive sleep apnea syndrome and ischemic heart disease: effects of continuous positive air pressure treatment. *J Am Coll Cardiol.* 1999 Nov 15;34(6):1744-9.

[103] Sullivan CE, Issa FG, Berthon-Jones M, Eves L. Reversal of obstructive sleep apnoea by continuous positive airway pressure applied through the nares. *Lancet.* 1981 Apr 18;1(8225):862-5.

[104] Basner RC. Continuous positive airway pressure for obstructive sleep apnea. *N Engl J Med.* 2007 Apr 26;356(17):1751-8.

[105] Derderian SS, Bridenbaugh RH, Rajagopal KR. Neuropsychologic symptoms in obstructive sleep apnea improve after treatment with nasal continuous positive airway pressure. *Chest.* 1988 Nov;94(5):1023-7.

[106] Zimmerman ME, Arnedt JT, Stanchina M, Millman RP, Aloia MS. Normalization of memory performance and positive airway pressure adherence in memory-impaired patients with obstructive sleep apnea. *Chest.* 2006 Dec;130(6):1772-8.

[107] Javaheri S. Effects of continuous positive airway pressure on sleep apnea and ventricular irritability in patients with heart failure. *Circulation.* 2000 Feb 1;101(4):392-7.

[108] Marin JM, Carrizo SJ, Vicente E, Agusti AG. Long-term cardiovascular outcomes in men with obstructive sleep apnoea-hypopnoea with or without treatment with continuous positive airway pressure: an observational study. *Lancet.* 2005 Mar 19-25;365(9464):1046-53.

[109] Pack AI, Platt AB, Pien GW. Does untreated obstructive sleep apnea lead to death? A commentary on Young et al. Sleep 2008;31:1071-8 and Marshall et al. Sleep 2008;31:1079-85. *Sleep.* 2008 Aug 1;31(8):1067-8.

[110] Veasey S. Treatment of obstructive sleep apnoea. Indian J Med Res. 2010 Feb;131:236-44.

[111] Newman AB, Foster G, Givelber R, Nieto FJ, Redline S, Young T. Progression and regression of sleep-disordered breathing with changes in weight: the Sleep Heart Health Study. *Arch Intern Med.* 2005 Nov 14;165(20):2408-13.

[112] Redenius R, Murphy C, O'Neill E, Al-Hamwi M, Zallek SN. Does CPAP lead to change in BMI? *J Clin Sleep Med.* 2008 Jun 15;4(3):205-9.

[113] Cartwright RD. Effect of sleep position on sleep apnea severity. *Sleep.* 1984;7(2):110-4.

[114] Kushida CA, Sherrill CM, Hong SC, Palombini L, Hyde P, Dement WC. Cervical positioning for reduction of sleep-disordered breathing in mild-to-moderate OSAS. *Sleep Breath.* 2001 Jun;5(2):71-8.

[115] Ferguson KA, Cartwright R, Rogers R, Schmidt-Nowara W. Oral appliances for snoring and obstructive sleep apnea: a review. *Sleep.* 2006 Feb 1;29(2):244-62.

[116] Chan AS, Lee RW, Cistulli PA. Non-positive airway pressure modalities: mandibular advancement devices/positional therapy. *Proc Am Thorac Soc.* 2008 Feb 15;5(2):179-84.

[117] Lundkvist K, Januszkiewicz A, Friberg D. Uvulopalatopharyngoplasty in 158 OSAS patients failing non-surgical treatment. *Acta Otolaryngol.* 2009 Nov;129(11):1280-6.

[118] Kushida CA, Nichols DA, Quan SF, Goodwin JL, White DP, Gottlieb DJ, et al. The Apnea Positive Pressure Long-term Efficacy Study (APPLES): rationale, design, methods, and procedures. *J Clin Sleep Med.* 2006 Jul 15;2(3):288-300.

[119] Rodway GW, Weaver TE, Mancini C, Cater J, Maislin G, Staley B, et al. Evaluation of sham-CPAP as a placebo in CPAP intervention studies. *Sleep*. 2010 Feb 1;33(2):260-6.

In: Current Advances in Cardiovascular Risk. Volume 2   ISBN: 978-1-62081-746-9
Editor: Sandeep Ajoy Saha   © 2012 Nova Science Publishers, Inc.

Chapter XVIII

Cardiovascular Risk Management in Rheumatoid Arthritis and other Types of Inflammatory Arthritis: Current Insights and Gaps?

Michael T. Nurmohamed[1,2,3,*]
Departments of Internal Medicine, [1]Rheumatology, [2]VU University Medical Centre, Jan van Breemen Research Institute,
[3]Amsterdam, The Netherlands

Abstract

There is, during the last decades, increasing evidence that inflammation plays an essential role in all stages of atherosclerosis, ranging from endothelial cell dysfunction, foam cell and fatty streak formation, plaque destabilization with rupture, thrombosis and infarction as the ultimate consequences. Therefore, it could be hypothesized that patients with chronic inflammatory diseases are more prone for (accelerated) development of cardiovascular disease in comparison to the general population. This would particularly hold for rheumatic disorders with a high inflammatory burden such as rheumatoid arthritis, ankylosing spondylitis and psoriatic arthritis. Indeed, there appears to be evidence for an increased, approximately doubled, cardiovascular risk in these inflammatory arthritis patients. Recent research indicated that "traditional" cardiovascular risk factors only partially explain this enhanced risk, and obviously, the other important reason is the underlying chronic inflammatory process that renders our patients more susceptible for the development of atherosclerosis.

In view of the amplified cardiovascular risk, cardiovascular risk management is mandatory and this should on one hand consist of assessment (and treatment if necessary) of the traditional cardiovascular risk factors and on the other hand of effective antirheumatic treatment.

---

[*] Address for correspondence: Dr. Michael T. Nurmohamed, rheumatologist. Departments of Internal Medicine and Rheumatology, VU University Medical Centre, PO Box 7057; tel:-31-20-4443432; fax:-31-20-4442138; E-mail: mt.nurmohamed@vumc.nl.

Keywords: Rheumatoid   Arthritis,   Cardiovascular   Risk,   Myocardial   Infarction, Cardiovascular Risk Management

Introduction

Patients with inflammatory rheumatic diseases suffer from an increased cardiovascular risk. This chapter summarizes pivotal epidemiological cardiovascular mortality and morbidity data of inflammatory arthritis patients as well as the contribution of "traditional" cardiovascular risk factors towards this increased risk. Nowadays, cardiovascular risk management is advocated for inflammatory arthritis patients, and this chapter will discuss the current insight and gaps of cardiovascular risk management in inflammatory arthritis patients.

Cardiovascular Mortality

The mortality in rheumatoid arthritis (RA) is elevated when compared with the general population and standardized mortality ratio's (SMR's) range from 1.3 to 3.0 [1]. This excess mortality is largely due to cardiovascular disease (CVD), particularly of atherosclerotic origin such as ischemic heart disease.

Mortality data in two other major chronic types of inflammatory arthritis belonging to the spondylarthropathies, i.e. ankylosing spondylitis (AS) and psoriatic arthritis (PsA), is much more limited than in RA, but it appears also to be increased particularly in patients seen at referral centers who are likely to suffer from more severe disease, and SMR's range between 1.5 and 1.9 for AS and between 1.1. and 2.1 for PsA [2,3].

Cardiovascular Morbidity

The last decades several studies have been published indicating an enhanced rate of cardiovascular (CV) diseases, i.e. myocardial infarction (MI), cerebrovascular disease, peripheral arterial disease and heart failure in patients with RA. In a prospective Dutch study, the magnitude was investigated by comparing prevalent CVD with that of diabetes, a well-established cardiovascular risk factor [5].This study included more than 350 patients (diagnosed between 1989 and 2001, aged between 50 and 75 years; the CARRÉ (Dutch acronym for " CARdiovascular disease in RhEumatoid arthritis") study), and participants of a Dutch population-based cohort study on CVD and its underlying risk factors (Hoorn study). Prevalent CVD was seen in 13% patients with RA, 5.0% in persons without diabetes and 12% in type 2 diabetes patients respectively. The odds ratios for CVD, adjusted for age and sex, were 3.1 in RA, and 2.3 in diabetes in comparison to the general population without diabetes. Correction for CV risk factors slightly decreased the odds ratios. The prospective part of this investigation demonstrated CV events in 9% of the RA patients and in 4% in the person without diabetes from the general population [6].The incidence rates were 3.1 per 100 patient/years for RA, and 1.5 per 100 person/years for the general population. The age- and sex-adjusted relative risk was 2.0 with almost no change after correcting for CV risk factors.

Altogether, this study suggests that the CV risk RA is increased to an extent that is comparable to that of diabetes. Very recently these data were confirmed by a nationwide Danish investigation [7]. The study population included the entire Danish population ≥ 16 years of age on January 1, 1997 (n=4,311,022). Patients with incident diabetes and RA were identified according to prescription claims, hospitalizations and outpatient clinics visits, by individual-level-linkage of nationwide administrative registers The population was followed until first MI or December 31, 2006. A total of 10,477 and 103,215 people developed RA and diabetes, respectively. The incidence rate ratio (IRR) of an MI after developing RA increased to 1.7 (95% confidence interval (CI) : 1.5 – 1.9), and this was completely comparable to the enhanced risk of MI after developing diabetes of 1.7 (1.6-1.8). Altogether, this investigation confirms that RA is an independent risk factor for myocardial infarction of similar magnitude as diabetes.

Although CV mortality is apparently enhanced in AS there are only a limited number of papers investigating CV morbidity in AS patients. A population-based cohort study from the United Kingdom General Practice Research Database, identified almost 5400 males with AS and a significantly higher rate of first-time myocardial infarction was shown in 11.000 matched controls (hazard ratio=1.4; 95% CI: 1.2-1.8) [8]. The rate of MIs was age-dependent and peaked at age 60 - 64 (hazard ratio: 2.4; 95% CI: 1.3-4.5). A recent, questionnaire based, study in 600 patients with AS showed a prevalence MI of 4.4% versus 1.2% in the general population. The age and gender adjusted odds ratio was 3.1 (95% C.I.:1.9 – 5.1) [9].

Data about CV morbidity PsA patients is also limited. A recent database investigation of 650 PsA patients showed a 2.5-fold increased prevalence of MI [10]. Another, questionnaire based , study in 750 patients with PsA demonstrated that the prevalence of ischemic CVD were comparable to that of RA [11].

Cardiovascular Risk Factors

It is well known that elevated levels of total cholesterol (TC), low-density-lipoprotein (LDL)-cholesterol (LDL-C) and a lowered level of high-density lipoprotein (HDL) cholesterol (HDL-C) are associated with an increased CV risk. The literature about lipid profiles in patients with RA points towards an inverse relationship between lipid levels and disease activity [12], i.e. a higher disease activity is related with a lower TC but even more depressed HDL-cholesterol, resulting in a higher (unfavorable) atherogenic index (TC/HDL-C ratio) [14].

During the last decades there is an increased interest in apolipoprotein A-1 (apo A-1), and apolipoprotein B (apo-B). Apo A-1 is the protein present on the HDL-C particles, whereas apo-B is found on the LDL-C, very low density lipoprotein (VLDL) and chylomicrons particles. Hence, assessment of plasma apo A-1 and plasma apo-B gives an assessment of the total number of anti-atherogenic and atherogenic particles, respectively.

There is evidence that apo-B is a better prognostic marker for CV events than LDL-C and that the apo-B/apo A-1 ratio is a more appropriate predictor for CV risk [14]. Actually, apo A-1 might protect against CV disease whereas apo-B might increase the susceptibility for the new CV disease. Confirming the expectations, disease activity in RA had an inverse relationship with apo-A1 and HDL-C levels [15].

Smoking is an important risk factor for CV disease in the general population. It is conceivable that smoking might play a (CV) role in RA as it increases the susceptibility for the development of RA as well its severity [16]. A recent study indicated a higher prevalence of smoking in RA patients, as well as an increased CV risk in these patients versus non-smoking RA-patients. However, the effect was less significant than in the control subjects (HR for CV disease 1.3 and 2.2, for smoking vs. non-smoking RA patients and smoking vs. non-smoking controls, respectively) [17]. Literature data about the prevalence of type II diabetes are not uniform but as there is accumulating evidence for insulin resistance in RA, it is conceivable that the prevalence of diabetes will be enhanced in RA. Moreover, some investigations, but not all, reveal that the metabolic syndrome occurs more frequently in RA patients versus controls, which appears to be inflammation driven [18-20].

Data regarding hypertension are contradictory, but a recent study revealed significant under-diagnosing as well as under-treatment in patients with RA [21]. No conclusions can be reached with respect the contribution of "body mass" index and physical fitness towards the CV risk in RA.

The literature data regarding the lipid profile in AS and PsA patients is contradictory which might be due to different disease activities in the studied populations [22-25]. Similar to RA it appears that the degree of inflammation plays a role in the magnitude of dyslipidemia in AS as well as PsA patients. We investigated in 92 AS patients, in whom tumor necrosis factor (TNF) blocking therapy was started, lipid levels, inflammation markers, as C-reactive protein and serum amyloid A (SAA), during anti-TNF treatment [26]. In a subgroup HDL-C composition was investigated with surface-enhanced laser desorption/ionization time-of flight (SELDI-TOF). During anti-TNF treatment all inflammatory markers decreased whereas TC, HDL-C and apo A-1 levels increased significantly. SELDI-TOF analysis revealed that at initiation of TNF-blocking therapy there were high concentrations of SAA within HDL-particles that decreased during anti-TNF therapy. This is important as SAA replaces apo A-1 in HDL particles thereby impairing the antiatherogenic properties of HDL-C. Hence, it is plausible that decreasing SAA concentration restores the atheroprotective effects of HDL-C.

A few small studies have shown that hypertension occurs more frequently in AS patients as well as PsA [27]. Data regarding insulin resistance and the metabolic syndrome in PsA are too limited reach firm conclusions.

Cardiovascular Risk Management

The CV risk in inflammatory arthritis patient is approximately doubled in comparison to the general population. In RA this risk appears to be similar to type 2 diabetes, a well-established CV risk factor for which CV risk management (CV-RM) is essential.

Traditional CV risk factors only partially explain this excess CV risk in RA and, as indicated, the other important factor is the, underlying, chronic inflammatory process. Therefore, RA, but also AS and PsA, should be seen as a new, independent, CV risk factors for which CV-RM is mandatory. Normally, this is done on the basis of the 10 years absolute risk for a (fatal) CV event, which is calculated from a CV risk formula, such as the Framingham risk calculator and the Systematic Coronary Risk Evaluation (SCORE), based on CV-risk factors. Lipid lowering agents and/or antihypertensive treatment is then only initiated above a certain threshold, e.g. a 10-year CV-mortality risk of 10% or more.

One could argue that intervention trials with statins and/or antihypertensives and CV endpoints in should be awaited before conclusions about their efficacy in inflammatory arthritis patients can be reached. However, it is not likely that the effect of statins and/or antihypertensives would be less in inflammatory arthritis patients in comparison to the general population. Actually, the effects might be more pronounced as statins, ACE inhibitors and angiotensin blockers have also anti-inflammatory properties.

Recently, the European League Against Rheumatism (EULAR) recommendations for CV-RM in inflammatory arthritis patients were published [28], that advocated yearly CV risk screening for inflammatory arthritis patients (Table 1) Drug treatment with statins and/or antihypertensives is then dependent on the calculated 10-years CV risk. For RA it is recommended to adapt existing risk functions, such as SCORE, by a multiplier of 1.5 to achieve a more precise estimation of the 10 years CV risk. Finally, effective suppression on the inflammatory process is necessary to further decrease the CV-risk.

Table 1. EULAR recommendations for the CV-RM in inflammatory arthritis patients risk management in RA, PsA and AS

Recommendations	Strength of recommendation
1. RA is associated with a higher risk for CV disease. This probably also applies to AS and PsA The increased risk is to both traditional CV risk factors as well as the chronic inflammation.	B
2. Disease activity control is essential to lower the CV risk.	B
3. CV risk assessment is recommended for all RA patients and should be considered for all AS and PsA patients.	C
4. Risk score models should be adapted for RA by a 1.5 multiplication factor. when the RA patient meets 2 of the following 3 criteria: • Disease duration of more than 10 years; • RF or anti-CCP positivity; • Presence of extra-articular manifestations.	C
5. TC/HDL cholesterol ratio should be used when SCORE is applied	C
6. Intervention(s) should be carried out according to national guidelines.	C
7. Statins, ACE-inhibitors and/or AT-II blockers are preferred treatment options in view of their pleiotrophic properties.	C-D
8. The role of COXIBs and most NSAIDs regarding the CV risk is not well established in infllammatory arthrtis patients and needs further investigation. Hence, they should be prescribed cautiously, particularly in patients with documented CV disease or in the presence of CV risk factors.	C
9. Corticosteroids: use the lowest dose possible	C
10. Stop smoking	C

The EULAR recommendations were based on the available literature until May 2008 and since then there have be some reports advocating to increase the age of a RA patient by 10 years to get a more precise cardiovascular risk estimate instead of using a multiplication factor. Obviously, this discussion can only be solved by a RA-specific cardiovascular risk prediction model, but it will take years before such models are available. The EULAR task force clearly noted this need as well as the necessity for cardiovascular endpoint trials with statins and/or antihypertensive agents. The EULAR task force decided not to wait until the results of these CV endpoint trials become available as it is unlikely that the efficacy of (preventive) cardiovascular drug treatment will be lower in RA in comparison to the general population. Other criticisms are also possible, [29] and most of them were already noted by the task force. In the (near) future ongoing research will result in improved RA-specific CV risk models and improvement of the EULAR guidelines.

Conclusion

Patients with inflammatory arthritis i.e. RA, AS and PsA should be viewed as being at an approximately doubled risk for CV disease. For RA this risk might be similar to that of diabetes. Traditional CV risk factors may be increased in inflammatory arthritis patients, but there is clearly a pivotal role for the underlying chronic inflammatory process. Altogether, RA, AS and PsA should be seen as a new, independent, CV risk factors for which CV-RM is mandatory. Regular CV-risk screening is required for inflammatory arthritis and CV-RM should focus on traditional CV risk factors as well as tight disease control.

References

[1]   Van Doornum S, McColl G, Wicks IP. Accelerated atherosclerosis: an extraarticular feature of rheumatoid arthritis? *ArthritisRheum.* 2002;46:862-73.
[2]   Lehtinen K. Mortality and causes of death in 398 patients admitted to hospital with ankylosing spondylitis. *Ann Rheum Dis.* 1993;52:174-76.
[3]   Ali Y, Tom BDM, Schentag CT, Farewell VT, Gladman DD. Improved survival in psoriatic arthritis with calendar time. *ArthritisRheum.* 2007;56:2708-14.
[4]   Peters MJ, van der Horst-Bruinsma I, Dijkmans BA, Nurmohamed MT. Cardiovascular risk profile of patients with spondylarthropathies, particularly ankylosing spondylitis and psoriatic arthritis. *SeminArthritisRheum.* 2004;34:585-92.
[5]   van Halm V, Peters MJ, Voskuyl AE, Boers M, Lems WF, Visser M et al. Rheumatoid arthritis versus diabetes as a risk factor for cardiovascular disease, a cross sectional study. The CARRE Investigation. *Ann Rheum Dis.* 2009;68:1395-400.
[6]   Peters MJ, van Halm VP, Voskuyl AE, Boers M, Lems WF, Visser M et al. Rheumatoid arthritis as important independent risk factor for incident cardiovascular disease. *ArthritisRheum.2009*;58:691-6.
[7]   Lindhardsen J, Ahlehoff O, Gislason GH, Madsen OR, Olesen JB, Torp-Pedersen C, Hansen PR The risk of myocardial infarction in rheumatoid arthritis and diabetes

mellitus: a Danish nationwide cohort study. *Ann Rheum Dis.* 2011 Mar 11. [Epub ahead of print]

[8]   Symmons DPM, Googson NJ, Cook MN, Watson DJ. Men with ankylosing spondylitis have an increased risk of myocardial infarction. *ArthritisRheum.* 2004;50 (Suppl):S477.

[9]   Peters MJ, Visman I, Nielen MM, van Dillen N, Verheij RA, van der Horst-Bruinsma IE et al. Ankylosing spondylitis; a risk factor for myocardial infarction? *Ann Rheum Dis.* 2010;69:579-81.

[10]   Gladman DD, Ang M, Su L, Tom BD, Schentag CT, Farewell VT. Cardiovascular morbidity in psoriatic arthritis. *Ann Rheum Dis.* 2009 Jul;68(7):1131-5.

[11]   Jamnitski A, Visman IM, Peters MJL, Boers M, Dijkmans BAC, Nurmohamed MT. Prevalence of cardiovascular disease in psoriatic arthritis resembles that of rheumatoid arthritis. *Ann Rheum Dis.* 2010 Oct 18. [Epub ahead of print]

[12]   White D, Fayez S, Doube A. Atherogenic lipid profiles in rheumatoid arthritis. *N Z Med J.* 2006;119:U2125.

[13]   Boers M, Nurmohamed MT, Doelman CJA, Lard LR, Verhoeven AC, Voskuyl AE et al. Influence of glucocorticoids and disease activity on total and high density lipoprotein cholesterol in patients with rheumatoid arthritis. Ann Rheum Dis. 2003;62:842-45.

[14]   Walldius G, Jungner I. The apoB/apoA-I ratio: a strong, new risk factor for cardiovascular disease and a target for lipid-lowering therapy--a review of the evidence. *J Intern Med.* 2006;259:493-519.

[15]   Park YB, Lee SK, Lee WK, Suh CH, Lee CW, Lee CH et al. Lipid profiles in untreated patients with rheumatoid arthritis. *J Rheumatol.* 1999;26:1701-4.

[16]   Källberg H, Ding B, Padyukov L, Bengtsson C, Rönnelid J, Klareskog L, Alfredsson L; EIRA Study Group. Smoking is a major preventable risk factor for rheumatoid arthritis: estimations of risks after various exposures to cigarette smoke. *Ann Rheum Dis.* 201 ;70:508-11

[17]   Gonzalez A, MaraditKremers H, Crowson CS, Ballman KV, Roger VL, Jacobsen SJ et al. Do cardiovascular risk factors confer the same risk for cardiovascular outcomes in rheumatoid arthritis patients as in non-rheumatoid arthritis patients? *Ann Rheum Dis.* 2008;67:64-69.

[18]   Karvounaris SA, Sidiropoulos PI, Papadakis JA, Spanakis EK, Bertsias GK, Kritikos HD et al. Metabolic syndrome is common among middle-to-older aged Mediterranean patients with rheumatoid arthritis and correlates with disease activity: a retrospective, cross-sectional, controlled, study. *Ann Rheum Dis.* 2007;66:28-33.

[19]   Dessein PH, Tobias M, Veller MG. Metabolic syndrome and subclinical atherosclerosis in rheumatoid arthritis. *J Rheumatol.* 2006;33:2425-32.

[20]   Chung CP, Oeser A, Solus JF, Avalos I, Gebretsadik T, Shintani A et al. Prevalence of the metabolic syndrome is increased in rheumatoid arthritis and is associated with coronary atherosclerosis. *Atherosclerosis.* 2008;196:756-63.

[21]   Panoulas VF, Douglas KMJ, Milionis HJ, Stavropoulos-Kalinglou A, Nightingale P, Kita MD et al. Prevalence and associations of hypertension and its control in patients with rheumatoid arthritis. *Rheumatology (Oxford).* 2007;46:1477-82.

[22]   Divecha H, Sattar N, Rumley A, Cherry L, Lowe GDO, Sturrock R. Cardiovascular risk parameters in men with ankylosing spondylitis in comparison with non-inflammatory control subjects: relevance of systemic inflammation. *ClinSci (Lond).* 2005;109:171-76.

[23] Tam LS, Tomlinson B, Chu TTW, Li M, Leung YY, Kwok LW et al. Cardiovascular risk profile of patients with psoriatic arthritis compared to controls--the role of inflammation. *Rheumatology (Oxford). 2008;47:718-23.*

[24] van Halm, V, van Denderen JC, Peters MJ, Twisk JW, van der PM, van der Horst-Bruinsma IE et al. Increased disease activity is associated with a deteriorated lipid profile in patients with ankylosing spondylitis. *Ann Rheum Dis.* 2006;65:1473-77.

[25] Jones SM, Harris CP, Lloyd J, Stirling CA, Reckless JP, McHugh NJ. Lipoproteins and their subfractions in psoriatic arthritis: identification of an atherogenic profile with active joint disease. *Ann Rheum Dis.* 2000;59:904-9.

[26] Van Eijk, I, de Vries MK, Levels JH, Peters MJ, Huizer EE, Dijkmans BA et al. Improvement of lipid profile is accompanied by atheroprotective alterations in high-density lipoprotein composition upon tumor necrosis factor blockade: A prospective cohort study in ankylosing spondylitis. *Arthritis Rheum.* 2009;60:1324-30.

[27] Han C, Robinson DWJ, Hackett MV, Paramore LC, Fraeman KH, Bala MV. Cardiovascular disease and risk factors in patients with rheumatoid arthritis, psoriatic arthritis, and ankylosing spondylitis. *J Rheumatol.* 2006;33:2167-72.

[28] Peters MJ, Symmons DP, McCarey D, Dijkmans BA, Nicola P, Kvien TK, et al EULAR evidence-based recommendations for cardiovascular risk management in patients with rheumatoid arthritis and other forms of inflammatory arthritis. *Ann Rheum Dis.* 2010;69:325-31.

[29] Crowson CS, Gabriel SE. Towards improving cardiovascular risk management in patients with rheumatoid arthritis: the need for accurate risk assessment. *Ann Rheum Dis.* 2011 Feb 22. [Epub ahead of print].

In: Current Advances in Cardiovascular Risk. Volume 2   ISBN: 978-1-62081-746-9
Editor: Sandeep Ajoy Saha   © 2012 Nova Science Publishers, Inc.

Chapter XIX

Psoriasis and Cardiovascular Disease

Enrico Vizzardi, Ivano Bonadei, Barbara Piovanelli,
Riccardo Rovetta, Filippo Quinzani,
Antonio D'Aloia, Antonio Curnis
and Livio Dei Cas
Department of experimental and applied medicine,
section of cardiovascular diseases,
University of Study of Brescia, Brescia, Italy

Abstract

Psoriasis is a chronic immune-mediated disorder that affects about 2-3% of the adult population. It is equally distributed between the genders. Psoriasis is the more frequently diagnosed T-cell mediated disease in humans, and is one of the most common autoimmune diseases characterized by chronic inflammation of the skin, but the disease is not limited to the skin.

The disease is characterized by erythematous, scaling lesions, with variable patterns and body distribution and with various distinct clinical phenotypes: vulgar, inverted, guttate, erythrodermic, and pustular. It can also affect the nails and joints in 5-20% of the cases.

Epidemiological studies show that psoriasis is associated with a greater risk of comorbidities and mortality. The comorbidities most commonly associated with psoriasis are psoriatic arthritis, chronic inflammatory intestinal disease, and psychiatric and psychosocial disorders. More recent studies have shown an increased prevalence of cardiovascular comorbidities secondary to the metabolic alterations associated with psoriasis-among these are diabetes, obesity, dyslipidemia, hypertension, and coronary disease. The risk of myocardial infarction is higher in younger patients with severe psoriasis.

The objective of the chapter is to review the pertinent literature and highlight pathogenic mechanisms shared between psoriasis and atherosclerosis that may represent potential targets for the prevention or therapy.

Introduction

Psoriasis (PS) is a papulosquamous disease with variable morphology, distribution, severity, and course. Papulosquamous diseases are characterized by scaling papules (raised lesions <1 cm in diameter) and plaques (raised lesions >1 cm in diameter). Other papulosquamous diseases that may be considered in the differential diagnosis include tinea infections, pityriasis rosea, and lichen planus. The lesions of PS are distinct from these other entities and are classically very well circumscribed, circular, red papules or plaques with a grey or silvery-white, dry scale. In addition, the lesions are typically distributed symmetrically on the scalp, elbows, knees, lumbosacral area, and in the body folds. PS may also develop at the site of trauma or injury, known as *Koebner's phenomenon.* If PS is progressive or uncontrolled, it can result in a generalized exfoliative erythroderma. Nail involvement may be present, particularly if psoriatic arthritis [1] is present.

Occasionally PS may involve the oral mucosa or the tongue. When the tongue is involved, the dorsal surface may have sharply circumscribed gyrate red patches with a white-yellow border. The patches may evolve and spread, changing on a daily basis, can assume distinct annular patterns and may resemble a map- hence the term 'geographic tongue'.

PS can be highly variable in morphology, distribution, and severity. Despite the classic presentation described above, the morphology can range from small tear-shaped papules (guttate psoriasis) to pustules (pustular psoriasis) and generalized erythema and scale (erythrodermic psoriasis). In addition, these different forms of psoriasis may be localized, or widespread and disabling. Further, psoriasis may have a variable course - presenting as chronic, stable plaques, or may present acutely with rapid progression and widespread involvement. PS may be symptomatic with patients complaining of intense pruritus or burning.

PS treatment is based on 4 broad therapeutic categories, dictated mainly by disease severity [2]: I) topical agents (the first – line for most patients); II) phototherapy and photochemotherapy (limited to patients with moderate and severe PS); III) systemic drugs (for more severe forms) such as methotrexate (MTX), cyclosporine, and acitretin; IV) systemic biologics (to target specific steps in immune pathways involved in the pathogenesis of PS), such as etanercept.

The Pathophysiology of Psoriasis

PS is an immune disease, characterized by inappropriate activation of the cellular immune system directed against self-antigens. For more than a decade, the fundamental pathophysiology has been thought to be related to Th1-mediated cellular dysfunction which produces systemic inflammation and a concurrent increase in cytokine production. In short, an antigen-presenting cell (APC) identifies and processes a yet-to-be identified antigen in the skin. APC then presents, in a major histocompatibility class II-restricted fashion, processed antigen and activates naive T cells in the local lymph nodes, resulting in a clonal expansion of the Th1 arm under the influence of IL - 2. These activated Th1 clones enter the circulation and through the process of diapedesis, permeate through the endothelium and cause an inflammatory reaction in the affected skin. The cytokines driving this response are, of course, those of the Th1 profile and include tumor necrosis factor alpha (TNF α), IL-2 and interferon gamma (IFN-γ). This, in turn, leads to the recruitment of other immune cells and expression of vascular endothelial growth factor (VEGF), leading to vascular proliferation [3-5]. Krueger and Bowcock characterized the process as 'many interactive responses between infiltrating leukocytes, resident skin cells, and an array of pro-inflammatory cytokines, chemokines, and chemical mediators produced in the skin under regulation of the cellular immune system' [6]. Heredity and environmental factors may interact with this complex inflammatory process to modify further the clinical expression of the disease. The more severe the inflammatory response, the more severe is the disease phenotype.

Comorbidities in PS

Comorbidities tend to arise in complex disorders, they are frequently multigenic and multifactorial, and most often demonstrate an inflammatory background. Several epidemiological studies have shown that, in PS patients, a distinct number of concomitant disease entities have been observed more frequently than expected [7-10] and they may be roughly divided into two types: (I) comorbidities due to common pathogenic mechanisms such as psoriatic arthritis and Crohn's disease; and (II) comorbidities following chronic severe inflammation characteristic for PS such as cardiovascular disorders and the metabolic syndrome (MBS). Although the disorders represent separate entities, they appear to follow overlapping pathogenic pathways [11]. Comorbidities often become clinically manifest years after onset of PS and are frequently seen in severe disease. Persistent low-grade inflammation with secretion of proinflammatory cytokines (e.g. TNF- α) favors the development of insulin resistance and metabolic syndrome. In addition, biochemical and immunologic observations point toward an inflammatory immune mechanism that uses tools of the innate defense armamentarium [11].

PS and Ischemic Heart Disease

PS has been known to be associated with cardiovascular (CV) diseases (CVDs) since 1978, when McDonald and Calabresi first published a study on 323 hospitalized patients linking PS to arterial and venous vascular diseases [12]; they showed that the risk of arterial end venous vascular diseases (e.g. Myocardial infarction (MI), thrombophlebitis, pulmonary embolization, and cerebrovascular accident) was 2.2 times higher among the 323 patients with PS compared with 325 controls with other dermatologic conditions; disease duration did not appear to have an effect on the risk, but extent of skin involvement was associated with a slightly higher risk in older age groups [12]. A number of observations followed this report, mainly focusing on coronary artery disease (CAD) and suggesting that atherosclerosis (ATS) is more frequent in PS patients, and that PS may predispose to ATS [13-16]. However, one limitation of the early epidemiologic studies examining cardiac risk in PS patients is that they generally sampled hospitalized or specialty clinic patients, and were therefore likely biased toward patient populations with more severe diseases. Since more PS patients have mild disease, generalizing from the inpatient population may overestimate cardiovascular risk. This limitation is important because several recent studies using healthcare databases have demonstrated that higher disease severity is associated with higher cardiovascular risk, as has been demonstrated in the arthritis population [17-18]. Further data were uncovered by the largest population – based cohort study on PS outpatients currently available, published by Gelfand et al. in 2006 [19]. They compared outcomes among patients with and without a diagnosis of PS, using data collected by general practitioners and stored in the General Practice Research Database between 1987 and 2002 (mean follow up 5.4 years). In total, 130,976 PS patients, of whom 3827 (2.9%) had a severe form (the majority of whom received methotrexate), were included and matched with 556,995 controls. PS patients were classified as severe if they had been treated with a systemic therapy in their lifetime. The study demonstrated that patients with PS were more likely to have diabetes, hyperlipidemia, hypertension, a history of MI, a higher body mass index, and be a current smoker; and the prevalence of such comorbidities was higher among those with the more severe form of PS. The incidence rates of MI in controls, mild PS patients and severe PS patients were 3.58, 4.04 and 5.13 per 1000 person-years respectively. Patients with PS had an increased adjusted relative risk for MI that varied by age, and the risk persisted after controlling for major MI risk factors. The authors concluded that psoriasis may act as an independent risk factor for acute MI [19]. The findings of the previously mentioned study were further confirmed by the analysis of two US health care databases (IMS Health and MarketScan®) used to identify adults with diagnostic codes for PS, which also showed an increased CV risk even in patients with mild PS [20]. In particular, odds ratios (OR) for ATS, congestive heart failure, type 2 diabetes, and peripheral vascular disease were > 1.20 for PS patients. In both data sets, higher disease severity increased the risk for chronic heart failure, type 2 diabetes mellitus, hypertension, and ischemic heart disease. Xiao et al. [21], in their prevalence study with PS inpatients, observed that the OR of having an MI was 1.72 and 2.01 respectively for mild and severe PS, adjusted for others CV risk factors and systemic treatment. In this study too, severe PS was defined by the use of at least one systemic treatment over the study period. Another study noted that while CVDs are more prevalent in psoriasis patients overall, the risk of CV mortality is only increased in patients admitted to hospital with severe disease and in those with earlier age at first admission [17]. However, a few observations [22-23] do not seem to confirm the results obtained by Gelfand et al. [19]. Wakee et al. [22] studied a large Dutch cohort of 43,397 subjects, of whom 15,820 (37%) had PS (12.5% with severe disease defined by type of treatment). They argued that PS may not be an independent risk factor for hospitalizations for acute ischemic heart disease, because the risk of ischemic heart disease and of acute MI were not significantly different in patients with PS (ischemic heart disease HR 1.10; 95% CI 0.99-1.23; incidence rates of acute myocardial infarction HR 0.99; 95% CI 0.84-1.17). However, the limitation of this study was that they only considered cases of acute ischemic disease that needed hospitalization. A study published in 2009 by Brauchli et al [24] analyzed patients and controls taken from the UK General Practice Research Database in a 1:1 ratio. They did not find a significant difference in the incidence rates of MI and transient ischemic attack between PS patients and controls. But in a nested sub-analysis, data showed an increased MI risk for PS patients with a severe form and aged less than 60 years, confirming the observations of Gelfand et al. [19].

Table 1. Studies about risk of dyslipidemia in psoriasis

References	OR Dyslipidaemia
Driessen 2008	1.17 (0.66-2.09)
Kimball 2008	1.26 (1.22-1.30)
Wu 2008	1.35 (1.11-1.63)
Neimann2006	1.28 (1.24-1.33)
Naldi 2008	1.1 (0.7-1.7)
Kaye 2008	1.17 (1.11-1.23)
Sommer 2006	2.09 (1.23-3.54)
Gelfand 2006	1.11 (1.07-1.16)
Gerdes 2008	1.55 (1.20-2.00)
Mallbris 2006	1.04 (1.0-1.09)
Cohen 2008	1.0 (1.0-1.3)
Gisondi 2007	2.0 (1.4-2.8)

Table 2. Studies about risk of diabetes in psoriasis

References	OR Diabetes
Sommer 2006	2.48 (1.70-3.61)
Gelfand 2006	1.61 (1.53-1.70)
Neimann 2006	1.27 (1.23-1.31)
Cohen 2008	2.80 (2.68-2.99)
Shapiro 2007	1.27 (1.1-1.48)
Kaye 2008	1.33 (1.25-1.42)
Driessen 2008	1.91 (0.91-4.04)
Brauchli 2008	1.31 (1.13-1.51)
Qureshi 2009	2.08 (1.60-2.69)
Gerdes 2008	2.27 (1.64-3.13)
Wu 2008	1.42 (1.10-1.84)
Naldi 2008	1.1 (0.6-2.0)
Gisondi 2007	0.9 (0.6-1.3)
Kimball 2008	1.27 (1.21-1.33)

Table 3. Studies about the risk of hypertension in psoriasis

References	OR
Sommer 2006	3.27 (2.41-4.43)
Gelfand 2006	1.26 (1.20-1.30)
Neimann 2006	1.16 (1.14-1.18)
Cohen 2008	1.3 (1.2-1.5)
Kaye 2008	1.09 (1.05-1.14)
Driessen 2008	1.93 (1.16-3.23)
Qureshi 2009	1.32 (1.19-1.45)
Gerdes 2008	1.93 (1.63-2.28)
Wu 2008	1.49 (1.23-1.80)
Naldi 2008	0.8 (0.5-1.3)
Gisondi 2007	1.06 (0.8-1.5)
Kimball 2008	1.20 (1.17-1.24)

PS and Cardiovascular Risk Factors

Patients with severe PS have a 3-4 year average decrease in their life expectancy, comparable with the estimated reduction in the longevity of patients with severe hypertension [25]. This shortened lifespan is likely due in part to increased prevalence of CAD, which is the most common cause of death in patients with PS. Conditions that are contributors to CAD, such as dyslipidemia, obesity, hypertension, and diabetes mellitus, are more prevalent in patients with PS than in the general population and patients with other dermatologic disorders [26-29] (Tables 1-5).

Table 4. Studies about risk of obesity in psoriasis

References	OR
Neimann 2006	1.29 (1.26-1.32)
Cohen 2008	1.7 (1.5-1.9)
Kaye 2008	1.18 (1.14-1.23)
Driessen 2008	5.49 (3.09-9.74
Naldi 2008	1.7 (1.1-2.6)
Gisondi 2007	1.19 (0.91-1.55)
Herron 2005	2.39 (1.98-2.90)

Table 5. Studies about risk of metabolic syndrome in psoriasis

References	OR
Gisondi 2007	1.66 (1.20-2.40)
Cohen 2008	1.3 (1.1-1.4)
Sommer 2006	5.92 (2.78-12.8)

A) Obesity

Several studies have shown a significant association between increased body mass index (BMI) and PS, suggesting that PS patients are more frequently overweight or obese than is the general population, and the severity of PS may be correlated to BMI [30-31]. More recent studies have established that obesity may occur prior to the onset of PS and serve as a risk factor for development of the disease. For example, a large cohort study of over 78,000 nurses from the United States demonstrated a positive correlation between obesity and the risk of developing incident PS [32]. Conversely, Neimann et al. [29] showed that the risk of obesity was significantly increased in PS patients compared with that in healthy controls and strongly associated with disease severity (ORs of 1.27 and 1.79 for patients with mild and severe PS respectively). In line with this finding, Herron et al found that PS patients were almost twice as likely to be obese compared with the general population (34% vs. 18%; p=0.001) [30]. Further support for obesity as a consequence of PS comes from recent case – control studies. Although no differences in BMI were observed in PS patients versus controls at disease onset, another study [33] identified obesity as an independent risk factor associated with PS, accounting for 16% of all PS cases at onset. Another study [31] observed the association between these two factors- patients with a BMI of 26-29 were found to have a 1.9-fold increased risk of developing PS. Interestingly, it has been reported that BMI negatively affects the short – term clinical response to systemic treatment of PS [34], and weight loss increases the responsiveness of obese PS patients to a suboptimal dose of cyclosporine [35].

B) Cigarette Smoking

The prevalence of habitual smoking in PS patients is remarkably higher than that in the general population, and smoking has been identified as a risk factor for the development of PS [36]. A cross – sectional questionnaire – based health study among 18,747 adults in Oslo reported that in current smokers, the odds-ratio for reporting PS was 1.49 for males and 1.48 for females compared with "never-smokers" [37]. In a cohort of 2,368 PS patients followed for 16 weeks in the PSOCARE observational study, the incidence of smokers was 41% [38], almost twice that of the age – standardized rate observed in the Italian adult population [39]. In a large prospective analysis of 887 incident cases of PS, the multivariate relative risk of developing PS was 1.78 for current smokers and 1.37 for past smokers compared with never – smokers. The risk of incident PS among former smokers decreased to nearly that of never – smokers after 20 years of cessation [40]. In the study by Gelfand et al [29], cigarette smoking was more common in patients with PS than in the general population (OR 1.31). Approximately 80% of patients with PS had smoked cigarettes before the onset of the disease [30]. Cigarette smoking also may trigger PS and contribute to its severity [28, 41].

C) Insulin Resistance/Type 2 Diabetes

A high prevalence of insulin resistance and/or type 2 diabetes in PS has long been recognized, but the extent and the potential mechanisms underlying this association are poorly understood. The increased prevalence of diabetes in patients with PS was independent of traditional diabetes risk factors such as obesity and dyslipidemia in a large, population – based cross – sectional study in the UK [29]. Impaired glucose intolerance based on glucose oral tolerance test was reported in 13.2% of 53 patients and 40% of 17 patients with early and late onset PS, respectively, both of which were significantly higher than that (2.5%) found in controls [42]. Boehncke et al observed a significant correlation between PS severity and insulin secretion and levels of serum resistin, a cytokine known to be increased in insulin resistance, supporting the concept that insulin resistance occurs as a consequence of severe chronic inflammation [43]. Indeed, Kaye and Jick found that PS itself confers a risk of developing diabetes, as the cumulative incidence of diabetes in the PS cohort was higher than that of the comparison group (HR 1.33) [44]. The association between PS and type 2 diabetes is further strengthened by numerous cross – sectional studies that have shown that PS, especially in the severe form, confers a higher risk (up to 2.48) for developing diabetes [29, 45]. A shared genetic background may also contribute to the susceptibility to both PS and diabetes [46].

D) Adverse lipid profile

PS is associated with adverse changes in the lipid profile and an imbalance of oxidants/antioxidants [47]. Although the confounding effect of obesity and insulin resistance should be taken into account in evaluating this association, Mallbris et al.

found that patients have an abnormal lipoprotein composition already at the onset of PS independently of established confounding factors including age, sex, BMI, smoking blood pressure, and alcohol consumption, which suggests that dyslipoproteinemia in PS might be genetically determined rather than acquired [33]. A cross − sectional study of patients treated with PUVA or oral retinoids demonstrated increased total cholesterol and triglycerides, decreased HDL, and no alteration in LDL in PS patients compared to controls [48]. In a hospital clinic based cross- sectional study in Iran, PS patients were shown to have significantly higher mean levels of triglycerides, total cholesterol, LDL, and VLDL but no alterations in HDL [49]. Despite several studies [29,50], no consistent associations between PS and dyslipidemia have been reported.

E) Hypertension

Previous large population studies have examined the relationship between PS and hypertension, and have focused on the frequency of hypertension occurrence in PS patients compared to non-PS patients [51-53]. In a prospective study among U.S. female nurses, Qureshi et al. [51] found that women with PS experienced an increased risk for developing hypertension (RR 1.17). In a case-control study using a health-maintenance organization database [52], investigators found modestly increased odds of having hypertension among psoriasis patients (OR 1.37). In a hospital − based study, Lindegard et al observed that PS was significantly associated with hypertension [54], while Henseler and Christophers also found that hypertension was twice as frequent in PS as in control subjects [26]. On the other hand, Inerot et al. reported no increased frequency of hypertension in a population of patients with mild form of PS sampled from a patient organization [55]. A large, population based cross-sectional study also did not observe a significant association between PS and hypertension when controlling for risk factors such as obesity and smoking [29]

F) Hyperhomocysteinemia

Hyperhomocysteinemia may constitute an independent risk factor for cardiovascular diseases [56]. Homocysteine promotes many processes involved in ATS and also affects the coagulation system, and is an independent risk factor for both arterial and venous thrombosis. Some studies reported hyperhomocysteinemia in PS patients compared with healthy volunteers or nonpsoriatic dermatologic outpatients [57-59]. Gisondi et al [60] observed that plasma homocysteine directly correlated with PS severity according to PS area and severity index (PASI) score, whereas it was inversely correlated with plasma folic acid levels, which were lower in PS patients than in the controls and lower than the normal range in 32.5% of PS patients.

G) Endothelial dysfunction and subclinical ATS

At present, a number of screening tests to detect asymptomatic patients at risk of ATS are available, such as measurement of carotid artery intima − media thickness (IMT), and plaque imaging by high − resolution B − mode ultrasound [61] which is a useful, non-invasive surrogate marker of macrovascular ATS that provides early information on ATS in subclinical stages of the disease [62]. Increased IMT of the common carotid artery is an indicator of generalized ATS. Carotid ATS goes hand − in − hand with coronary ATS and hence the incidence of carotid plaques or increased

IMT is more in patients prone to CAD [63]. On this basis, a number of observations have emerged focusing on specific and often subclinical aspects of the ATS process in PS patients, further supporting the association between the two conditions. Ludwing et al. [64] found a significantly increased prevalence (59.4 vs. 28.1, p=0.015) and severity of calcification in the coronary arteries in patients with PS, and multiple linear regression calculations identified PS as a likely independent risk factor for coronary artery calcification. A different study showed an increased IMT in patients (with no other CV risk factors) with chronic PS (0.9 ± 0.2 mm vs. 0.7 ± 0.1 mm of controls , p < 0.001), suggesting a possible correlation between the disease and subclinical ATS [65]; carotid IMT positively correlated with patients age, duration of the disease and severity of PS based on PASI score. Analogous data were shown by Balci et al. [66]; they also demonstrate that PS patients had impaired endothelial function, measured by flow – mediated dilatation (FMD) and nitroglycerin – induced dilatation (NTD) of the brachial artery. Also, FMD was significantly reduced in PS patients compared to healthy controls in the reports of Ulusoy et al. [67] (13.9 ± 0.5 vs. 32.6 ± 6.3, p< 0.001) and Karadag et al. (5.6 ± 2.0 % vs. 10.9 ± 1.9 %, p< 0.001), but, in this latter case, there was no significant correlation between PASI and FMD [68]. On the other hand, Martyn – Simmons et al. [69] did not show a statistically significant difference in endothelial dysfunction, measured by FMD, between PS patients (without CV risk factors) and healthy controls. A cross – sectional study assessed arterial stiffness by measuring carotid – femoral and carotid – radial pulse wave velocity in 39 adult patients with moderate – to – severe PS and 38 controls [70]. The carotid – femoral pulse wave velocity was found significantly higher in PS patients than in controls, even after adjustment for age, gender, and CV risk factors, confirming the results of similar experiences [71-72]. Moreover, a positive correlation was noted between pulse wave velocity and PS duration, but not with PS severity [70], suggesting that PS duration could be a risk factor for arterial stiffness and thus ATS.

The Role of Inflammation as a Possible Link between PS and CAD

As mentioned above, IMIDs (Immune-mediated inflammatory diseases) are part of a spectrum of chronic diseases in which inflammation plays an important role in pathogenesis. Central to this pathogenesis is an imbalance in inflammatory cytokines. Inflammation also plays an important role in the pathogenesis of ATS which is an important risk factor for vascular disease. In addition, ATS has also been found to be more common in patients with rheumatoid arthritis and systemic lupus erythematosus than in healthy controls [73]. Inflammation may be an important link between PS and CAD. In order to understand this relationship, it is critical to examine the pathophysiology of PS and ATS. First, immune cells predominate in the development of psoriatic and atherosclerotic lesions, and their effector molecules are primarily responsible for the progression of these lesions [3] [74]. In fact, the upregulation of Th1-mediated cytokine cascades (IFN-γ, TNF-α, IL-1, IL-6) and subsequent inflammation appear to be a likely trigger for destabilization of those lesions [74]. In addition, both diseases have a common pattern of T-cell activation, including chemokines [3], local and systemic expression of adhesion molecules [3], and endothelins [75], C-reactive protein and Toll-like receptor [75]. Although inflammatory cytokines such as TNF-α have been extensively studied, emerging data have recently demonstrated the central role of IL-20 and IL-17 in the pathogenesis of PS [76]. IL-17 is secreted by a new subclass of CD4 + cells, the Th17 cells, and plays an important role in the pathogenesis of PS and broadly activates inflammation in a variety of organ systems [77-78]; for example, IL-17 is also elevated in the sera of patients with unstable CAD [79].

Perhaps more important is the observation that treatment of severe PS (such as other IMIDs), including the use of drugs associated per se with adverse effects on the cardiovascular system, may lead to the amelioration of ATS and reduction in mortality. In particular, the use of methotrexate and anti-TNF-α agents has been shown to reduce cardiovascular mortality and the incidence of myocardial infarction in rheumatoid disease, especially in patients who respond well in terms of reduced systemic inflammation, while cyclosporin and etretinate, known to cause hypertension and dyslipidemia, respectively, at the very least do not seem to increase the risks of cardiovascular-related death in PS [1,19,80-82]. More recently, Boehncke et al. examined currently available evidence favoring the concept of a causal link between PS and ATS; they concluded that PS is a systemic inflammatory disease that may cause insulin resistance, which in turn triggers endothelial cell dysfunction, leading to ATS and finally myocardial infarction or stroke [84].

The effect of systemic anti-inflammatory therapy for PS on the future risk of CVD also needs to be determined. Pending further investigation, individuals who develop psoriasis at a younger age, those with long-standing psoriasis, should consider addressing modifiable CVD risk factors.

According to these results, it is clear the importance of an early treatment of CVD risk factors in patients with PS, a condition that could increase the risk of developing CAD, especially in patient with severe PS: the clinician's role is to reduce the CVD risk with drug therapy and non-drug therapy. It is also important to provide patients with PS information about their CVD risk, especially in patients with other CAD risk factors such as abdominal obesity, high blood pressure or diabetes.

Patients with PS and an abnormal serum lipid level or elevated value of C-reactive protein (CRP) should follow a multifaceted lifestyle approach to reduce CAD risk. Weight loss and physical activity in patients with elevated LDL cholesterol values should be undertaken. In the presence of only one CAD risk factor and LDL cholesterol >160 mg/dl, the goal should be the reduction of cholesterol at value <160 mg/dl. For two or more risk factor it is necessary the reduction of cholesterol at value < 130 mg/dl, with the target value of 100 mg/dl. In the presence of CVD, the target level is < 100 mg/dl with the target of < 70 mg/dl if CVD is associated with diabetes mellitus (DM), metabolic syndrome, or heavy cigarette smoking.

Drug therapy for elevated LDL cholesterol should be prescribed in patients with PS and high cholesterol levels in whom the lifestyle changes don't permit the achievement of target level. Statins reduce LDL cholesterol and also may have favorable effect on plaque psoriasis and on plasma level of PCR [89-90]. Statins should be used with caution in patients treated with methotrexate and are contraindicated in patients with active or chronic liver diseases. Also niacin can be used, for its role on the elevation of HDL cholesterol, and have the same contraindication of statins. Fibrates are contraindicated in patient with active liver diseases and should be used with caution in patients treated with cyclosporine or methotrexate. Gemfibrozil has been linked to exacerbations of PS [91].

Another point is the reduction of blood pressure. The target value is < 140/90 mmHg in all patients with PS and ≤ 2 CAD risk factors and < 130/80 mmHg in patients with previous CVD, DM, chronic renal disease or ≥ 3 CAD risk factors. A correct lifestyle with a diet high in potassium and calcium, low in sodium and moderation of alcohol intake, increase the efficacy of antihypertensive drug therapy and allows to decrease the CAD risk. All patients with PS and elevated blood pressure not controlled to target level with a correct lifestyle should be treated with pharmacologic therapy. All the classes of drugs can be used in patient with PS such as thiazide-type diuretics, angiotensin-converting enzyme inhibitors (ACEi), angiotensin receptor blockers (ARB), direct renin inhibitor, β-blockers (BB) and calcium channel blockers. There is no evidence that one class of anti-hypertensive drug is more or less effective than another in patient with PS. There are a few cases reported in literature in which BB, ACEI or ARB may rarely precipitate psoriatic flare-ups [92-93], so patients that receive these drugs should be monitored for exacerbations of PS. It may be important also to early identify patients with PS and metabolic syndrome, in order to start CAD prevention strategies: systemic inflammation is a common feature of both these diseases, and it could be an important way to stop the progression of the disease at its beginning. The metabolic syndrome is diagnosed when ≥ 3 of these criteria are present:

1. Increased waist circumference ≥ 102 cm in men and 88 cm in women
2. Elevated serum level of triglycerides ≥ 150 mg/dl
3. Reduced serum level of HDL cholesterol: < 40 mg/dl in men and < 50 mg/dl in women
4. Elevated blood pressure ≥ 130/85 mmHg
5. Elevated fasting glucose ≥ 100 mg/dl

Particular attention should be used in patients in treatment with cyclosporine. In this patients an increase of the levels of LDL cholesterol and blood pressure may be seen. Also patients in treatment with corticosteroids can have an increased CAD risk due to elevation of blood pressure. There is no evidence in the literature on the utility of ultraviolet phototherapies or biological drugs such as anti-TNFα drugs on CAD risk factors. Biological drugs should be used with caution in patient with heart failure because they could exacerbate symptoms of HF [94], although other studies underline the improvement of symptoms [95].

Conclusion

The association between CAD and PS is limited to retrospective analyses of large patient data sets. However epidemiologic data may contribute to support an association of PS with several risk factors for cardiovascular disease and for ATS with coronary artery diseases. Patients with PS should be screened for diabetes, hypertension and hyperlipidemia. Certainly, any cardiac symptoms should be taken seriously and evaluated appropriately. Clinicians should pay close attention to cardio-vascular risk factors in patient with PS, particularly in those with moderate to severe forms, starting an early treatment. Physicians managing cardiovascular risk factors in patients with PS should adhere to standard ATS prevention and treatment guidelines. Attention also should be put on a proper and aggressive early treatment of the PS itself.

References

[1] Prodanovich S, Ma F, Taylor JR et al. Methotrexate reduces incidence of vascular diseases in veterans with psoriasis or rheumatoid arthritis. *J Am Acad Dermatol 2005*; 52: 262–7.

[2] Menter A, Griffiths EM. Current and future management of psoriasis. *Lancet* 2007;370:272–284.

[3] Schon MP, Boehnke W - H.Psoriasis. *N Engl J Med* 2005; 352:1899-912.

[4] Krueger G, Ellis CN. Psoriasis - recent advances in understanding its pathogenesis and treatment. *J Am Acad Dermatol* 2005; 53 (1 Suppl. 1): S94-100.

[5] Lee MG, Cooper AJ. Immunopathogenesis of psoriasis. *Aust J Dermatol* 2006; 47:151-9.

[6] KruegerJG, Bowcock A. Psoriasis pathophysiology: current concepts of pathogenesis. *Am Rheum Dis* 2005; 64 (Suppl.2):ii 30 - 6.

[7] B., Lindegard. Diseases associated with psoriasis in a general population. *Dermatologica* 1986;172:298-304.

[8] Naldi L, Parazzini F, Brevi A, et al. Family history, smoking habits,alcohol consumption and risk of psoriasis. *Br J Dermatol* 1992;127:212-7.

[9] Christophers E, Henseler T. Contrasting disease patterns in psoriasis and atopic dermatitis. *Arch Dermatol Res* 1987;297:48-51.

[10] Henseler T, Christophers E. Disease concomitance in psoriasis. *J Am Acad Dermatol* 1995;32:98.

[11] Christophers E. Nov-Dec, Comorbidities in psoriasis. *Clin Dermatol.* 2007 and 25(6):529-34.

[12] Mc Donald Cj, Calabresi P. Psoriasis and occlusive vascular disease. *Br J Dermatol* 1978: 99: 469-475.

[13] Ena P, Madeddu P, Glorioso N, Cerimele D, Rappelli A. High prevalence of cardiovascular diseases and enhanced activity of the renin-angiotensin system in psoriatic patients. *Acta Cardiol* 1985: 40: 199–205.

[14] B., Lindegard. Diseases associated with psoriasis in a general population of 159,200 middle-aged, urban, native Swedes. *Dermatologica* 1986: 172: 298–304.

[15] Krueger GG, Duvic M. Epidemiology of psoriasis: clinical issues. *J Invest Dermatol* 1994: 102: 14S–18S.

[16] Henseler T, Christophers E. Disease concomitance in psoriasis. *J Am Acad Dermatol* 1995: 32: 982–986.

[17] Mallbris L, Akre O, Granath F, Yin L, Lindelöf B, Ekbom A, Ståhle-Bäckdahl M. Increased risk for cardiovascular mortality in psoriasis inpatients but not in outpatients. *Eur J Epidemiol.* 2004;19(3):225-30.

[18] Crown WH, Bresnahan BW, Orsini LS, et al. The burden of illness associated with psoriasis:cost of treatment with systemic therapyand phototherapy in the US. *Curr Med Res Opin* 2004; 20: 1929–1936.

[19] Gelfand JM, Neimann AL, Shin DB, Wang X, Margolis DJ,Troxel AB. Risk of myocardial infarction in patients with psoriasis. *JAMA* 2006: 296: 1735–1741.

[20] Kimball AB, Robinson D Jr, Wu Y, et al. Cardiovascular disease and risk factors among psoriasis patients in two US healthcare databases, 2001–2002. *Dermatology* 2008: 217:27–37.

[21] J. Xiao, L-H Chen, Y-T Tu, X.H Deng, J Tao. Prevalence of myocardial infarction in patients with psoriasis in central China. *JEADV* 2009, 23, 1311-1315.

[22] Wakkee M, Herings RM, Nijsten T. Psoriasis may not be an independent risk factor for acute ischemic heart disease hospitalizations: results of a large population-based Dutch cohort. *J Invest Dermatol* 2009 Oct 8.

[23] Schmitt J, Ford DE.Psoriasis is independently associated with psychiatric morbidity and adverse cardiovascular risk factors, but not with cardiovascular events in a population based sample. *J Eur Acad Dermatol Venereol* 2009 Dec 10.

[24] Brauchli YB, Jick SS, Miret M, Meier CR.Psoriasis and risk of incident myocardial infarction, stroke or transient ischaemic attack: an inception cohort study with a nested case-control analysis. *Br J Dermatol* 2009: 160: 1048–1056.

[25] Gelfand JM, Troxel AB, Lewis JD, Kurd SK, et al. The risk of mortality in patients with psoriasis. *Arch Dermatol* 2007; 143:1493-1499.

[26] Henseler T, Christophers E. Disease concomitance in psoriasis. *J Am Acad Dermatol* 1995; 32:982-986.

[27] Kremers HM, Mc Evoy MT, Dann FJ et al. Heart diseases in psoriasis. *J Am Acad Dermatol* 2008; 58:347-352.

[28] Wakke M, Thio HB, Prens EP, et al.Unfavorable cardiovascular risk profiles in untreated and treated psoriasis patients. *Atherosclerosis* 2007; 190: 1-9.

[29] Neimann AL, Shin DB, Wang X, et al. Prevalence of cardiovascular risk factors in atients wih psoriasis. *J Am Acad Dermatol* 2006; 55: 829 - 35.

[30] Herron MD, Hinckley M, Hoffman MS, et al. Impact of obesity and smoking on psoriasis presentation and management. *Arch Dermatol* 2005; 141:1527-1534.

[31] Naldi L, Chatenoud L, Linder D et al. Cigarette smoking, body mass index, and strefful life events as risk factors for psoriasis: resuts from an Italian case - control study. *J Invest Dermatol* 2005; 125:61-67.

[32] Setty AR, Curhan G, Choi HK.Obesity, waist circumference, weight change, and the risk of psoriasis in women: Nurses' Health Study II. *Arch Int Med* 2007; 167:1670 - 1675.

[33] Mallbris L, Granath F, Hamstem A, et al.Psoriasis is associated with lipid abnormalities at the onset of skin disease. *J Am Acad Dermatol* 2006;54:614-621.

[34] Naldi L, Addis A, Chimenti S, et al. Impact of body mass index and obesity on clinical response to systemic treatment for psoriasis. Evidence from the Psocare project. *Dermatology* 2008; 217:365-373.

[35] Gisondi P, Del Giglio M, Di Francesco V, Zamboni M, Girolomoni G. Weight loss improves the response of obese patients with moderate - to - severe chronic plaque psoriasis to low - dose cyclosporine therapy: a randomized, controlled, investigator - blinded clinical trial. *Am J Clin Nutr* 2008; 88:1242-1247.

[36] L, Naldi. Cigarette smoking and psoriasis. *Clin Dermatol* 1998; 16:571-574.

[37] Bo K, Thoresen M, Delgard F. Smokers report more psoriasis, but not atopic dermatitis or hand eczema: results from a Norwegian population survey among adults. *Dermatology* 2008; 216:40-45.

[38] G, Favato. High incidence of smoking habit in psoriatic patients. *Am J Med* 2008; 121:e17.

[39] ISTAT. http://www.istat.it/sanita/Healt. [Online] [Cited: Febr 20, 2009.]

[40] Setty AR, Curhan G, Choi HK. Smoking and the risk of psoriasis in women: Nurses' Health Study II. *Am J Med* 2007; 120:953-9.

[41] Fortes C, Mastroeni S, Leffondrè K, et al. Relationship between smoking and the clinical severity of psoriasis. *Arch Dermatol* 2005;141:1580 - 1584.

[42] Ucak S, Ekmekci TR, Basat O, et al.Comparison of various insulin sensitivity indices in psoriatic patients and their relationship with type of psoriasis. *J Eur Acad Dermatol Venereol* 2006;20:517-522.

[43] Boehneke S, Thaci D, Beschmann H, et al. Psoriasis patients show signs of insulin resistance. *Br J Dermatol* 2007; 157:1249-1251.

[44] Kaje JA, Li L, Jick SS. Incidence risk factors for myocardial infarction and other vascular diseases in patients with psoriasis. *Br J Dermatol* 2008;159:895-902.

[45] Shapiro J, Cohen AD, David M, et al.The association between psoriasis, diabetes mellitus and atherosclerosis in Israel: a case - control study. *J Am Acad Dermatol* 2007; 56:629-634.

[46] Wolf N, Quaranta M, Prescott NJ, et al. Psoriasis is associated with pleiotropic susceptibility loci identified in type II diabetes and Chron disease *J Med Genet* 2008;45:114-116.

[47] 47.Rocha - Pereira P, Santos - Silva A, Rebelo I, et al.Dislipidemia and oxidative stress in mild and severe psoriasis as a risk for cardiovascular disease. *Clin Chim Acta* 2001; 303:33-39.

[48] Cohen AD, Sherf M, Vidavsky L, et al.Association between psoriasis and the metabolic syndrome. *Dermatol* 2008; 216:152-155.

[49] Akhyani M, Ehsani AH, Robati RM, Robati AM.The lipid profile in psoriasis: a controlled study. *J Eur Acad Dermatol Venereol* 2007; 21:1330-1332.

[50] Farshchian M, Zamanian A, Farshcian M et al. Serum lipid level in Iranian patients with psoriasis. *J Eur Acad Dermatol Veneorol* 2007; 2007: 802 - 805.

[51] Qureshi AA, Choi HK, Setty AR, Curhan GC. Psoriasis and the risk of diabetes and hypertension: a prospective study of US female nurses. *Arch Dermatol.* 2009 Apr;145(4):379-82.

[52] Cohen AD, Weitzman D, Dreiher J. Psoriasis and hypertension: a case-control study. *Acta Derm Venereol.* 2010;90(1):23-6.

[53] Mehta NN, Azfar RS, Shin DB, Neimann AL, Troxel AB, et al. Patients with severe psoriasis are at increased risk of cardiovascular mortality: cohort study using the General Practice Research Database. *Eur Heart J 2010*;31:1000-1006.

[54] B, Lindegard. Diseases associated with psoriasis in a general population of 159,200 middle - aged, urban, native Swedes. *Dermatologica* 1986;172:298-304.

[55] Inerot A, Enerback C, Enlund F, et al.Collecting a set of psoriasis material through a patient organisation; clinical characterisation and presence of additional disorders. *BMC Dermatol* 2005;5-10.

[56] Vizzardi E, Bonadei I, Zanini G, et al.Homocysteine and heart failure: an overview. *Recent Pat Cardiovasc Drug Discov.* 2009 Jan;4(1):15-21.

[57] Malerba M, Gisondi P, Radaeli A, Sala R, Calzavara Pinton PG, Girolomoni G. Plasma homocysteine and folate levels in patients with chronic plaque psoriasis. *Br J Dermatol* 2006;155:1165-1169.

[58] Karabudak O, Ulusoy RE, Erikci AA, et al. Inflammation and hypercoagulable state in adult psoriatic men. *Acta Derm Venereol* 2008;88:337-340.

[59] Vanizor Kural B, Orem A, Cimit G, et al.Plasma homocysteine and its relationship with atherothrombotic markers in psoriatic patients *Clin Chim Acta* 2003;332:23-30.

[60] Gisondi P, Girolomoni G Psoriasis and atherothrombotic diseases: disease-specific and non-disease-specific risk factors.. *Semin Thromb Hemost.* 2009 Apr;35(3):313-24.

[61] Naghavi M, Falk E, Hecht HS et al.From vulnerable plaque to vulnerable patient - part III: executive summary of the screening for heart attack prevention and education (SHAPE) task force report. *Am J Cardiol* 2006; 98 (2): 2 - 15.

[62] Kimbal AB, Gladman D, Gelfand GM et al. National psoriasis foundation clinical consensus on psoriasis comorbidities and recommendations for screening. *J Am Acad Dermatol* 2008; 58 (6): 1031 - 1042.

[63] Celermajer DSW, Sorensen KE, Gooch VM et al. Non - invasive delection of endothelial dysfunction in children and adults at risk of atherosclerosis. *Lancet* 1992; 340: 1111 - 1115.

[64] Ludwig RJ, Herzog C, Rostock A, Ochsendorf FR, Zollner TM et al. Psoriasis: a possible risk factor for development of coronary artery calcification. *Br J Dermatol* 2007: 156, 271 - 276.

[65] El -Mongy S, Fathy H, Abdelaziz A, et al. Subclinical atherosclerosis in patients with chronic psoriasis: a potential association. *Vols. J Eur Acad Dermatol Venereol 2010*, 24, 661 - 666.

[66] Balci DD, Balci A, Karazincir S et al. Increased carotid artery intima - media thikness and impaired endothelial function in psoriasis. *JEADV* 2009, 23 1-6.

[67] Ulusoy Eralp, Karabudak O, Yokusoglu M, et al.Non invasive assesment of impaired endothelial function in psoriasis. *Rheumatol Int* (2010) 30:479-483.

[68] Karadag AS, Yavuz B, Ertugrul DT et al. Is psoriasis a pre - atherosclerotic disease? Increased Insulin resistance and impaired endothelial function in patients with psoriasis. *Int J Der* 2010, 49. 642 - 646.

[69] Martyn - Simmons CL, Ranawaka RR, Chowienczyk P et al. A prospective case - controlled cohort study of endothelial function in patients with moderate to severe psoriasis. *Brit J Derm* 2011; 164, 26 - 32.

[70] Gisondi P, Fantin F, Del Giglio M, et al. Chronic plaque psoriasis is associated with increased arterial stiffness. *Dermatology* 2009; 218:110-113.

[71] Soy M, Yildiz M, Sevki Uyanik M, et al. Susceptibility to atherosclerosis in patients with psoriasis and psoriatic arthritis as determined by carotid - femoral (aortic) pulse wave velocity measurement. *Rev Esp Cardiol* 2009: 62: 96 - 99.

[72] Yiu KH, Yeung CK, Chan HT, et al. Increased arterial stifness in patients with psoriasis is associated with active systemic inflammation. *Brit J Dermat* 2011: 164, 514 - 520.

[73] Hahn BH, Grossman J, Chen W, McMahon M.The pathogenesis of atherosclerosis in authoimmune rhumatic diseases: roles of inflammation and dyslipidemia. *J Autoimmun* 2007; 28:69-75.

[74] Hansson GK. Inflammation, atherosclerosis, and coronary artery disease. *N Engl J Med.* 2005;352:1685-1695.

[75] Alexandroff AB, Pauriah M, Camp RD et al. More than skin deep – atherosclerosis as a systemic manifestation of psoriasis. *Br J Dermatol* 2009; 161: 1–7.

[76] Wei CC, Hsu YH, Li HH, et al IL-20: biological functions and clinical implications. *J Biomed Sci* 2006; 13:601–612.

[77] Arican O, Aral M, Sasmaz S, Ciragil P.Serum levels of TNF-alpha, IFN-gamma,IL-6, IL-8, IL-12, IL-17, and IL-18 in patients with active psoriasis and correlation with disease severity. *Mediators Inflamm* 2005; 2005:273–279.

[78] Sabat R, Phillip S, Hoflich C, et al. Immunopathogenesis of psoriasis. *Exper Dermatol* 2007; 16:779–798.

[79] Hashmi S, Zeng QT. Role of interleukin-17 and interleukin-17-induced cytokines interleukin-8 in unstable coronary artery disease. *Coron Artery Dis* 2006; 17:699–706.

[80] 80.Van den Borne BE, Landewe RB, Houkes I et al.No increased risk of malignancies and mortality in cyclosporin A-treated patients with rheumatoid arthritis. *Arthritis Rheum* 1998; 41: 1930–7 1998.

[81] Stern RS, Fitzgerald E, Ellis CN et al.The safety of etretinate as long-term therapy for psoriasis: results of the etretinate follow-up study. *J Am Acad Dermatol* 1995; 33: 44–52.

[82] Dixon WG, Watson KD, Lunt M et al.Reduction in the incidence of myocardial infarction in patients with rheumatoid arthritis who respond to anti-tumor necrosis factor alpha therapy: results from the British Society for Rheumatology Biologics Register. *Arthritis Rheum* 2007; 56: 2905–12.

[83] Louden BA, Pearce DJ, Lang W, Feldman SR. A Simplified Psoriasis Area Severity Index (SPASI) for rating psoriasis severity in clinic patients. *Dermatol Online J.* 2004 Oct 15;10(2):7.

[84] Zheng Y, Danilenko DM, Valdez P, et al. cytokine, mediates IL-23-induced dermal inflammation and acanthosis. Vols. *Nature.* 2007;445:648-651.

[85] Nickoloff BJ.Med.2007, Cracking the cytokine code in psoriasis. *Nat and* 13:242-244.

[86] Willerson JT, Ridker PM. Inflammation as a cardiovascular risk factor. Vols. *Circulation.* 2004;109:II2-10.

[87] hazizadeh R, Shimizu H, Tosa M and Ghazizadeh M. G Pathogenic mechanisms shared between Psoriasis and Cardiovascular Disease. *Int J Med Sci* 2010; 7 (5):284-289.

[88] Boehncke WH, Boehncke S, Tobin AM and Kirby B.The 'psoriatic march': a concept of how severe psoriasis may drive cardiovascular comorbidity. *exper Derm,* 20, 303-307.

[89] McCarey DW, McInnes IB, Madhok R et al. Trial of Atorvastatin in Rheumatoid Arthritis (TARA): double-blind, randomized placebo controlled trial. *Lancet* 2004; 363:2015-2021.

[90] Shirinsky IV, Shirinsky VS. Efficacy of simvastatin in plaque psoriasis: a pilot study. *J Am Acad Dermatol* 2007; 57:529-531.

[91] Wolf R, Schiavo AL, Russo A, de Angelis F, Ruocco V. Effects of gemfibrozil on in vitro cultured normal human skin explants. *Int J Dermatol* 1999; 38:65-69.

[92] Fry L, Baker BS. Triggering psoriasis: the role of infections and medications. *Clin Dermatol* 2007; 25 : 606-15.

[93] Wakefield PE, Berger TG, James WD. Atenolol- induced pustular psoriasis. *Arch Dermatol* 1990; 126 : 968-69.

[94] Kwon HJ, Cotè TR, Cuffe MS, Kramer JM, Braun MM. Case report of heart failure after therapy with tumor necrosis factor antagonist. *Ann Intern Med* 2003; 138: 807-11.

[95] Wolfe F. Michaud K. Heart failure in rheumatoid arthritis: rates, predictors, and effects of anti-tumor necrosis factor therapy. *Am J Med* 2004; 116: 305-11.

In: Current Advances in Cardiovascular Risk. Volume 2   ISBN: 978-1-62081-746-9
Editor: Sandeep Ajoy Saha   © 2012 Nova Science Publishers, Inc.

Chapter XX

Management of Cardiovascular Risk in Patients with Periodontal Diseases

F. Graziani [1,2,*] and M. Tonetti [3]
[1]Department of Surgery, Section of Oral Surgery,
University of Pisa, Pisa, Italy
[2]Eastman Dental Institute, Department of Periodontology,
University College of London, UK
[3]European Research Group on Periodontology (ERGOPERIO),
Berne, Switzerland

Abstract

Periodontitis is a chronic infectious disease characterized by progressive inflammatory loss of the tooth's supporting tissues. It is a major public health issue as it affects in severe forms >10% of the adult population and it is the major cause of tooth loss and oral disability. It is caused by a bacterial biofilm harboring gram negative anaerobes and microaerophilic pathogens. Bacteria, however, are necessary but not sufficient for clinical manifestation of the disease. Indeed, the host inflammatory response has a pivotal role in determining tissue damage. The variance on the individual responsiveness of inflammation is modulated by environmental, acquired and genetic factors.

Periodontitis has been associated not just with local tissue damage but also with a moderate systemic inflammatory response, representing a chronic source of systemic inflammation which, together with the bacteremia due to periodontal infection, may constitute the biological rationale of cardiovascular connections.

Indeed Periodontitis has been connected with an increased risk of cardiovascular events. Nevertheless, the nature of the association is unclear since both periodontitis and atherosclerosis share numerous risk factors. Causality of this association may be explored through intervention trials. Early systematic reviews and a definitive intervention clinical trial indicate that intensive periodontal therapy results in decrease in systemic

---

* Corresponding Author: Filippo Graziani DDS, MCD, PhD. Dept. of Surgery, Section of Dentistry and Oral Surgery; f.graziani@med.unipi.it. University of Pisa, Via Roma 55, 56126, Pisa.

inflammation and improvement of endothelial dysfunction in systemically healthy subjects.

Evidence to date is consistent with the notion that severe generalized periodontitis may play a determinant role in the development of systemic inflammation and endothelial dysfunction. Periodontitis has effects that reach beyond the oral cavity and their treatment and prevention may contribute to prevention of atherosclerosis. Periodontal treatment of cardiovascular patients should also be performed with careful assessment of hemostasis. Indeed treatment may constitute a serious hazard in patient with a bleeding tendency. Finally, the most recent infective endocarditis prevention guidelines are reported.

Abbreviations

CV   Cardiovascular
CVD   Cardiovascular Diseases
Pg   Porphyromonas gingivalis
Tf   Tannerella forsythia
Aa   Aggregatibacter actinomycetemcomitans
LPS   Lipopolysaccharide
IL   Interleukin
TNF   Tumour Necrosis Factor
NSAIDS   Non-Steroidal Anti-Inflammatory Agents
PMN   Polimorphonucleates
CRP   C-reactive protein
LDL   Low-density lipoprotein
CPTIN   Community Periodontal Index of Treatment Needs
SAA   Serum Amyloid A
FMD   Flow-mediated dilatation
IMT   Thickness of the intima-media
ARIC   Atherosclerosis Risk in Community
Ig   Immunoglobulin
BP   Blood Pressure
PAVE   Periodontitis and Vascular Events
APR   Acute-phase response
INR   International Normalised Ratio
GH   Gingival hyperplasia
IE   Infective endocarditis
NBTE   Non-bacterial thrombotic endocarditis
NICE   National Institute for Health and Clinical Excellence

1. Periodontal Diseases

Periodontal diseases are clinical pathologies affecting tooth-supporting tissues. They are usually subdivided in gingivitis and periodontitis according to the presence of tissue destruction. Among these periodontitis has been linked to cardiovascular diseases (CVD) for a variety of different reasons connected to both pathogenic and therapeutic factors. Cardiovascular diseases are amongst the most prevalent and significant diseases in developed countries showing a high rate of mortality.

Periodontitis is a multi-factorial chronic infectious disease characterized by loss of the connective tissue attachment to the teeth and resorption of the alveolar bone that may ultimately determines tooth exfoliation [1]. The accumulation of dental plaque biofilm near the gingival margin triggers the pathogenic process [2;3]. It is a very common disease as moderate forms of periodontal disease are thought to be universal for their high prevalence (50-60% of the adult population) whereas severe forms affect only a minority of adults (5-15%) [4;5].

1.2. Bacterial Load: Periopathogens

Microbial plaque is considered the decisive factor in the initiation of the gingival inflammation despite the etio-pathogenesis of periodontitis is not yet fully understood [6]. Supra- and subgingival plaque, once colonized by specific gram negative bacterial species (mainly *Porphyromonas gingivalis (Pg), Tannerella forsythia (Tf), Aggregatibacter actinomycetemcomitans(Aa), Campylobacter rectus, Prevotella intermedia* and some spirochetes) can potentially initiate and perpetuate periodontal damage. These bacteria have been described as periodontopathogens o periopathogens. Subgingival microbial plaque behaves as a biofilm [7]. Accordingly, bacterial populations closely adhere to each other and to other surfaces to reach a higher virulence rather than in their planktonic state [8]. These associations in the biofilm are not random but to some extent follow a specific pathway. In patients suffering from periodontitis bacteria tend to assemble themselves in groups which have been shown to be usually six. These groups have been named: the complexes [9]. Two of these complexes (named orange and red) include the majority of the putative periopathogens.

1.3. Host Response

The individual host response is the other essential component in the pathogenesis of periodontitis. An over-reacting inflammatory response is needed to determine periodontal tissue destruction as, despite the infectious nature of periodontitis, bacteria proved to be essential but not sufficient to cause disease. Periopathogens and/or their toxic products (LPS) within the gingival sulcus may gain access to the gingival tissue and elicit a local inflammatory response characterized by neutrophils, lymphocytes and macrophages [10]. Local macrophage activation results in production of pro-inflammatory cytokines such as IL-1α and β, TNF-α and IL-6 in order to contain the bacterial challenge [2;11-13]. Connective tissue destruction occurs as the result of matrix metalloproteinase activation in response to cell stimulation by pro-inflammatory cytokines [2]. This inflammatory response is associated with connective attachment loss and migration of the gingival epithelial attachment along the root surface [14]. Disruption of attachment of tooth supporting tissues represents the pathognomonic lesions of periodontitis. Ultimately, the amount of destruction may expand on the entire tooth length and subsequently determine tooth loss.

Local production and accumulation of inflammatory mediators is the major mechanism leading to periodontal attachment loss and bone loss [15]. A series of studies in experimental animals and humans has shown that the administration of Non-Steroidal Anti-Inflammatory Agents (NSAIDS) significantly blocks periodontal destruction in subjects with naturally occurring periodontitis. Indeed, local levels of inflammatory mediators have been used as markers for active periodontal breakdown.

1.4. Risk Factors for Periodontitis

Periodontal destruction is therefore due to an excessive inflammatory response to a gram negative bacteria assault. The amount of hyper-responsiveness of the inflammatory defense is influenced by environmental, acquired and genetic risk factors. Cigarette smoking, diabetes, stress, nutrition, HIV infection, obesity and osteoporosis have all been considered to be environmental and acquired risk factors for periodontitis [3]. Particularly, smokers are more likely to develop disease and to have an impaired clinical healing after periodontal therapy when compared with non-smokers [16]. Subjects with uncontrolled diabetes type 1 and type 2 (if adults) have more severe periodontal disease than non affected individuals [17].

Evidence derived from twin studies suggests that genetic factors may also play a determinant role in the onset and progression of periodontitis among populations [18]. Furthermore, inflammatory genes polymorphisms which may influence individual production of local inflammatory mediators including IL-1 and TNF-α have been associated with periodontitis [19;20]. Similarly genetic variants for Fcγ receptor for the constant (Fc) region of immunoglobulin G are likely to play a role in the pathogenesis of periodontitis [20]. Hyper-responding individuals or subjects with deficiencies in immune function (leucocytes PMN activity) also manifest with clinically more advanced disease [21].

2. Periodontal Diseases and Cardiovascular Diseases: A Link through Systemic Inflammation and Atherosclerosis?

In the last 50 years, cardiology has witnessed tremendous progress in the understanding of the risk factors for atherosclerosis and cardiovascular diseases. In spite of such enormous progress, a decade ago it was highlighted that almost one out of two heart attacks are occurring in subjects without the classic Framingham study cardiovascular risk factors: high lipids, hypertension, diabetes and smoking [22]. The recognition that much is still to be learnt about the pathogenesis of atherosclerosis has given strength to research approaches into alternative causes of atherosclerosis.

As it is understood today, atherosclerosis occurs in response to injury of the vascular endothelium [23]. Furthermore, the nature of the process is inflammatory [24]. An important hypothesis in cardiology has been that chronic infections may contribute to atherogenesis. The validity of such hypothesis has been confirmed by studies indicating that subjects exposed to chronic infections have 2-3 higher odds of having carotid atherosclerosis [25]. Chronic obstructive pulmonary disease with infectious exacerbations, chronic bronchitis, chronic sinusitis, chronic/recurrent urinary tract infections – but also an amorphous group of "other" infections - were all associated with higher odds of carotid atherosclerosis. Pathogens sustaining these chronic infections were considered to either have a direct effect on the vasculature or to exert an effect acting as a source of systemic inflammation that in turn would trigger the atherosclerotic process. Indeed epidemiological studies linking systemic inflammation, atherosclerosis and cardiovascular events have shown consistent associations between levels of systemic inflammatory markers and increases in carotid intima-media thickness, myocardial infarction and non-hemorrhagic stroke.

Interest for the infectious/inflammatory hypothesis of atherosclerosis led a group of cardiologists in Finland to look into the relationship between oral health and myocardial infarction [26]. Since those early reports, debate has been raging with regards to the existence and nature of an association between periodontal disease and atherosclerotic cardiovascular disease.

2.1. Biological Plausibility

Several well-designed preclinical studies have indicated possible mechanistic explanations for the association between periodontal infections and atherosclerotic cardiovascular disease [27]. There are mainly two types of mechanism involved: bacteria from periodontal disease may enter the circulation and contribute directly to the development of atherogenesis and contribution of systemic inflammation, due to periodontitis, to CVD. The following scientific evidence further explains a possible connection.

There are some biological suggestions of a potential role of periopathogens on the atherosclerotic plaque formation. Oral and systemic inoculation of P.gingivalis in apolipoprotein E deficient (i.e. more susceptible to atherosclerosis) animal models have shown that altogether with infection of periodontal tissues measured as alveolar bone loss, a systemic response towards P.gingivalis was mounted [28;29]. Higher aortic expression of vascular cell adhesion molecule-1 and tissue factor was also noted in the P.g. inoculated animals [29]. Moreover atherosclerotic lesions of the proximal aortas and aortic trees are more advanced and occurred earlier in P.g.-challenged animals [28]. Conversely, atherosclerotic lesions did not appear in the control animals despite their higher susceptibility.

a. DNA of periopathogens has been localized within atherosclerotic plaque. Human specimens of 50 endoarterectomy showed that in at least the 44% of the samples DNA of some target periopathogens, among T.f, P.g and A.a was present [30]. Further studies confirmed these findings [31;32].

b. *Periopathogens are able to invade endothelial cells.* P.gingivalis has shown the capability to invade several cell lines and the majority of P.gingivalis strains may invade vascular tissues [33].

c. *Periopathogens may trigger platelet aggregation on their membrane.* Platelet aggregation is characteristic of athcromas. It has been shown that *P. gingivalis* may facilitate platelet aggregation through its fimbriae and through its vesicles (membrane evaginations projecting to the outer environment) may determine a potent platelet aggregation-inducing activity [34].

d. *P.gingivalis accelerates macrophages transition to foam cells.* An important feature in the development of early atherosclerotic lesions is cholesterol uptake into macrophages to form foam cells. Murine macrophages could be stimulated by *P. gingivalis* to accumulate low-density lipoproteins (LDL) to form foam cells [35].

e. *Periopathogens have been linked to an increased host inflammatory reaction.* Systemic inflammation is closely linked to the onset of atherosclerosis [36]. Subjects affected by periodontal disease develop an intense local production of pro-inflammatory cytokines that may enter the blood stream as shown by the high levels of inflammatory bio-markers in both gingival tissues and serum [37;38]. This triggers a systemic acute-phase systemic inflammatory response, characterized by increased levels of acute phase proteins such as C-reactive protein (CRP) and vascular dysfunction [39-41].

The association is therefore biologically plausible and thus emphasis has been generally given to the strength and the consistency of the findings. Therefore, to sum up a plausible biological mechanism would suggest that bacteria or their toxic products may easily gain access to the circulatory system. Indeed episodes of bacteremia have been detected after normal activity such as chewing or brushing. Similar to bacterial dissemination, an excessive local production of pro-inflammatory cytokines may get access to the blood stream and trigger a systemic acute-phase response. Thus periodontal subjects when compared with matched periodontal healthy subjects show higher levels of CRP, IL-6, lower number of erythrocytes and hemoglobin concentrations, higher values of haptoglobin, moderate leukocytosis and increased cholesterol, LDL and glucose levels [42]. These differences were also significant when the analyses accounted for a series of possible confounding factors (age, sex, smoking, socioeconomic status, diabetes, body mass index, alcohol use).

2.2. Epidemiological Evidence

Since the first case-controlled studies in 1989, significant positive associations between various cardiovascular diseases (myocardial infarction, hospitalization, cardiac sudden death and peripheral vascular disease) and measures of oral health (alveolar bone loss, the Community Periodontal Index of Treatment Needs, etc.) have been reported.

The majority of epidemiological studies have indeed shown the presence of a significant association between periodontitis and myocardial infarction and stroke. Such studies usually report moderately increased risk of CVD in subjects with periodontitis (odds ratios, relative risks or hazard ratios ranging between 1.2 and 3.9) [43;44]. More recently [45] a meta-analytic data indicated that prevalence and incidence of coronary heart disease are significantly increased in periodontitis as OR varied from 1.14 to 2.22 according to the quality level of the studies included. The effect of tooth loss was also evaluated with a meta-regression analysis. Indeed it was shown that an inverse relationship between the number of teeth and the relative risk of CVD may exist. Lower risk has in general been presented in models corrected for other known risk factors such as age, gender, smoking and other confounders [46]. Certainly among them the role of cigarette smoking perhaps represents the strongest confounder [47].

Since these epidemiologic data were reported, the debate was centered on whether or not the association is: 1. real or due to residual confounding (e.g. by cigarette smoking: a common risk factor for both CVD and periodontitis) and 2. causal in nature (i.e. Periodontitis contributes to the causal path leading to atherosclerosis and/or cardiovascular events). Both issues can only be fully addressed by intervention trials: randomized controlled clinical experiments that seek to obtain an attenuation of the effect (atherosclerosis, cardiovascular events) through the elimination of the "cause" or exposure (periodontitis).

3. Effect of Periodontal Therapy on Cardiovascular Risks

Periodontal treatment has multiple treatment facets which have to be adapted to each single patient. Nevertheless, it is possible to design a therapeutic tree in which the majority of the cases can be included.

In general the objective of periodontal therapy is "to alter or eliminate the microbial etiology and contributing risk factors for periodontitis, thereby arresting the progression of the disease and preserving the dentition in a state of health, comfort, and function with appropriate aesthetics; and to prevent the recurrence of periodontitis" (American Academy of Periodontology).

In order to do accomplish these goals, as the cause of the disease is primarily infectious in nature, in the early stages of the treatment particular care should be devoted to the control of such infection. Thus instruction, reinforcement, and evaluation of the level of dental plaque of the patient are mandatory. Subsequently a causative phase, *i.e.* a therapeutic phase aiming at removal of subgingival deposit of plaque, must be performed. This phase is called supra- and subgingival scaling and root planing. Nevertheless, periodontal treatment does often comprise surgical corrective sessions following the causative phase of treatment. Ultimately, being in the majority of the cases a chronic disease, the long term success will be achieved when a supportive continuous therapy will be provided.

3.1. Short Term Effects of Periodontal Therapy on Markers of Cardiovascular Risk

Physiological reaction within the post-operative 72 hours has shown interesting features. Intensive nonsurgical periodontal therapy produced an acute inflammatory response as shown by the dramatic increase of blood markers of inflammation in the early days after treatment [48]. Non surgical periodontal therapy has been associated with a significant acute-phase response (APR) as assessed by changes in serum levels of C-reactive protein, fibrinogen, interleukin-6 [49;50] and serum amyloid A (SAA) [51] within the first days after treatment. Moreover, a significant effect on parameters of vascular health was also noted as significant perturbation of the endothelial and hemostatic system was registered [52]. D-dimer increases up to about 70% within the first week, significant increases of plasma soluble E-selectin and von-Willebrand factor did also increase showing marked post-therapy endothelial cell activation and therefore an increase tendency of inflammation and coagulation. The mechanisms underlying could be that both the bacteremia and the tissue damage following subgingival instrumentation [53] determine an increase of pro-inflammatory mediators [54] and acute-phase proteins [55]. Systemic inflammation may determine subsequently a reduction of vascular function.

Endothelial function may also be impaired as measured through flow-mediated dilatation (FMD) of the brachial artery [56]. Systemically healthy subjects not taking medications with severe generalized periodontitis were randomized to a control treatment (oral hygiene instructions and supra-gingival ultrasonic debridement) or an intensive periodontal therapy (oral hygiene instruction, scaling and root planing and extraction of hopeless teeth). In the intensive groups a significant worsening of the function was noted as FMD decreases within the first 24 hours.

Interestingly the analysis of systemic effects after surgical treatment did not yield the amount of expected inflammation [57]. Increases in CRP and SAA serum levels following surgical periodontal sessions were lower in magnitude than those detected after non-surgical therapy. This is somehow in contrast with the clinical perception of periodontal surgical procedure being a "trauma" of a greater magnitude when compared with non-surgical therapy. Possible speculations may suggest that, during periodontal surgery, the traumatized surface area is smaller than whole-mouth non-surgical periodontal treatment. Thus, a smaller postoperative wound could be responsible for a systemic inflammatory response of a lesser degree. Secondly, subgingival instrumentation of the entire dentition would be associated with a greater bacteremia as opposed to periodontal surgery because of a reduction in the quantity and quality of periodontal pathogens found in the periodontal pockets due to the host habitat modifications that have already taken place after non-surgical therapy [58].

The exact implications of the inflammatory changes taking place after periodontal treatment are yet to be determined. Inflammation could lead to an acute state of vascular dysfunction [56;59] and a possible increased risk of vascular events. In healthy individuals, however, the host response to inflammatory stimuli often resolves without complications. It is plausible to believe, however, that in other individuals perhaps already suffering from a vascular dysfunctional state, invasive therapy associated with substantial systemic inflammation could alter the integrity of the vasculature.

A recent case series [60] suggests that adults who underwent invasive dental procedures had an increased risk for myocardial infarction or stroke in the 4 weeks after the procedures compared with during other times (incidence ratio, 1.50 [95% CI, 1.09 to 2.06]). Further study is needed to determine whether this transient increase is due to acute dental inflammation, physiologic stress, or other mechanisms. The authors however stated that the absolute risks are minimal, and the long-term benefits on vascular health will probably outweigh the short-lived adverse effects. Further research is needed for a better understanding of these findings.

3.2. Long Term Effects of Periodontal Therapy

An initial cohort study showed that periodontal therapy consisting of oral hygiene instructions, scaling and root planing and extraction of hopeless teeth can result in a dose-dependent improvement in systemic IL-6 and CRP: the better the clinical outcome of periodontal therapy, the larger the magnitude of the decrease in systemic markers of inflammation [48].

Such initial data led to the performance of two small pilot trials to optimize the treatment regimen for maximal improvement of systemic parameters. Intensive periodontal therapy – defined as the combined application of oral hygiene instructions, extraction of hopeless teeth, scaling and root planing under local anesthesia performed over a 24 hour period and local controlled delivery of minocycline at all pockets 4 mm or deeper – gave better and earlier improvements as compared to conventional mechanical debridement alone [42;61].

A recent meta-analysis of these pilot intervention trials has indicated that periodontal therapy resulted in a weighted mean reduction in serum CRP of 0.5 mg (95% CI 0.08-0.93 mg). These data are in agreement with the notion that periodontitis contributes to the systemic inflammatory burden and that periodontal treatment leads to clinically relevant improvements in systemic inflammation [62] . These findings are important because increased levels of serum CRP (but also of other inflammatory parameters) are excellent predictors of the development of atherosclerosis and myocardial infarction [63-65].

On the other hand, these data must be interpreted with caution as they refer to systemically healthy subjects with severe generalized periodontitis. It is unclear what the impact of less severe and widespread forms of periodontitis is or how clinically significant cardiovascular disease interferes with these findings.

3.2.1. Periodontitis and Endothelial Dysfunction

Endothelial dysfunction is considered to be the first inflammatory change of the vascular endothelium leading to arteriosclerosis. An early case-control study indicated that subjects with periodontitis had higher levels of endothelial dysfunction measured as flow mediated dilatation of the brachial artery that matched controls [66]. Two pilot studies reported that periodontal therapy seemed to lead to changes in endothelial dysfunction [59;67].

A recent definitive trial sought to assess the effect of intensive periodontal therapy on FMD of the brachial artery [56]. Systemically healthy subjects not taking medications with severe generalized periodontitis were randomized to a control treatment (oral hygiene instructions and supra-gingival ultrasonic debridement) or an intensive periodontal therapy (oral hygiene instruction, scaling and root planing and extraction of hopeless teeth). No changes in FMD were observed over a 6-month period in the controls; after intensive treatment, however, there was a biphasic change in FMD: in the first days following treatment there was a worsening of the systemic outcome followed by an improvement compared to baseline and the control group. At the end of the trial FMD in the test group was significantly better than in the control but also significantly better than at baseline indicating that periodontal therapy led to an improvement of endothelial dysfunction in these subjects. The effect of treatment was dose-dependent: there was a significant correlation between the reductions in the number of periodontal pockets and bleeding on probing and the improvement in endothelial function. In parallel to the changes in endothelial function, periodontal therapy led to changes in inflammatory and cardiovascular biomarkers further strengthening the results of the trial with the indication of plausible mechanisms. This trial was the first confirmation of a causal link between an early functional cardiovascular parameter and periodontitis. It is important to highlight that these results were obtained in a subject population that was systemically healthy and affected by severe generalized periodontitis: the effect of systemic conditions or the impact of less widespread and severe periodontitis are still to be determined.

3.2.2. Periodontitis and Carotid Atherosclerosis

Among parameters of atherosclerosis that can easily be measured, carotid atherosclerosis Early atherosclerosis of the carotid is frequently measured as increase in the thickness of the intima-media (IMT) of the arterial wall. Measurement of these parameters has received considerable attention as it is highly correlated with disease in the coronary arteries as well as the cerebral arteries and thus is a good predictor of both cardiovascular and cerebrovascular ischemic events.

In the context of the Atherosclerosis Risk in Community (ARIC) Study, subjects with severe generalized periodontitis had higher odds (OR 1.3 95% CI 1.03-1.66) of having carotid intima-media thickness (IMT) of 1 mm or more after correcting for other known factors. Interestingly the study reported that subjects with severe generalized periodontitis had higher risk than those with less widespread disease suggestion the possibility of a dose dependent effect of the exposure [68]. In a follow-up study of the same material with better definition of bacterial exposure using serum IgG antibodies against oral micro-organisms, higher chances of having carotid atherosclerosis were observed among subjects with elevated antibody titers to Campylobacter rectus and Peptostreptococcus micros [69]. Interestingly this association was present in both smokers and never smokers suggesting that smoking did not act as confounder or effect modifier in this association.

A recent pilot study reported the effect of periodontal therapy on changes in carotid IMT [70]. A group of otherwise healthy individuals affected by mild to moderate periodontitis was treated with root debridement. Six and 12 months afterwards, IMT was significantly decreased at different locations in the carotid artery. These pilot observations indicate that changes in IMT following periodontal therapy are possible in systemically healthy subjects and provide important information for the design of properly designed and sized intervention trials.

3.3.3. Periodontitis and Cardiovascular Events

Periodontitis is associated with cardiovascular events and non-hemorrhagic stroke. Intervention trials aimed at assessing whether or not periodontal therapy decreases the risk for cardiovascular pose formidable challenges in terms of size of the study, length of follow-up (with associated ethical issues), co-morbidity, concomitant medications, delivery of effective treatment and supportive periodontal care. To effectively address some of the issues, the Periodontitis and Vascular Events (PAVE) study was designed and executed in pilot form. PAVE was a secondary cardiac prevention trial enrolling 303 subjects with periodontal disease and a previous history of recent cardiovascular events. It enriched the probability of cardiovascular events by recruiting subjects who had suffered from a first myocardial infarction or who had symptoms of angina and in these subjects aimed at reducing the risk of a future event [71;72]. The study was aimed at assessing the feasibility to perform a definitive study with such a design in a co-ordinated cardiac and dental center setting. Subjects in the study randomly received either community care or scaling and root planing according to protocol. The results of the study indicated that the intervention did not perform well in terms of periodontal outcomes: no significant differences could be demonstrated between the test and the control groups. Furthermore, the level of improvement fell short of established clinical standards and thus highlighting the challenges of secondary cardiac prevention trial designs [73]. No improvement of CRP levels could be seen throughout the study irrespective of the allocation: CRP baseline levels of about 3 mg/l remained stable during the first six months. Obviously failure of the intervention requires careful interpretation of negative results of intervention trials: lack of attenuation of the effect may not be expression of lack of a cause and effect relationship between periodontitis and atherosclerotic diseases [74].

3.4.3. Periodontitis and Blood Pressure

Treatment of periodontitis may also determine some beneficial effects on blood pressure. A recent trial evaluating the renal effects of non-surgical periodontal treatment found that both systolic and diastolic blood pressure diminished significantly [57]. The extent of reduction was on 5-6 mmHg reduction. A positive effect on blood pressure of the same magnitude was already noticed [42]. Interestingly the decrease in systolic BP at 2 months correlated with the degree of reduction in gingival bleeding which is a sensitive clinical marker of periodontal inflammation and infection. In fact systolic BP has been positively associated with the severity of periodontitis [75].

Possible explanations of this finding are merely speculative. It may be due to the decrease of patient anxiety during treatment as multiple sessions are needed. Nevertheless, it may also be due to the effect of treatment on the reduction of systemic inflammation and the effect of this reduction on vascular function [59]. This extremely interesting topic definitely deserves further research.

4. Periodontal Treatment in Cardiovascular Patients

Periodontal treatment, both non-surgical and surgical, comprises invasive procedures which may determine a significant tissutal trauma. Intervention therapies such as surgery are major oral healthcare hazards to the patient with a bleeding tendency. Therefore, one of the major considerations in providing periodontal treatments in CV patients is to ensure that hemostasis is achieved. Most bleeding tendencies are from the use of anticoagulants [76] usually prescribed to treat CVD.

4.1. Periodontal Patients Undertaking Anticoagulants

Anticoagulant therapy is often administered to CVD patients in the form of warfarin (coumarin) or heparin. Despite interruption of continuous anticoagulant therapy have been recommended for dental surgery to prevent intra and postoperative bleeding, no well-documented cases of serious bleeding after dental surgery in patients receiving warfarin or heparin have been identified. Conversely, there are some documented cases of thromboembolic complications in patients whose warfarin therapy was stopped for dental treatment [77]. For patients within the therapeutic range of INR of 3.5 or below, warfarin/heparin therapy has been suggested not be modified or discontinued for simple oral surgical intervention [78]. More complicated and invasive oral surgical procedures would represent an exception to this recommendation for patients with an INR on the high end of the scale, and they should be discussed with the physician managing the condition requiring anticoagulants. Nevertheless, the clinician's judgment must always be considered for all treatment decisions.

Surgical periodontal treatment does often comprise removal of granulation tissues. Increased inflammation of the oral tissues in patients on anticoagulants can contribute to excessive bleeding even with minor surgical procedures. Therefore, the following precautions, should be considered [76-81]:

4.1.1. Presurgical Recommendation

1. Additional drugs tending to promote bleeding should be avoided (e.g. aspirin and other non-steroidal anti-inflammatory drugs).
2. Properly investigate co-morbidities which may enhance intra-surgical bleeding (liver disease, malabsorption, renal disease, leukemia, etc.).
3. For patients whose INR is within the therapeutic range, bleeding after a simple surgical intervention such as a tooth extraction can usually be controlled locally. The high end of the therapeutic range of INR is 2.5, threshold of an increased risk of bleeding. Patients showing an INR greater than 2.5 should be referred to their physician for dose adjustment before invasive dental procedures.
4. As INR may vary largely, values should be obtained within 24 hours before the periodontal procedure. When this is not available clinician should rely on an INR obtained the week before surgery. An excessive interval of time among INR and surgery should be discouraged.

4.1.2. Surgical Recommendation

1. Intrapapillary and/or intraligamentary injections should be preferred as nerve block anesthesia may cause bleeding into fascial spaces of neck and obstruct airway.
2. Care should be taken to minimize the surgical field. Thus, when feasible, buccal flap elevation should be preferred and lingual tissues in the lower molar regions should preferably be left undisturbed as uncontrolled hemorrhage may endanger the airway.
3. Surgical procedures should be performed in the morning and during the first days of the week in order to allow more time for hemostasis and to avoid problems at the weekend.
4. Minimal bone should be removed and the teeth should be sectioned for removal where possible.
5. Meticulous curettage of granulation tissues should always be performed in order to avoid local causes of post-surgical bleeding.
6. Bleeding should be assessed intraoperatively. Hemostatic agent such as oxidized regenerated cellulose; resorbable gelatin sponge; collagen or fibrin glues, which consist mainly of fibrinogen and thrombin may be used to enhance hemostasis and tissue sealing.
7. Extraction of periodontally affected teeth may results in postoperative bleeding.
8. Careful suturing should be advised in order to stabilize flaps and to prevent postoperative disturbance of wounds.
9. After suturing gauze pressure (possibly with an antifibrinolytic agent) should be applied and, after 10 minutes hemostasis should be assessed.

10. The occurrence of additional risk factors for bleeding should prompt the treating clinician to be more cautious (*i.e.* to place more sutures and to prescribe in advance the use of an antifibrinolytic agent, such as tranexamic acid or epsilon aminocaproic acid).

4.1.3. Post-surgical Recommendation

1. If bleeding is controlled, the patient should be dismissed and given a 7-day follow-up appointment. Meticulous and thorough instructions on bleeding should be provided.

2. Subjects should be instructed about that some bleeding from the wound during the first 24-48 post-operative hours is expected and to try to contain it with pressure of antifibrinolytic agent-soaked gauze.

3. Ice bags should be applied in the first postoperative hours in order to reduce swelling and enhance vasoconstriction.

4. Antibiotic should be given to reduce the risk of postoperative infection which may determine bleeding tendency.

5. Aspirin and non-steroidal anti-inflammatory drugs should be avoided. Postoperative pain may be controlled with acetaminophen (Paracetamol) which does not affect platelets.

4.2. Periodontal Patients Undertaking Acetylsalicylic Acid

Aspirin is the most commonly used preventive and therapeutic agent for vascular ischemic events. It has been reported not to be stopped for minor oral surgical intervention as during clinical trials no episodes of uncontrolled intraoperative bleeding or postoperative bleeding were noted in the group undertaking aspirin [79;80]. Local measures for bleeding control are usually effective in managing patients undertaking aspirin [81].

4.3. Periodontal Patients Undertaking Calcium Channel Blockers

Calcium channel blockers do present an unpleasant gingival effect which has been extensively documented: gingival hyperplasia. Gingival hyperplasia (GH) is a thick and fibrotic enlargement due to an overgrowth of gingival tissues.

Among these drugs, nifedipine is the most documented. Nevertheless, not all patients undertaking nifedipine develop gingival overgrowth, indeed there are some other important risk factors such as age, gender (males appear to be three times more likely to develop GH), nifedipine serum levels, concomitant administration of cyclosporine, presence of plaque and gingival inflammation and some kind of genetic predisposition [82].

The first phase of treatment comprises a thorough non surgical debridement and improvement/motivation to reach a high standard of dental plaque control. Whilst this is efficacious in treating very limited and mild form of GH, the treatment for the majority of the lesions is surgical in nature with either laser or gingivectomy/flaps techniques [83].

Usually surgical treatment is efficacious in containing GH, nevertheless relapse may occur. When GO tends to recur a drug substitution may be considered from the physician. In fact, despite all calcium channel blockers have shown to potentially determine GH, some drugs such as isradipine are less prone to develop the overgrowth.

4.4. Prophylaxis of Infective Endocarditis

Infective endocarditis (IE) is a serious and possible life-threatening. Its complex pathogenesis involves a sequence of events. Endothelial damage caused by turbulent blood flow seen in congenital or acquired heart disease causes platelets and fibrin deposition leading to formation of non-bacterial thrombotic endocarditis (NBTE). In this setting an episode of bacteremia could result in bacterial adherence to NBTE, bacterial proliferation within the NBTE, and formation of vegetations, the typical lesions of infective endocarditis.

In the last six decades guidelines for preventing infective endocarditis have been formulated. Guidelines were mainly empiric in nature and based on the concept that patients with possible endothelial damage and bacteremia during medical procedures were considered at a high risk of developing IE. Thus, prevention of bacteremia with antibiotics, despite conflicting results on their efficacy in reducing bacteremia, became the ultimate target to minimize the risk of IE. Nevertheless, trials have indicated that the usage of antibiotics may not necessarily decrease the incidence of IE.

Tooth extraction causes evident bacteremia. However, bacteremia in periodontal patients is present even after tooth-brushing, flossing or chewing. Thus the cumulative bacterial effect in one year is much higher than the one resulting after dental extraction [84]. Only a small portion of IE is thought to be originated from dental procedures. Interestingly, studies which show reduction in bacteremia do not show reduction in infective endocarditis [85]. On these premises societies of cardiology have tried over the last decade to develop a more evidence based approach [86].

The American Heart Association infective endocarditis prophylaxis recommendations (2007) now recognizes some condition in which prophylaxis is deemed as reasonable. These are (i) presence of prosthetic cardiac valve or prosthetic material used for cardiac valve repair; (ii) history of previous infective endocarditis; (iii) some congenital heart disease; (iv) post-cardiac transplant valvulopathy [87]. According to these guidelines periodontal surgery in a subject affected by one of the above mentioned conditions is one of the therapeutic acts which may require prophylaxis.

In 2008 the National Institute for Health and Clinical Excellence (NICE) released some new guidelines with a more radical distance from the classic empiric ones as it was stated that antibiotic prophylaxis is not any longer recommended for people undergoing dental procedures. This was further stressed by a Cochrane review showed no evidence of usage of penicillin prophylaxis for preventing IE in risk subjects undergoing an invasive dental procedure [88].

Conclusion

This chapter has a two-fold aim. On one hand it discussed the impact of periodontal disease and periodontal treatment on CVD onset and progression and, on the other hand, focused on periodontal treatment on subjects undergoing pharmacological treatment for their CVD.

Periodontal disease has been suggested to be linked to CVD through the effect of systemic inflammation showed by subjects affected by this disease. Despite numerous confounding factors which may distort the strength of this association, intervention trials have further reinforced the causality of a possible link. Therefore clinicians should carefully assess the possible impact of periodontal disease treatment on CVD conditions.

Subjects affected by CVD usually take drugs that may have an effect on i) periodontal treatment or ii) periodontal disease such as the impact of calcium channel blockers on gingival enlargement. Critical focus on precautions and suggestions to manage the bleeding tendency of CVD subjects during periodontal treatment is provided. Lastly, the effects of possible post-therapeutical bacteremia on infective endocarditis are discussed and summary of the most recent guidelines are delivered.

Interesting findings in the last decade have suggested that periodontology may significantly contribute in managing CVD risk. Nonetheless, future long-term intervention trials assessing true CVD outcomes are needed to carefully evaluate the possible role of periodontal treatment in routine CVD risk management.

References

[1]   Williams RC. Periodontal disease. *N Engl J Med* 1990 Feb 8;322(6):373-82.
[2]   Page RC. The role of inflammatory mediators in the pathogenesis of periodontal disease. *J Periodontal Res* 1991 May;26(3 Pt 2):230-42.
[3]   Pihlstrom BL, Michalowicz BS, Johnson NW. Periodontal diseases. *Lancet* 2005 Nov 19;366(9499):1809-20.
[4]   Papapanou PN. Periodontal diseases: epidemiology. *Ann Periodontol* 1996 Nov;1(1):1-36.
[5]   Papapanou PN. Epidemiology of periodontal diseases: an update. *J Int Acad Periodontol* 1999 Oct;1(4):110-6.
[6]   De NE. The role of inflammatory and immunological mediators in periodontitis and cardiovascular disease. *Ann Periodontol* 2001 Dec;6(1):30-40.
[7]   Page RC, Offenbacher S, Schroeder HE, Seymour GJ, Kornman KS. Advances in the pathogenesis of periodontitis: summary of developments, clinical implications and future directions. *Periodontol 2000* 1997 Jun;14:216-48.
[8]   Costerton JW, Lewandowski Z, DeBeer D, Caldwell D, Korber D, James G. Biofilms, the customized microniche. *J Bacteriol* 1994 Apr;176(8):2137-42.
[9]   Socransky SS, Haffajee AD, Cugini MA, Smith C, Kent RL, Jr. Microbial complexes in subgingival plaque. *J Clin Periodontol* 1998 Feb;25(2):134-44.
[10] Socransky SS. Microbiology of plaque. Compend Contin Educ Dent 1984;*Suppl* 5:S53-S56.
[11] Kinane DF, Adonogianaki E, Moughal N, Winstanley FP, Mooney J, Thornhill M. Immunocytochemical characterization of cellular infiltrate, related endothelial changes and determination of GCF acute-phase proteins during human experimental gingivitis. *J Periodontal Res* 1991 May;26(3 Pt 2):286-8.

[12] Lamster IB, Novak MJ. Host mediators in gingival crevicular fluid: implications for the pathogenesis of periodontal disease. *Crit Rev Oral Biol Med* 1992;3(1-2):31-60.

[13] Ebersole JL, Singer RE, Steffensen B, Filloon T, Kornman KS. Inflammatory mediators and immunoglobulins in GCF from healthy, gingivitis and periodontitis sites. *J Periodontal Res* 1993 Nov;28(6 Pt 2):543-6.

[14] Offenbacher S, Collins JG, Arnold RR. New clinical diagnostic strategies based on pathogenesis of disease. *J Periodontal Res* 1993 Nov;28(6 Pt 2):523-35.

[15] Williams RC, Jeffcoat MK, Howell TH, Rolla A, Stubbs D, Teoh KW, et al. Altering the progression of human alveolar bone loss with the non-steroidal anti-inflammatory drug flurbiprofen. *J Periodontol* 1989 Sep;60(9):485-90.

[16] Bergstrom J. Tobacco smoking and chronic destructive periodontal disease. *Odontology* 2004 Sep;92(1):1-8.

[17] Taylor GW. Bidirectional interrelationships between diabetes and periodontal diseases: an epidemiologic perspective. *Ann Periodontol* 2001 Dec;6(1):99-112.

[18] Michalowicz BS, Diehl SR, Gunsolley JC, Sparks BS, Brooks CN, Koertge TE, et al. Evidence of a substantial genetic basis for risk of adult periodontitis. *J Periodontol* 2000 Nov;71(11):1699-707.

[19] Page RC, Kornman KS. The pathogenesis of human periodontitis: an introduction. *Periodontol* 2000 1997 Jun;14:9-11.

[20] Loos BG, John RP, Laine ML. Identification of genetic risk factors for periodontitis and possible mechanisms of action. *J Clin Periodontol* 2005;32 Suppl 6:159-79.

[21] Genco RJ. Current view of risk factors for periodontal diseases. *J Periodontol* 1996 Oct;67(10 Suppl):1041-9.

[22] Braunwald E. Shattuck lecture--cardiovascular medicine at the turn of the millennium: triumphs, concerns, and opportunities. *N Engl J Med* 1997 Nov 6;337(19):1360-9.

[23] Ross R. Atherosclerosis--an inflammatory disease. *N Engl J Med* 1999 Jan 14;340(2):115-26.

[24] Libby P. Inflammation in atherosclerosis. *Nature* 2002 Dec 19;420(6917):868-74.

[25] Kiechl S, Egger G, Mayr M, Wiedermann CJ, Bonora E, Oberhollenzer F, et al. Chronic infections and the risk of carotid atherosclerosis: prospective results from a large population study. *Circulation* 2001 Feb 27;103(8):1064-70.

[26] Mattila KJ, Nieminen MS, Valtonen VV, Rasi VP, Kesaniemi YA, Syrjala SL, et al. Association between dental health and acute myocardial infarction. *BMJ* 1989 Mar 25;298(6676):779-81.

[27] Brodala N, Merricks EP, Bellinger DA, Damrongsri D, Offenbacher S, Beck J, et al. Porphyromonas gingivalis bacteremia induces coronary and aortic atherosclerosis in normocholesterolemic and hypercholesterolemic pigs. *Arterioscler Thromb Vasc Biol* 2005 Jul;25(7):1446-51.

[28] Li L, Messas E, Batista EL, Jr., Levine RA, Amar S. Porphyromonas gingivalis infection accelerates the progression of atherosclerosis in a heterozygous apolipoprotein E-deficient murine model. *Circulation* 2002 Feb 19;105(7):861-7.

[29] Lalla E, Lamster IB, Hofmann MA, Bucciarelli L, Jerud AP, Tucker S, et al. Oral infection with a periodontal pathogen accelerates early atherosclerosis in apolipoprotein E-null mice. *Arterioscler Thromb Vasc Biol* 2003 Aug 1;23(8):1405-11.

[30] Haraszthy VI, Zambon JJ, Trevisan M, Zeid M, Genco RJ. Identification of periodontal pathogens in atheromatous plaques. *J Periodontol* 2000 Oct;71(10):1554-60.

[31] Fiehn NE, Larsen T, Christiansen N, Holmstrup P, Schroeder TV. Identification of periodontal pathogens in atherosclerotic vessels. *J Periodontol* 2005 May;76(5):731-6.

[32] Aimetti M, Romano F, Nessi F. Microbiologic analysis of periodontal pockets and carotid atheromatous plaques in advanced chronic periodontitis patients. *J Periodontol* 2007 Sep;78(9):1718-23.

[33] Dorn BR, Burks JN, Seifert KN, Progulske-Fox A. Invasion of endothelial and epithelial cells by strains of Porphyromonas gingivalis. *FEMS Microbiol Lett* 2000 Jun 15;187(2):139-44.

[34] Sharma A, Novak EK, Sojar HT, Swank RT, Kuramitsu HK, Genco RJ. Porphyromonas gingivalis platelet aggregation activity: outer membrane vesicles are potent activators of murine platelets. *Oral Microbiol Immunol* 2000 Dec;15(6):393-6.

[35] Kuramitsu HK, Qi M, Kang IC, Chen W. Role for periodontal bacteria in cardiovascular diseases. *Ann Periodontol* 2001 Dec;6(1):41-7.

[36] Ridker PM. Intrinsic fibrinolytic capacity and systemic inflammation: novel risk factors for arterial thrombotic disease. *Haemostasis* 1997;27 Suppl 1:2-11.

[37] Offenbacher S, Farr DH, Goodson JM. Measurement of prostaglandin E in crevicular fluid. *J Clin Periodontol* 1981 Aug;8(4):359-67.

[38] Hutter JW, van d, V, Varoufaki A, Huffels RA, Hoek FJ, Loos BG. Lower numbers of erythrocytes and lower levels of hemoglobin in periodontitis patients compared to control subjects. *J Clin Periodontol* 2001 Oct;28(10):930-6.

[39] Wu T, Trevisan M, Genco RJ, Falkner KL, Dorn JP, Sempos CT. Examination of the relation between periodontal health status and cardiovascular risk factors: serum total and high density lipoprotein cholesterol, C-reactive protein, and plasma fibrinogen. *Am J Epidemiol* 2000 Feb 1;151(3):273-82.

[40] Slade GD, Offenbacher S, Beck JD, Heiss G, Pankow JS. Acute-phase inflammatory response to periodontal disease in the US population. *J Dent Res* 2000 Jan;79(1):49-57.

[41] Joshipura KJ, Wand HC, Merchant AT, Rimm EB. Periodontal disease and biomarkers related to cardiovascular disease. *J Dent Res* 2004 Feb;83(2):151-5.

[42] D'Aiuto F, Parkar M, Nibali L, Suvan J, Lessem J, Tonetti MS. Periodontal infections cause changes in traditional and novel cardiovascular risk factors: results from a randomized controlled clinical trial. *Am Heart J* 2006 May;151(5):977-84.

[43] Janket SJ, Baird AE, Chuang SK, Jones JA. Meta-analysis of periodontal disease and risk of coronary heart disease and stroke. *Oral Surg Oral Med Oral Pathol Oral Radiol Endod* 2003 May;95(5):559-69.

[44] Khader YS, Albashaireh ZS, Alomari MA. Periodontal diseases and the risk of coronary heart and cerebrovascular diseases: a meta-analysis. *J Periodontol* 2004 Aug;75(8):1046-53.

[45] Bahekar AA, Singh S, Saha S, Molnar J, Arora R. The prevalence and incidence of coronary heart disease is significantly increased in periodontitis: a meta-analysis. *Am Heart J* 2007 Nov;154(5):830-7.

[46] Humphrey LL, Fu R, Buckley DI, Freeman M, Helfand M. Periodontal disease and coronary heart disease incidence: a systematic review and meta-analysis. *J Gen Intern Med* 2008 Dec;23(12):2079-86.

[47] Hyman JJ, Winn DM, Reid BC. The role of cigarette smoking in the association between periodontal disease and coronary heart disease. *J Periodontol* 2002 Sep;73(9):988-94.

[48] D'Aiuto F, Parkar M, Andreou G, Suvan J, Brett PM, Ready D, et al. Periodontitis and systemic inflammation: control of the local infection is associated with a reduction in serum inflammatory markers. *J Dent Res* 2004 Feb;83(2):156-60.

[49] D'Aiuto F, Nibali L, Mohamed-Ali V, Vallance P, Tonetti MS. Periodontal therapy: a novel non-drug-induced experimental model to study human inflammation. *J Periodontal Res* 2004 Oct;39(5):294-9.

[50] D'Aiuto F, Parkar M, Tonetti MS. Periodontal therapy: a novel acute inflammatory model. *Inflamm Res* 2005 Oct;54(10):412-4.

[51] Graziani F, Cei S, La FF, Vano M, Gabriele M, Tonetti M. Effects of non-surgical periodontal therapy on the glomerular filtration rate of the kidney: an exploratory trial. *J Clin Periodontol* 2010 Jul;37(7):638-43.

[52] D'Aiuto F, Parkar M, Tonetti MS. Acute effects of periodontal therapy on bio-markers of vascular health. *J Clin Periodontol* 2007 Feb;34(2):124-9.

[53] Lofthus JE, Waki MY, Jolkovsky DL, Otomo-Corgel J, Newman MG, Flemmig T, et al. Bacteremia following subgingival irrigation and scaling and root planing. *J Periodontol* 1991 Oct;62(10):602-7.

[54] Birkedal-Hansen H. Role of cytokines and inflammatory mediators in tissue destruction. *J Periodontal Res* 1993 Nov;28(6 Pt 2):500-10.

[55] Gabay C, Kushner I. Acute-phase proteins and other systemic responses to inflammation. *N Engl J Med* 1999 Feb 11;340(6):448-54.

[56] Tonetti MS, D'Aiuto F, Nibali L, Donald A, Storry C, Parkar M, et al. Treatment of periodontitis and endothelial function. *N Engl J Med* 2007 Mar 1;356(9):911-20.

[57] Graziani F, Cei S, Tonetti M, Paolantonio M, Serio R, Sammartino G, et al. Systemic inflammation following non-surgical and surgical periodontal therapy. *J Clin Periodontol* 2010 Sep;37(9):848-54.

[58] Haffajee AD, Teles RP, Socransky SS. The effect of periodontal therapy on the composition of the subgingival microbiota. *Periodontol 2000* 2006;42:219-58.

[59] Seinost G, Wimmer G, Skerget M, Thaller E, Brodmann M, Gasser R, et al. Periodontal treatment improves endothelial dysfunction in patients with severe periodontitis. *Am Heart J* 2005 Jun;149(6):1050-4.

[60] Minassian C, D'Aiuto F, Hingorani AD, Smeeth L. Invasive dental treatment and risk for vascular events: a self-controlled case series. *Ann Intern Med* 2010 Oct 19;153(8):499-506.

[61] D'Aiuto F, Nibali L, Parkar M, Suvan J, Tonetti MS. Short-term effects of intensive periodontal therapy on serum inflammatory markers and cholesterol. *J Dent Res* 2005 Mar;84(3):269-73.

[62] Paraskevas S, Huizinga JD, Loos BG. A systematic review and meta-analyses on C-reactive protein in relation to periodontitis. *J Clin Periodontol* 2008 Apr;35(4):277-90.

[63] Albert CM, Ma J, Rifai N, Stampfer MJ, Ridker PM. Prospective study of C-reactive protein, homocysteine, and plasma lipid levels as predictors of sudden cardiac death. *Circulation* 2002 Jun 4;105(22):2595-9.

[64] Ridker PM, Cannon CP, Morrow D, Rifai N, Rose LM, McCabe CH, et al. C-reactive protein levels and outcomes after statin therapy. *N Engl J Med* 2005 Jan 6;352(1):20-8.

[65] Sabatine MS, Morrow DA, Jablonski KA, Rice MM, Warnica JW, Domanski MJ, et al. Prognostic significance of the Centers for Disease Control/American Heart Association

high-sensitivity C-reactive protein cut points for cardiovascular and other outcomes in patients with stable coronary artery disease. *Circulation* 2007 Mar 27;115(12):1528-36.

[66] Amar S, Gokce N, Morgan S, Loukideli M, Van Dyke TE, Vita JA. Periodontal disease is associated with brachial artery endothelial dysfunction and systemic inflammation. *Arterioscler Thromb Vasc Biol* 2003 Jul 1;23(7):1245-9.

[67] Elter JR, Hinderliter AL, Offenbacher S, Beck JD, Caughey M, Brodala N, et al. The effects of periodontal therapy on vascular endothelial function: a pilot trial. *Am Heart J* 2006 Jan;151(1):47.

[68] Beck JD, Elter JR, Heiss G, Couper D, Mauriello SM, Offenbacher S. Relationship of periodontal disease to carotid artery intima-media wall thickness: the atherosclerosis risk in communities (ARIC) study. *Arterioscler Thromb Vasc Biol* 2001 Nov;21(11):1816-22.

[69] Beck JD, Eke P, Lin D, Madianos P, Couper D, Moss K, et al. Associations between IgG antibody to oral organisms and carotid intima-medial thickness in community-dwelling adults. *Atherosclerosis* 2005 Dec;183(2):342-8.

[70] Piconi S, Trabattoni D, Luraghi C, Perilli E, Borelli M, Pacei M, et al. Treatment of periodontal disease results in improvements in endothelial dysfunction and reduction of the carotid intima-media thickness. *FASEB J* 2009 Apr;23(4):1196-204.

[71] Beck JD, Couper DJ, Falkner KL, Graham SP, Grossi SG, Gunsolley JC, et al. The Periodontitis and Vascular Events (PAVE) pilot study: adverse events. *J Periodontol* 2008 Jan;79(1):90-6.

[72] Couper DJ, Beck JD, Falkner KL, Graham SP, Grossi SG, Gunsolley JC, et al. The Periodontitis and Vascular Events (PAVE) pilot study: recruitment, retention, and community care controls. *J Periodontol* 2008 Jan;79(1):80-9.

[73] Offenbacher S, Beck JD, Moss K, Mendoza L, Paquette DW, Barrow DA, et al. Results from the Periodontitis and Vascular Events (PAVE) Study: a pilot multicentered, randomized, controlled trial to study effects of periodontal therapy in a secondary prevention model of cardiovascular disease. *J Periodontol* 2009 Feb;80(2):190-201.

[74] Armitage GC. Effect of periodontal therapy on general health--is there a missing component in the design of these clinical trials? *J Clin Periodontol* 2008 Dec;35(12):1011-2.

[75] Taguchi A, Sanada M, Suei Y, Ohtsuka M, Lee K, Tanimoto K, et al. Tooth loss is associated with an increased risk of hypertension in postmenopausal women. *Hypertension* 2004 Jun;43(6):1297-300.

[76] Scully C, Cawson R. *Medical Problems in Dentistry*. 4th ed. Oxford, London and Boston: Butterworth-Heinemann; 1997.

[77] Wahl MJ. Dental surgery in anticoagulated patients. *Arch Intern Med* 1998 Aug 10;158(15):1610-6.

[78] Scully C, Wolff A. Oral surgery in patients on anticoagulant therapy. *Oral Surg Oral Med Oral Pathol Oral Radiol Endod* 2002 Jul;94(1):57-64.

[79] Ardekian L, Gaspar R, Peled M, Brener B, Laufer D. Does low-dose aspirin therapy complicate oral surgical procedures? *J Am Dent Assoc* 2000 Mar;131(3):331-5.

[80] Madan GA, Madan SG, Madan G, Madan AD. Minor oral surgery without stopping daily low-dose aspirin therapy: a study of 51 patients. *J Oral Maxillofac Surg* 2005 Sep;63(9):1262-5.

[81] Aframian DJ, Lalla RV, Peterson DE. Management of dental patients taking common hemostasis-altering medications. *Oral Surg Oral Med Oral Pathol Oral Radiol Endod* 2007 Mar;103 Suppl:S45-11.

[82] Seymour RA, Ellis JS, Thomason JM. Risk factors for drug-induced gingival overgrowth. *J Clin Periodontol* 2000 Apr;27(4):217-23.

[83] Pilloni A, Camargo PM, Carere M, Carranza FA, Jr. Surgical treatment of cyclosporine A- and nifedipine-induced gingival enlargement: gingivectomy versus periodontal flap. *J Periodontol* 1998 Jul;69(7):791-7.

[84] Roberts GJ. Dentists are innocent! "Everyday" bacteremia is the real culprit: a review and assessment of the evidence that dental surgical procedures are a principal cause of bacterial endocarditis in children. *Pediatr Cardiol* 1999 Sep;20(5):317-25.

[85] Roberts GJ, Radford P, Holt R. Prophylaxis of dental bacteraemia with oral amoxycillin in children. *Br Dent J* 1987 Mar 7;162(5):179-82.

[86] Gopalakrishnan PP, Shukla SK, Tak T. Infective endocarditis: rationale for revised guidelines for antibiotic prophylaxis. *Clin Med Res* 2009 Sep;7(3):63-8.

[87] Wilson W, Taubert KA, Gewitz M, Lockhart PB, Baddour LM, Levison M, et al. Prevention of infective endocarditis: guidelines from the American Heart Association: a guideline from the American Heart Association Rheumatic Fever, Endocarditis, and Kawasaki Disease Committee, Council on Cardiovascular Disease in the Young, and the Council on Clinical Cardiology, Council on Cardiovascular Surgery and Anesthesia, and the Quality of Care and Outcomes Research Interdisciplinary Working Group. *Circulation* 2007 Oct 9;116(15):1736-54.

[88] Oliver R, Roberts GJ, Hooper L, Worthington HV. Antibiotics for the prophylaxis of bacterial endocarditis in dentistry. *Cochrane Database Syst Rev* 2008;(4):CD003813.

Chapter XXI

Depression and Coronary Artery Disease

Gita Ramamurthy and Mantosh Dewan
Dept of Psychiatry, Upstate Medical University, Syracuse, NY, US

Abstract

The presence of depression is associated with a higher future incidence of CAD. Depression may also predict a worse medical outcome in established CAD. Proposed mediators of the association between CAD and depression include both behavioral and biological variables. Questions remain as to whether depression is a true risk factor for CAD, or merely a confounder, for another biomedical or psychosocial variable.

Evidence for the association of CAD and depression is strong enough to recommend screening for primary and secondary prevention. Exercise improves mood and medical outcomes in depressed CAD patients. Referral to cardiac rehabilitation with a psychosocial component should be considered for depressed patients with CAD.

Treatment options for depression in CAD patients include watchful waiting, psychotherapy and/or antidepressants. If prescribed, SSRIs should be the first choice of antidepressants. Research into the safety of SSRIs in CAD patients has yielded contradictory findings. TCAs are cardiotoxic, and should be avoided. Noradrenergic drugs may worsen prognosis, particularly in the presence of arrhythmias, or left ventricular dysfunction. Because depression often spontaneously remits soon after an MI, immediate treatment may not be needed. Rather, a reasonable strategy might include watchful waiting, with close follow-up to identify high risk patients with persistent depression. Persistent post-MI depression, particularly when treatment –unresponsive, predicts a poor medical prognosis.

Neither antidepressants and/or psychotherapy improved depression or mortality, except for the COPES intervention, which was studied in persistent post-MI depression. The COPES intervention is a collaborative stepped approach, emphasizing patient satisfaction and choice between problem-solving psychotherapy and/or pharmacotherapy.

Introduction

> *"Deprived by Tristan of this our solitary,*
> *swiftly fleeting, final earthly joy?*
> *-His wound, though - where?*
> *Can I not heal it?*
>   *...*
> *Together, at least, let fade life's enfeebled fire!"*
>
> *- Richard Wagner, 1865, from Tristan und Isolde [1]*

Medical models of pre-scientific cultures did not differentiate psyche from soma. For example, ancient Egyptians believed the heart was the source of consciousness[2]. The scientific method, articulated by Rene Descartes and others, led to the ascension of mind-body dualism [3]. The "body as machine" approach opened the way to unprecedented medical advancements. However, reductionism may have neglected the importance of mind-body interactions, which so influenced pre-modern understanding [3].

These classical beliefs still influence our language. We routinely refer to psychosomatic ideas in metaphor. These metaphors often reference the heart in connection to subjective feelings, as illustrated by common expressions, such as "warm-hearted", "heartless", etc.

Expressions, such as "dying of a broken heart," reflect the widespread belief that emotion influences health. The idea that extreme sadness can be fatal is a common theme throughout the classics. At the end of Wagner's opera, *Tristan und Isolde*, Isolde cannot bear the death of her lover. Overwhelmed by grief, she dies, collapsing over Tristan's body.

Antonio Damasio, a leading neuroscientist, asserts that feelings are not solely created by the brain, but rather are the result of an interaction between the brain and body [4]. Some proponents of the emerging field of embodied cognition argue that language is not only a manipulation of abstract symbols, but may be influenced by sensorimotor brain maps [5].

Thus, the endurance of psychosomatic ideas from classical times may reflect an intuitive awareness of the interaction between the body, brain and our subjective experiences. The hypothesis that depression worsens the incidence and prognosis of coronary artery disease is one of the most extensively studied areas in psychosomatic medicine.

The Association between Depression and Coronary Artery Disease

In a 2005 review article, Rudisch and Nemeroff estimated that 17% to 27% of CAD patients have major depression, and a significantly larger percentage have subsyndromal symptoms of depression. The INTERHEART study of 24767 participants, from 52 countries, compared cases with an incident acute MI to age-, sex- and site-matched controls free of heart disease. Compared to controls, patients with coronary artery disease had a higher prevalence of depression: 17.6% in controls vs. 24.0% in cases with CAD.

Evidence for the association of depression with the incidence of CAD is strong, as documented by several systematic reviews [6-9]. Based on two meta-analyses, depression increases the relative risk of CAD incidence by 64% (RR = 1.64) [6-7].

Less evidence supports an association of depression with CAD prognosis. Although research was extensive, many studies had inadequate statistical power. According to two systematic reviews, only about half of the studies reported a significant association between depression and adverse CAD outcomes [8, 10]. In a 2006 meta-analysis, the pooled adjusted relative risk of adverse CAD outcomes from depression was 1.53 [11]. In their systematic review, Frasure-Smith and Lesperance noted that all of the negative studies were too underpowered to detect a difference, indicating that these studies may have had falsely negative results [8].

In summary, there is robust evidence for the correlation of depression with future incidence of CAD. Studies of the association between depression and the prognosis of established CAD show less consistent results, but suggest a link.

That CAD risk may be increased by depression is concerning. The current treatment of depression, which often takes place in primary care offices [12], has been critiqued as needing improvement [13-14].

The Basis for the Association – Confounders

Does an association indicate that depression causes CAD? Is there another explanation?

A statistically valid, replicated association alone does not demonstrate causation, but rather, can be the result of confounding. Depression is not a confounder for CAD risk factors, such as diabetes mellitus, hypertension or high cholesterol. Depression remained associated with CAD after adjustment for multiple demographic and biomedical covariates. The association of depression with CAD was not explained by traditional risk factors, with one exception - smoking. As discussed below, depression may increase the risk of smoking, a known coronary risk factor.

Fewer studies made adjustments for nontraditional cardiac risk factors. Perhaps, depression is a confounder for emerging CAD risk factors, such as anxiety, low social support or other psychosocial factors.

What if depression and ischemic heart disease resulted from the same patho-physiological process(es)? For example, inflammation, or a shared genetic factor, increases the risk of both depression and coronary atherosclerosis [15-17]. However, the contribution of either factor to the association between CAD and depression appears modest [18-21].

Inflammation and depression may have a bidirectional relationship. That is, inflammation may cause depression, and vice versa. As discussed below, inflammation has also been proposed to mediate the effect of depression on CAD [22].

Researchers have suggested [23-24] that atherosclerosis could cause both depression and coronary heart disease. Atherosclerosis, a systemic process, could affect the blood supply of not only the myocardium, but also the frontal lobe, causing depression [23-24].

The association between depression and CAD may be bidirectional [18]. CAD is estimated to increase the hazard risk of depression over subsequent years by 175% whereas the presence of depression increases the risk of CAD over subsequent years by 120% [18].

The Basis for the Association - Mediators

If depression is a risk factor for CAD, what mediates the risk? Both behavior, such as physical inactivity, and biomedical mediators, such as heart rate variability (HRV), play a mediating role.

Heart rate variability (HRV), the variability in the interval between beats, is primarily mediated by parasympathetic tone [25]. Diminished HRV predicts death and arrhythmias in the presence of CAD [25]. Reduced HRV, from autonomic dysfunction in depression, has been proposed to mediate worse CAD outcomes [22].

Low HRV may explain the CAD risk of depression in diabetics, but not in the general population. In a study of type I diabetics, decreased HRV and insulin sensitivity partly mediated the increased CAD incidence among depressed patients [26]. In contrast, HRV did not mediate CAD risk in a general population study [27]. Perhaps, among diabetics, pre-existing low HRV from autonomic neuropathy [28] increases susceptibility to a further decrease in HRV.

The Heart and Soul trial was specifically designed to identify mediators of the effect of depression on CAD prognosis [29]. 1017 patients with stable CAD were followed for about 5 years. Depressive symptoms predicted a higher rate of cardiovascular events (HR = 1.31). Behavior, particularly physical inactivity, and, to a lesser extent, smoking and non-adherence, played the most important role in mediating the relationship.

Of possible biological factors, only inflammation (CRP) mediated the association, albeit modestly [29]. Noninvolved variables included the use of SSRIs or TCAs, HRV, or serotonin, omega-3 fatty acids, norepinephrine or cortisol.

Curiously, "other antidepressants" (i.e. not SSRIs or TCAs) reduced the effect size of depression by 8.8%. "Other antidepressants" included noradrenergic medications [30], which may be cardiotoxic, as discussed below. The authors also proposed that the "other antidepressants" category might be a confounder for treatment resistant depression.

Some biomedical risk factors may carry a higher CAD risk in the presence of depression.

For example, Ladwig found that inflammation predicted future CAD events only in depressed patients [31]. i.e. Depression may behave as a cofactor that permits inflammation to negatively affect CAD outcomes.

In summary, evidence indicates that behaviors and biomedical factors mediate the effect of depression on CAD. Behaviors include smoking, sedentary living [32] and poor treatment adherence [33-35]. Inflammation is a likely biomedical mediator [36-37]. Other possible mediating factors include insulin resistance [38-39], altered endothelial function, [40-41], platelet activation [42-43] and changes in autonomic function [44-45] including reduced heart rate variability (HRV) [26, 46].

Psychosocial Comorbidity

Psychosocial factors other than depression have been linked to an increased incidence and/or worse prognosis of CAD. These include anxiety [26, 47], PTSD [48], hostility [49], and poor social support [50]. Another such factor is Type D personality, a personality prone to negative emotions and inhibition of emotional self-expression [51].

That these psychosocial variables correlate with traditional and emerging coronary risk factors supports their prognostic importance. Anxiety is linked to inflammation [52], low HRV [53] and nonadherence to treatment [54]. Anger traits correlate with low HRV [55] and metabolic syndrome [56]. Psychosocial stress has been associated with decreased HRV [57], and increased inflammation [58-59].

Given their correlation with intermediate variables that promote CAD, how can one know whether anxiety, anger or depression is the true risk factor? A systematic review revealed a consistent association of anxiety and depression with increased CAD incidence [60]. Based on the positive studies, anxiety increased the relative risk of CAD incidence in a range from 2.40 to 7.80. The reviewers concurred with a 2002 meta-analysis revealing that depression increased the average relative risk of CAD incidence by 1.64 [7]. The average relative risk of CAD prognosis from anxiety or depression was not reported, because evidence for a correlation was mixed. The review also reported a weak and inconsistent association between anger and CAD.

How important are different psychosocial factors relative to each other? Research has yielded inconsistent answers. Depression has been reported to be a confounder for anxiety [26, 61], PTSD [48], perceived stress [26], denial [62], and type D personality [51]. Other research contradicts these findings. For example, when anger, anxiety and depression scores were entered into regression analysis, only depression significantly correlated with progression of carotid atherosclerosis [63]. This latter study implies that anger and anxiety are confounders, whereas depression is the "true" risk factor.

Perhaps the CAD risk from anger, anxiety and depression is due to a common factor [60].

All three emotions include the experience of distress. Does this common factor, distress, cause the CAD risk of these emotions? Alternatively, is CAD risk the result of unique aspect(s) of anxiety, anger, or depression?

Kubzansky et al used factor analysis to identify common aspects of anxiety, depression and anger, reflecting "general distress," and their unique aspects [64]. CAD incidence was predicted by "general distress" and by the unique aspects of anxiety and anger. Considered simultaneously, only general distress, and a unique aspect of anxiety carried CAD risk. Thus, some unique and common elements of anger, anxiety and depression predicted CAD incidence.

Some evidence even suggests that anxiety mitigates the adverse effect of depression. In the WISE study (Women's Ischemia Syndrome Evaluation), adverse medical outcomes were predicted by depression with low co-morbid anxiety, but not with high co-morbid anxiety [65].

In a consensus, seven prospective studies reported that low social support predicts adverse CAD outcomes among depressed patients [50, 66-73]. The studies differed in their report of the relative prognostic importance of social support and depression. In four studies, depression predicted adverse medical outcomes independently of social support [50, 67, 71-72]. Two reported that depression was a confounder, whereas social support was the true risk factor [68, 73]. One study reported no impact from either factor alone; only the joint presence of social isolation and depression predicted CAD progression [66].

In summary, it does appear likely that among depressed patients with CAD, low social support predicts worse medical outcomes. Anxiety, like depression, is strongly associated with CAD incidence, and may be associated with CAD prognosis. There is weak evidence for anger as a CAD risk factor.

Given that their prognostic relevance is not fully defined, should a clinician address psychological concerns co-morbid with depression? We agree with the 2008 AHA science advisory [74], which recommends that patients with likely depression (PHQ-9 score $\geq$ 10) should be referred to providers who can identify and treat co-morbid mental disorders.

Addressing several psychosocial factors does not require multiple interventions. Some treatments address multiple psychosocial concerns, including depression. Cardiac rehabilitation with a psychotherapy component, or the Ornish intervention, can improve multiple psychological concerns, as discussed later. SSRIs, which reduce depression, also treat anxiety [75-76] and may reduce aggression [77].

The Prognostic Impact of Depression: Subgroups of Interest

Why is the evidence linking depression to adverse CAD outcomes inconsistent? One explanation is that the prognostic effect is restricted to specific patient subgroups, or particular depressive symptoms.

Depression manifests as a set of somatic, cognitive and affective symptoms. Each group of symptoms has been examined for its particular contribution to prognosis. Many studies have assessed whether the timing of depression onset (before vs. after an MI, new vs. recurrent onset) changes treatment response and/or outcomes. The prognosis of post MI patient subgroups with different trajectories of depressive symptoms (recurrent, transient, treatment-refractory) has also been investigated.

Somatic, Affective and Cognitive Dimensions of Depression

Each dimension of depression - cognitive, affective or somatic - may have a unique contribution to prognosis.

Anorexia, fatigue, and other somatic symptoms are core manifestations of depressive disorders, and are often included in depression scales. However, medical conditions, such as heart failure, also have somatic features, such as fatigue. Thus, somatic symptoms from medical illness can falsely elevate depression scores. High scores on a depression scale may reflect severe depression, or mild depression with severe medical illness.

If the somatic symptoms alone predict adverse outcomes, then what does the prognostic risk of high depression scores mean? Do poor outcomes result from severe depression or from the nonspecific burden of severe medical illness?

Medical illness at baseline probably does not explain the prognostic risk of depression.

Most researchers statistically adjusted for biomedical covariates, such as diabetes or ejection fraction. Furthermore, when depression scales were divided into their somatic and affective components, depression retained an adverse prognostic risk independent of its somatic component [78-79].

Negative affect is a component of depression which carries an adverse risk independent of its somatic dimension [79]. Symptoms that reflect the affective component of [80-81], such as anhedonia [82] or hopelessness [79, 83] predict adverse cardiac outcomes independently of biomedical and other variables.

Affective symptoms alone, however, do not completely explain the association between depression and adverse cardiac prognosis. Even after adjustment for the affective dimension, the Beck Depression Inventory (BDI) scores still predicted cardiac mortality [84]. Thus, the prognostic power of the BDI was due both to negative affectivity, and to some unique property measured by the scale. Although somatic symptoms alone do not mediate the CAD risk of depression either, their contribution to CAD outcomes appears distinct from that of affective or cognitive depression symptoms.

In the Heart and Soul study [85], somatic symptoms (appetite problems, sleeping difficulty, psychomotor changes and fatigue) predicted (HR = 1.46, p=0.05) adverse cardiovascular events whereas cognitive symptoms (depressed mood, lack of interest, worthlessness, concentration problems and suicidal ideation) only showed a statistical trend (HR = 1.08, p =0.09)

The prognostic value of somatic symptoms was independent of biomedical factors, including history of MI, diabetes, ejection fraction, smoking, BMI and medications. Thus, it is unlikely that the risk carried by somatic depressive symptoms merely reflects severe medical illness. Rather, the somatic dimension of depression likely carries unique prognostic importance.

Researchers have combined cognitive, somatic and affective groups of symptoms into sets to examine which symptom sets are most predictive of outcomes. A cognitive-affective combination (cognitive with affective symptoms) and a somatic-affective combination (combining somatic with affective symptoms) were compared. Most of the evidence indicates that the somatic-affective set has greater prognostic value [86-88].

Specific symptom groups, cognitive, affective or somatic, may be associated with particular biological markers. For example, in the Heart and Soul study, somatic depressive symptoms, but not cognitive symptoms, are associated with lower heart rate variability [89]. In the future, defining which symptom clusters predict poor outcomes may facilitate the identification of biological markers that mediate the risk.

Timing of Depression Onset: Post-MI vs. Pre-MI, New vs. Recurrent

Several researchers have examined whether the timing of depression onset affects treatment response or prognosis. Does it matter whether the depression episode begins after the MI (post-MI onset) or before (pre-MI onset)? Is there a difference in outcomes associated with incident depression, defined by no past depression history, compared to recurrent depression?

According to the SADHART trial [90] and the CREATE trial [91], two characteristics of depression, incident or new onset (i.e. no prior episodes) or post-MI onset, predicted a lower likelihood of depression response from SSRIs over placebo.

Do these two characteristics, incident depression and post-MI onset, also influence medical outcomes? Neither impacted prognosis, according to the SADHART study [92]. In contrast, three studies reported that post-MI depression carried a worse prognosis than "pre-MI" depression [93-95].

Six studies compared outcomes from incident depression and recurrent depression. Three studies [95-97] reported a worse outcome from incident depression, one from recurrent depression [98], and two reported no difference [92, 94].

In summary, patients with depression of new onset, or post-MI onset, may benefit less from SSRIs over placebo. Post-MI depression may carry a worse prognosis than "pre-MI" depression. It is unknown whether incident depression carries a worse prognosis than recurrent depression.

The Course of Post-MI Depression

Does the course of post-MI depression influence prognosis? Possible trajectories for depression include remission, persistence, and new onset of depression. Seven studies monitored the course of depression, over a 6-12 month period, beginning soon after the MI [92, 94, 99-103]. The research examined the medical outcomes predicted by each trajectory of depression.

Persistent depression was an adverse prognostic factor, independent of other demographic and cardiac risk factors, in four intervention trials (ENRICHD [102], MIND-IT [100], M-HART [101], SADHART [92]).

These trials reported that persistent depression predicted an adverse prognosis whenever there was an intervention, whether the treatment was psychotherapy, pharmacotherapy, or, even to placebo [92, 100-102]. In the SADHART Placebo arm, depression persistence may have reflected unresponsiveness to the placebo effect, and/or to the benefit of regularly scheduled staff support [92]. In three trials, Control patients received "usual care" [100-102]. Persistent depression was an adverse risk in Intervention arm patients, Placebo arm patients, but not among patients receiving usual care.

Why does depression persistence predict high risk in patients with receiving psychotherapy, pharmacotherapy or placebo treatment, but not among patients given usual care?

Carney and Freedland [104] have proposed that when depression persists *specifically from treatment resistance,* there is a poor prognosis; overall depression persistence is not high risk. That is, the whole group of patients with persistent depression does not have worse outcomes. However, after treatment, patients with persistent depression can be divided into two subgroups - responders and nonresponders. Only unresponsive, treatment-resistant depression predicts poor outcomes. In the context of usual care, without depression treatment, the nonresponders cannot be identified. When blended together in a single group, the high risk carried by the treatment resistant patient subgroup is diluted by the lower risk of treatment responders. The overall composite risk of persistent depression in the usual care group is not elevated.

The MIND-IT, ENRICHD and M-HART trials support the idea that depression persistence carries an adverse prognosis among treated patients only. In other words, the risk associated with depression persistence reflects the adverse prognosis predicted by nonresponse to an intervention.

However, other studies indicate that depression persistence without treatment does carry an adverse risk. In two trials, among patients receiving usual care, persistent post-ACS depression predicted worse medical outcomes [94, 99]. In these studies, compared to nondepressed patients, only those with persistent depression had increased mortality. There was no significant difference in prognosis between the nondepressed patients and those with transient depression.

Milani and Lavie monitored the course of depression in enrollees of a cardiac rehabilitation program with a behavioral component [103]. Most of the time, depressive symptoms improved or remitted. In some patients, depression persisted, or developed de novo (new onset) during treatment. The worst all-cause mortality rate was predicted by new onset depression (25%) or persistent depression (15%), compared to remitted depression (6%) and nondepressed control patients (5%). Persistence of depression, and possibly new onset of depression after the MI, could have reflected treatment resistance.

Thus, considerable evidence indicates that recalcitrance to depression treatment, whether involving psychotherapy, medication or cardiac rehabilitation, is a marker for poor post-MI health outcomes. Persistent depression may predict adverse health outcomes. Transient depression may carry less/ no increased risk. New onset depression that begins months after the MI may also carry a higher adverse risk.

Whether due to treatment resistance, persistence, or to new onset after the MI, depression that is present months after an MI indicates a high risk. Psychological and biomedical cardiac risk factors should be addressed. Enrollment into cardiac rehabilitation with a behavioral component, or the Ornish intervention, should be encouraged, as discussed later. Strong consideration should be given to the COPES intervention (see below), which was demonstrated to improve mood and prognosis in patients with persistent depression.

Screening

Evidence for the association of CAD and depression is strong enough to recommend screening for primary and secondary prevention.

Screening for Primary Prevention of CAD

Depressed patients without coronary disease should be advised of their elevated relative risk of CAD, estimated as RR=1.64 [6-7]. They should be referred to their primary care providers, to review CAD symptoms and risk factors. Risk factors include age, male gender, hypertension, high lipids, family history of early coronary disease, metabolic syndrome/diabetes mellitus, smoking, obesity, physical inactivity, and possibly inflammatory markers, such as C-reactive protein.

Screening for Secondary Prevention of CAD

Science Advisories of the AHA (American Heart Association)[74] and AAFP (American Association of Family Physicians) [105] recommend that patients with CAD should be screened for depression.

The AAFP does not specify a specific psychometric scale, but does recommend that post-MI patients should be screened at hospitalization during an MI, and then at regular intervals.

Table 1. Comparison of Depression Scales

Depression Scale	Cut-off Score to Diagnose MDD	Sensitivity/ Specificity *	Predictive Value *- Positive/Negative	Other Characteristics
2-STEP (PHQ-2 +/- PHQ-9) [107]	≥ 2 for PHQ2 & ≥ 6 for PHQ9	75/84	57 /92	6. Shortest Screening Time 7. Recommended by AHA
PHQ-9 [108]	≥ 5	91/75	45/98	
	≥ 10**	54/91	58/90	
BDI [109]	≥ 8	82 /79	NR	
	≥ 10**	54/91	NR	
HADS [108]	≥5	86/75	44/96	• No somatic items
	≥8**	46/92	55/88	• Measures anxiety & depression

"2-STEP" measurement involves only assessing for depression with PHQ-9, if there is a positive PHQ-2 during screening. *Sensitivity, Specificity and Predictive Values in the diagnosis of MDD among patients with CAD, and rounded to no decimal point. **generally accepted cut-offs Abbreviations: Scales: BDI = Beck Depression Scale, HADS = Hospital Anxiety and Depression Scale, PHQ=Patient Health Questionnaire; NR = Not Reported in Cardiac Patients.

The AHA suggestions are as follows: At minimum, clinicians should use the Patient Health Questionnaire (PHQ-2), which asks about the presence of low mood or anhedonia. If the PHQ-2 is positive, the AHA recommends further assessment with the PHQ-9. Patients with low-grade depressive symptoms (PHQ-9 <10) should have repeat testing in one month. Patients with PHQ-9 scores over 10, or with persistent low-grade depressive symptoms (two serial PHQ-2 scores ≥ 2, regardless of PHQ-9), should be referred to a professional qualified to diagnose and address depression.

Is the two step screening recommended by the AHA a better test for depression than screening with other measures? As noted in table 1, this two step test has similar validity in diagnosing MDD as other depression scales, such as the HADS, BDI and PHQ-9, but takes much less time to complete. Although the two step screening is comparable to other measures in assessing MDD, it is unknown how it compares in identifying depressed patients with a poor prognosis. Unlike the HADS, the BDI and PHQ-9 measure somatic depressive symptoms, which, as discussed earlier, are known to be of prognostic importance. On the other hand, the HADS may have better prognostic value: The HADS also measures depression and anxiety, both of which are associated with prognosis.

As discussed in earlier, evidence is suggestive, but not conclusive for an association for depression with adverse CAD prognosis. The risk of screening involves the time cost, patient distress from a mental health diagnosis, and the possibility of harm from treatment. When depression is identified and successfully treated, there is at minimum, a benefit from improved quality of life, but whether there are better medical outcomes is uncertain.

Given the ambiguity about whether depression treatment improves medical outcomes, some researchers argued, in 2009, that systematic depression screening overuses resources [106]. Furthermore, the scarcity of mental health providers increases the danger of misdiagnosis and/ or overmedication with antidepressants, by providers unqualified in mental health treatment.

New evidence that depression treatment, such as the COPES intervention, may improve outcomes (as discussed below) strengthens the argument for screening. Furthermore, screening allows identification of subgroups, such as patients with treatment resistant/persistent depression, suspected to carry a particularly adverse prognosis.

In summary, the AAFP recommends that screening post-MI patients for depression, but does not identify specific measures, perhaps because of inadequate evidence of the optimal screening test. The AHA recommends a short two step screening of all CAD patients with the PHQ-2, followed by the PHQ-9 only if the PHQ-2 is positive. The various screening tools discussed above are summarized in Table 1.

Among patients recovering from an acute coronary syndrome (MI/unstable angina), we recommend that screening take place soon after the MI and then be repeated every 3 months for a year.

Patients with depression should receive psychoeducation about depression diagnosis and treatment, its possible role as cardiac risk factor, and factors that may underlie the risk, such as medication nonadherence, smoking and physical inactivity. Patients should also be advised to identify and address co-morbid concerns such as low social support, anxiety, and, perhaps, hostility. Patients can be offered a referral to cardiac rehabilitation and/or a mental health provider.

Patients in whom depression persists or appears after three months post-ACS should be diagnosed with persistent/recalcitrant depression, a subgroup which likely carries a worse prognosis. Such patients should be followed up closely. Particular consideration should be given to cardiac rehabilitation and referral to a mental health provider.

Impact of Cardiac Rehabilitation on Depression and its Associated Mortality

The American Heart Association recommends cardiac rehabilitation programs in the treatment of CAD [110]. This multidisciplinary approach to overall risk reduction provides nutritional counseling, risk factor management, psychosocial interventions, promotion of adherence, and exercise training [110]. Multiple biomedical [111] and psychological concerns [112], such as depression, anxiety, and hostility are addressed.

The Exhaustion Intervention trial (EXIT) reported psychological benefits, but an unclear medical impact of a multidisciplinary intervention after a percutaneous coronary intervention (PCI) for CAD with a multidisciplinary intervention [113]. Specifically, patients in the intervention arm participated in group therapy focusing on stressors leading to exhaustion, and on support for recovery by promoting rest and making rest more efficient. Recovery was promoted by discussing the optimal duration for rest, doing relaxation exercises, physical exercise, and by assigning homework. Patients were offered optional meetings with a cardiologist, dietitian, and a health educator to address questions about medical aspects, nutrition, and smoking. Patients with major depression who did not improve were advised to consult their family physicians about an antidepressant.

The intervention reduced the odds of being depressed at 18 months by 51% [114]. Controlling for antidepressants did not significantly change the result. Exhaustion severity was only reduced in patients without prior CAD [114]. Hostility was not reduced, but other psychological variables, including anxiety (in women) and health-related quality of life, improved [114].

After the EXIT intervention, patients showed decreased anxiety and exhaustion, but 6 month cardiac events, increased (RR = 1.78; p = .02) [113]. How could a multidisciplinary intervention of exercise, smoking cessation, etc, that successfully improved distress increase 6 month rates of revascularization and ACS? The researchers suggested that Intervention patients may have found it easier to ask for revascularization. Cardiac procedure rates are soft endpoints, because they are prone to subjective influences, such as patient requests. The study appeared underpowered to assess changes restricted to hard endpoints, such as MI or death.

Although 6 month cardiac outcome rates worsened, the intervention did not change the 2 year event rate of the overall population [113]. In the patient subgroup with prior CAD, improved exhaustion predicted 60% fewer new cardiac events [113]. This effect was not seen in patients without prior CAD.

Another trial studied showed that even a short 8 week multidisciplinary intervention can improve mental well-being after an MI/CABG [115]. The control arm received usual care and exercise. The intervention, which combined stress management and health education, reduced hostility and type A behavior. Depression scores did not change, perhaps because of low baseline scores. 9 month cardiac event rates were unchanged, but the study was underpowered.

A study by Milani and Lavie demonstrated the benefit of a 3 month cardiac rehabilitation program in 338 patients with CAD and depression. There was no control arm. Patient data from before, and after, the intervention was compared. After cardiac rehabilitation, depressed patients showed marked improvements in depression as well as reduced anxiety, somatization, and hostility. Depressed patients also showed improved exercise capacity, percentage of body fat, triglyceride levels and HDL. The absence of a control arm prevents definitive conclusions. Nonetheless, the study supports the value of cardiac rehabilitation in depressed patients.

The same authors did a retrospective review of patients enrolled in a rehabilitation program. Patients who completed rehabilitation were compared to a control group who had not completed the program [103]. The intervention involved 36 educational and exercise sessions over 12 weeks. Education consisted of lectures and group sessions around heart disease, coronary risk factors, and psychosocial adaptations to the disease.

Among depressed patients, those who completed rehabilitation had a significantly reduced prevalence of depression (by 63%) and mortality (by 73%) than the control group of noncompleters. Multivariate analysis identified the following independent predictors of death among those who underwent cardiac rehabilitation: peak VO2, age, ejection fraction, and depressive symptoms.

Completers of rehabilitation were assigned to the intervention group, and non-completers to the control group. Thus, clear conclusions cannot be drawn. Although cardiac rehabilitation may have decreased mortality, other possible differences between completers and noncompleters, such as medication adherence, could explain improved outcomes.

Baseline differences between the control and intervention group complicate the interpretation of results. However, it is valid to compare patient subgroups within the Intervention arm. As discussed below, subgroup comparisons were made on the basis of depression trajectory, and on whether exercise capacity improved.

Patients with transient depression, which resolved during cardiac rehabilitation, had similar survival rates to the subgroup without depression. In contrast, there were high mortality rates in patients with unimproved baseline depression or with new onset depression persisting to the end of the program (15% and 25%, respectively). As reviewed earlier, it is likely that persistent, worsening or treatment recalcitrant depression carries a particularly adverse prognosis.

The study also strongly supported the medical and psychological benefit of exercise. Gains in exercise capacity, whether modest or robust, predicted improved depression (from a baseline of 18% to 4-5% prevalence) and enhanced survival. Decreased exercise capacity was associated with unchanged depression. Patient subgroups with a decrease, modest gain, and robust gain in exercise capacity had mortality rates of 15%, 6%, and 4% respectively.

These results emphasize the importance of adherence to an exercise regime. Modest and robust gains in exercise capacity predicted comparable improvement in mood and survival. Thus, CAD patients need not become exceptional athletes to benefit from exercise.

The above studies support the use of cardiac rehabilitation in treating depression, and other possible behavioral risk factors, such as anxiety or hostility. The above investigations, which specifically study depressed patients, lack enough power to definitively conclude whether mortality is improved. However, a systematic Cochrane review of studies of cardiac rehabilitation reported improved cardiac survival rates by about 30% [116].

Referral to cardiac rehabilitation with a psychosocial component should be considered for depressed patients with CAD. Providers should emphasize the value of exercise to optimize mood and medical outcomes.

The "Ornish" Intervention – Lifestyle Change

The Lifestyle Heart Trial, by Ornish et al, was a randomized control trial which demonstrated that coronary artery disease could be reversed by intensive lifestyle change without lipid lowering drugs [118]. The "Ornish" intervention (Table 2), involving exercise, a low fat vegetarian diet, stress management and group support, reversed CAD: coronary artery stenosis was reduced by 4.5% after 1 year and 7.9% after 5 years [119]. At follow-up, the control group, which received usual care, had worse atherosclerosis (12 % worse than baseline after 5 years), and over twice as many cardiac events (RR = 2.47). After 1 year, controls also had greater psychological distress. By the fifth year, only patients who were highly adherent to the Ornish program continued to show improvements in measures of psychological distress.

The researchers indicated that the psychological component of the program contributed to improvement. Adherence to stress management, involving hatha yoga and meditation, was related to decreased stenosis at 1 year and 5 years.

Some lifestyle changes predicted improved behavioral measures. Decreased fat intake correlated with reduced psychological distress; adherence to stress management was associated with less trait anger and weight loss [119].

The M-CLIP (Multisite Cardiac Lifestyle Intervention Program) study enrolled 1152 CAD patients in the "Ornish" intervention [120]. After three months, multiple coronary risk

MDD predicted increased 1 year adverse postoperative events (HR = 2.3) [130] and higher 10 year mortality rates (HR = 1.8) [131]

The CABG may cause adverse neurological sequelae, possibly from microembolic cerebral ischemia associated with a bypass [132]. Thus, depression that begins after a CABG may be a neurological postoperative complication. Cognitive deficits from mild impairment to frank delirium are common after a CABG [133-134]. We recommend bedside cognitive testing (such as a mini-mental status exam ™) in patients suspected of post-CABG depression, to assess concomitant cognitive deficits, and to rule out delirium in the differential diagnosis.

Evidence for the effect of antidepressants on post-CABG prognosis is quite limited. In a study of 309 post-CABG patients that linked depression to adverse medical outcomes, antidepressants did not significantly affect prognosis. [130].

Serotonin reuptake inhibitors have been linked to platelet dysfunction [135], and to increased blood loss in patients undergoing orthopedic surgery [136]. However, SSRIs/SNRIs, did not predict increased bleeding events (RR = 1), up a month post-CABG [137], even with adjustment for covariates, such as age, gender, comorbidity, and the use of platelet inhibitors, such as aspirin. Although 30 day mortality rates were unaffected, power was not adequate to assess risk.

A few studies have prospectively examined the effect of depression treatment of post-CABG patients on mood and postoperative medical outcomes. Two important trials are the "Bypassing the Blues" trial [135] and the Post-CABG trial [138].

The Bypassing the Blues trial examined the impact of telephone-delivered collaborative care of depression after a CABG [139]. Over 8 months, nurse care managers regularly phoned Intervention patients to monitor depression scores, provide psychoeducation and encourage adherence. Nurse care managers provided watchful waiting for mild depressive symptoms, and when appropriate, referral to a primary care physician or a mental health specialist. Most patients received 2 trials of SSRIs, starting with citalopram, before considering a drug with norepinephrine reuptake inhibition.

At 2 and at 8 months, Intervention patients were significantly less depressed. Medical prognosis, measured by rehospitalization rates, was unchanged. Subgroup analysis of rehospitalization rates in the Intervention arm showed a nonsignificant decrease among depressed men (p=0.07), and increase among depressed women (p=0.22).

In the Post-CABG trial, 1319 participants who were 1 to 11 years post-CABG, were randomized to an aggressive or a moderate lipid-lowering strategy [138]. Participants underwent coronary angiography at enrollment and after 4 years. Among patients in the moderate lipid-lowering strategy (LDL goal: 130-140 mg/dl), depression scores were associated with substantial graft progression. This association was not significant among participants receiving aggressive lipid-lowering therapy. Thus, aggressive lowering of LDL to 60-85 mg/dl may reduce the risk of atherosclerotic progression from depression. Of note, although an LDL goal of 60-85 was not compared to the generally recommended ATPIII (Adult Treatment Panel III, National Cholesterol Education Project) LDL goal of below 100.

Post-CABG patients have worse medical outcomes when depressed. Citalopram has been shown to help depression. There are no known safety concerns or benefits to prognosis with SSRIs, but evidence is quite limited. Interestingly, aggressive lowering of LDL to 60-85 mg/dl may reduce the risk of CAD progression from depression.

When post-CABG depression is suspected, we recommend that patients undergo bedside cognitive testing (such as a mini-mental status exam ™) to assess concomitant cognitive deficits, and to rule out delirium in the differential diagnosis.

Psychotherapy and Established Coronary Disease

Thou art discontent, thou art sad and heave: but why? On what ground?... Rule thyself then with reason...wean thyself from such fond conceits, vain fears, strong imaginations, restless thoughts. ... If ... our judgment be so depraved, our reason overruled... that we cannot seek our own good...the best way for ease is to impart our misery to some friend, not smother it up in our breast...grief concealed strangles the soul; but when as we shall but impart it to some discreet, trusty, loving friend, it is instantly removed...

Richard Burton, 1621 - from "The Anatomy of Melancholy [140]

Four major randomized trials have investigated the benefit of psychotherapy for depression and medical prognosis in coronary disease: the M-HART (Montreal Heart Attack Readjustment) trial, the ENRICHD (Enhancing Recovery in Coronary Heart Disease) trial, the CREATE trial (Canadian Cardiac Randomized Evaluation of Antidepressant and Psychotherapy Efficacy), and the COPES trial (Coronary Psychosocial Evaluation Studies)

The M-HART trial [141-143] randomized 1376 depressed and/or anxious subjects after recent MIs into a "usual care" control arm and an intervention arm. The intervention involved monthly phone calls, and, at times of distress, home visits from nurses. Nurses, supervised by mental health providers, offered support, cognitive restructuring, education and, if needed, psychiatric referrals.

The intervention did not significantly improve depression or change overall survival over the usual care group. Increased distress during treatment predicted higher mortality rates. Women, and patients with repressive coping styles, had reduced survival rates, possibly because of a higher prevalence of distress despite treatment. Better survival rates seen in men with high anxiety were mediated by reduced depression scores.

Other studies did not reproduce results indicating that psychotherapy was harmful to women, or uniquely beneficial to highly anxious men. The study results do emphasize the importance of monitoring patient response to whatever treatment is chosen. If patient distress is unimproved, the risk of adverse outcomes is higher, and providers should discuss other treatment options.

Even without intervention, repressive coping styles already predict worse post MI outcomes (death or MI) [144]. Unfortunately, psychological treatment may cause further harm. As noted by the M-HART researchers [142], patients with a repressive coping style avoid information that is potentially threatening. The authors cited a small study reporting that repressors who retained high levels of information about their illness had more distress and post-MI complications [145].

In a 2010 review [146], Myers noted that repressors with CAD likely carry a poor prognosis, particularly when confronting psychological aspects of their illness and/or gaining knowledge about their condition.

The ENRICHD trial examined whether cognitive behavioral therapy (CBT) for depression and/or poor social support improved mood and cardiac prognosis after a recent MI [70]. Patients were randomized to receive CBT, or usual care, in the control arm. In both arms, some patients received antidepressants. Depression scores of "control" patients were sent to their primary care providers. CBT arm patients with severe depression, or inadequate mood improvement, received antidepressants.

After 2.5 years, depression improved from CBT, though only modestly more than from usual care; "control" patients had a high spontaneous remission rate.

CBT had no effect on overall survival. The patient subgroup with depression unresponsive to CBT (with/without antidepressants) had worse survival rates (HR = 0.37) than those receiving usual care. Adding group therapy to individual CBT showed a trend (p=0.11) towards 23% fewer adverse medical events compared to patients in usual care [147]. While interesting, this result cannot be generalized because group treatment was not randomly assigned.

The CREATE study randomized patients with established CAD into four intervention arms: 1. Citalopram, 2. placebo, 3. IPT + placebo and 4. IPT + citalopram. All groups received clinical management, which included psychoeducation.

Adding IPT to clinical management provided no mood benefit, whether with placebo or citalopram. Medical outcomes from IPT were not reported.

Among patients with low social support, adding IPT predicted less mood improvement than clinical management alone. The authors cited an NIMH (National Institute of Mental Health) depression trial, which reported that high social dysfunction predicted a poor IPT response [148]. According to the authors, addressing both interpersonal and cardiac concerns may have been too difficult for patients with low social support. The lower demands of psychoeducation and medical management may allow better treatment.

In summary, IPT was not better than clinical management alone in depression treatment. This does not indicate that CBT works, albeit modestly, whereas IPT does not improve post-ACS depression. Clinical management was not equivalent to "usual care," as it consisted of support and psychoeducation. Depression improved with support and psychoeducation, whether or not there was also IPT.

Possibly, patients with low social support are best treated without IPT, and rather, with psychoeducation and support alone ; however, definitive recommendations require further evidence.

If post-MI spontaneous remission rates are high, should depression soon after an MI be aggressively treated right away? Would watchful waiting be a better strategy? In the ENRICHD trial and the SADHART study, patients receiving "usual care" or placebo had a high spontaneous remission rate of depression after an MI.

In the CREATE trial, the rate of spontaneous remission could not be measured; all patients received clinical management. If each arm had a high rate of spontaneous remission, the benefit of adding IPT, or of any treatment, would have been diluted.

The COPES trial (Coronary Psychosocial Evaluation Studies Randomized Controlled Trial) [149] examined the effectiveness of an intervention similar to the IMPACT program [150] over usual care.

The IMPACT program involves the collaboration of mental health specialists with primary care providers in a stepped approach to treat older adults with depression.

The study enrolled patients with depression persisting for three months post-ACS (unstable angina/ MI/ revascularization). Thus, patients whose depression spontaneously improved, or responded to conventional treatment, were excluded. Persistent or treatment refractory post-ACS depression likely predicts a particularly poor cardiac prognosis.

The M-HART trial reported that patients whose distress increased after psychotherapy had a worse prognosis than the controls. COPES researchers emphasized the importance of an effective intervention that avoided iatrogenic harm. The IMPACT intervention [150] supports patient preference and satisfaction with depression treatment in chronic illness care [150].

The COPES intervention involved patient choice of brief problem-focused psychotherapy (PST) and/or pharmacotherapy [151]. Stepped-care decisions were guided by serial depression scores. [151]. Patients without improvement were offered the choice of switching treatments (c.g. psychotherapy to medications), adding other treatments, or intensifying the original treatment choice [151].

At the end of the six month trial, patients in the intervention arm were significantly more satisfied with depression treatment, and less depressed than the controls, who received usual care. There were significantly more major adverse cardiac events in the intervention arm (10 patients) than the controls (3 patients).

The COPES trial showed improved cardiac outcomes in the depression treatment arm.

In summary, the high rate of spontaneous remission after an MI may have reduced the added benefit from CBT or IPT. Some patients become more distressed by psychotherapy. Patients with repressive coping styles may worsen with psychotherapy, particularly if confronted with information that they find threatening. Patients with low social support benefited more from psychoeducation than from IPT. In general, because some depressed patients are unimproved, or feel worse with psychotherapy, serial monitoring of mood is important. If depression does not respond, clinicians should consider changing treatment strategies.

As reviewed elsewhere, none of the antidepressant and/or psychological treatments improved both depression and mortality, except for the COPES intervention.

The rate of remission suggests psychotherapy may not be needed in depression that occurs soon after an MI. Rather, a reasonable strategy might include watchful waiting, with close follow-up to identify high risk patients with persistent depression.

The COPES trial results suggest that the high risk patient subgroup with persistent/recalcitrant depression should be offered the COPES intervention. The emphasis on patient satisfaction may have reduced the risk of worse distress, and thus resulted in better medical outcomes.

Antidepressants and Coronary Disease

How useful and safe are antidepressants in patients with CAD?

A number of randomized controlled trials have compared depression treatment outcomes from antidepressants to either usual care or placebo. Paroxetine was compared to nortriptyline, but not to placebo, or usual care [152].

Table 3. Summary of findings from randomized placebo-controlled antidepressant trials

Drug / Trial	Number of subjects	Population	Years of fu	Overall Group Depression Improvement Compared to Placebo	Subgroups with *NO Antidepressant Benefit* over placebo	Overall Group: *Antidepressant Effect* on Outcome Measures:	Subgroups with Worse Prognosis
Sertraline / SADHART	369	1 month post ACS	1 yr (mortality followed for 7 yrs)	Superior to Placebo	Mild/ Moderate depression (not severe) first depressive episode post-ACS onset (except severe depression) All 3 of above	*No Significant Change* vitals EKG intervals (incl. QTc) echocardiogram parameters cardiac events 1 y mortality 7 y mortality	Persistent depression (28% 7 yr mortality) Severe depression (26% 7 yr mortality) Both of above (32% 7 yr mortality)
Citalopram / CREATE	284	Established CAD	0.25 yr	Superior to Placebo	first depressive episode post-ACS onset (within 6 months) ACE inhibitor use	*No Significant Change* Vitals EKG parameters medical events	–
Fluoxetine	54	3-12 months after a first MI	0.5 yr		Moderate/Severe Depression (HAM-D > 21)	*No Significant Change* cardiac hospitalizations serious noncardiac diseases survival vitals EKG parameters *Possible Change (but unlikely)* interferes with post-MI ventricular remodeling? (unlikely)	–
Mirtazapine	94	3-12 months post MI	1 ½ yr	Superior to placebo	-	*No Significant Change* Vitals EKG intervals, incl QTc cardiac events	Unresponsive depression*

Drug / Trial	Number of subjects	Population	Years of fu	Overall Group Depression Improvement Compared to Placebo	Subgroups with *NO Antidepressant Benefit* over placebo	Overall Group: *Antidepressant Effect* on Outcome Measures:	Subgroups with Worse Prognosis
MIND-IT						*Significant Change* Weight gain (1.7 kg)	

* In the MIND-IT intervention arm, depression unresponsive to mirtazapine was treated with citalopram. Unresponsive depression was defined as depression.

Abbreviations: *ACS – acute coronary syndrome, EKG = electrocardiograph, fu = follow up, MI = myocardial infarction, yr= year.*

All of the antidepressant trials, except the CREATE trial, enrolled patients after a recent acute coronary event (see table 3). The CREATE trial of citalopram enrolled patients with stable CAD, only some of whom had a recent ACS [153]. The findings are summarized in table 3.

Antidepressant Efficacy

> Granatus, a precious stone so called, because it is like the kernels of a Pomegranate, an imperfect Ruby...if hung about the neck, or taken in drink, it much resisteth sorrow, and recreates the heart.
>
> Richard Burton, 1621 - from "The Anatomy of Melancholy" [140]

All of the antidepressants, sertraline [154], citalopram [91], fluoxetine [155]and mirtazapine [156], were superior to placebo in depression treatment of the overall study population. The studies identified patient subgroups with treatment refractory depression, or a poor medical prognosis.

In the subgroup of patients with a first episode of depression (i.e. no prior episodes), citalopram or sertraline offered no treatment advantage over placebo. Although statistically insignificant, 33% of responders and 16% of nonresponders to mirtazapine had prior episodes of depression [100].

That a new episode of depression predicts antidepressant unresponsiveness is concerning, because new onset depression may carry a particularly adverse prognosis.

Citalopram also offered no antidepressant benefit over placebo in the subgroup of patients with a recent ACS (within 6 months) [91]. In contrast, depression in post-ACS patients did respond to sertraline, fluoxetine and mirtazapine. Post-hoc analysis indicated that only fluoxetine only improved mild depression, not moderate or severe depression.

Depression severity did not influence whether mood improved with citalopram or mirtazapine. Mild or moderate depression predicted a lower likelihood of depression response to sertraline.

In the SADHART trial, patients with mild-moderate depression began *after* an acute coronary event had a high spontaneous remission rate.

This may reflect resolution of a grief reaction that began after a diagnosis of coronary disease, a result that parallels findings of the ENRICHD trial [70]. The low efficacy of sertraline with post-ACS onset was unchanged whether or not there were prior depressive episodes. However, if post-ACS depression was severe, sertraline was more effective than placebo, and thus, was more likely to be needed.

Three characteristics predict no benefit from sertraline over placebo: first episode, mild-moderate depression (HAM-D > 20) and onset after ACS.

Patients with recurrent, severe depressive episodes that began before ACS are 70% more likely to improve with sertraline than placebo [90].

Antidepressant Safety - Intervention Trials

> Cured yesterday of my disease, I died last night of my physician.
> – from "The Remedy Worse than the Diseaes" by Matthew Prior (1714)

None of the antidepressant intervention trials had enough power to assess their safety. It has been estimated that about 4000 subjects would be required to detect a 20% reduction in risk [154]. Furthermore, the safety of citalopram and sertraline is even less defined in patients meeting exclusionary criteria, such as severe angina, uncontrolled hypertension, severe bradycardia and nonatherosclerotic coronary disease.

The studies followed vitals, EKG intervals, including the QTc, and serious medical events (see table 3). In the overall study population, sertraline and citalopram had no significant effect on outcome measures. The only safety concern noted with mirtazapine was weight gain of 1.7 kg (3.7 lbs). Compared to placebo, fluoxetine had no significant adverse outcomes, except for a question as to whether fluoxetine impedes the recovery of the stroke volume.

After 6 months (week 25), the ATVI (Aortic Time Velocity Integral), an indirect index of stroke volume, improved by 4% in the placebo arm. There was no change in the fluoxetine arm. Does fluoxetine interfere with post-MI ventricular remodeling? This is unlikely: The difference was corrected by statistical adjustments for differences between the size of MI at baseline. Thus, the authors concluded that the difference is more likely related to patients in the fluoxetine group having had larger MIs than the placebo group. Without replication in other studies, no clinical conclusions can be extrapolated from this finding.

In both the SADHART trial, of sertraline, and the MIND-IT trial, of mirtazapine, persistent, unresponsive depression predicted lower survival rates [92, 100]. Patients in the SADHART trial received sertraline or placebo. In the MIND-IT intervention arm, depression unresponsive to mirtazapine was treated with citalopram. Both trials defined unresponsive, persistent depression as a nonresponse to any antidepressant, or to placebo.

In the sertraline trial, severe depression at baseline predicted a 26% higher 7 year mortality rate (26%). Patients with persistent depression, that was severe at baseline, carried a particularly high seven year mortality rate (32%).

Paroxetine has been compared to nortriptyline, a tricyclic antidepressant (TCA) in a 6 week randomized study of CAD patients [152]. With no placebo arm, this study could not compare the benefit/risk of paroxetine to no treatment. Rather, the trial compares its safety and efficacy to a TCA, a class of antidepressants believed to be cardiotoxic (see below).

Both paroxetine and nortriptyline improved depression. During the 6 week follow up, nortriptyline caused significantly more adverse cardiac effects, including an 11% increase in pulse, and decreased HRV. Of the ten patients who discontinued nortriptyline, three had noncardiac adverse events, and seven had cardiac events, including sinus tachycardia, severe angina and an asymptomatic increase in PVCs. Paroxetine had no clinically significant effects on vital signs or on cardiac conduction. One patient on paroxetine developed unstable angina. This trial reinforces the safety superiority of SSRIs over TCAs [152].

To our knowledge, there are no longitudinal placebo controlled studies of tricyclic antidepressant on patients with coronary artery disease. Several review articles [158] [159] have recommended avoiding tricyclic antidepressants in patients with myocardial ischemia because they are class I antiarrhythmics, a class of drugs which increases the risk of post-MI sudden death [69].

Tricyclic antidepressants have other cardiotoxic effects, including reduced heart rate variability, slowed intracardiac conduction, wider QTc, increased heart rate, and tachyarrhythmias [160-161]. For this reason, when possible, tricyclic antidepressants should be avoided in patients with heart disease [162].

Antidepressant Safety – Longitudinal Trials

Aside from being underpowered, most antidepressant intervention trials of depressed CAD patients could not assess long term safety; endpoints were measured after six months or less. The MIND-IT trial, which evaluated mirtazapine, and the SADHART trial, which assessed sertraline, followed patients for a longer duration, 18 months, and 7 years, respectively. Extended follow up is particularly important in post MI patients because antidepressants could theoretically disrupt cardiac remodeling. Cardiac remodeling impacts left ventricular dysfunction, a key long term prognostic indicator [163].

Given these limitations of the medication intervention trials, it is worthwhile examining other studies relevant to the safety of antidepressants.

Several researchers have proposed that the correlation between depression and adverse outcomes may be partly mediated by antidepressant toxicity.

Several longitudinal studies, the Nurse's Health Study [164], the Women and Ischemia Syndrome Evaluation (WISE) study [165], Women's Health Initiative (WHI) [166] and the Heart and Soul Study [29], reported that antidepressants partly mediated the link between depression and adverse cardiovascular events. This association persisted after multivariate analysis adjustment for depression and other covariates associated with adverse prognosis.

The Nurse's Health Study, of 63459 women without CAD, reported an association of sudden cardiac death both with SSRIs (HR= 5.07) and non-SSRI antidepressants (HR = 3.19) [164]. In the WHI study, of136293 women without CAD, both TCAs and SSRIs were associated with increased risk of stroke and all-cause mortality [166].

The WISE study, which followed 519 women suspected of CAD, revealed an association between psychotropic medications (combined anxiolytics or antidepressants) with cardiovascular events [165]. This association was not present with either anxiolytics or antidepressants alone, which may have reflected low power. Specific antidepressant classes were not identified.

The authors of the Nurse's Health Study, WHI, and WISE studies cautioned that although these results suggest antidepressant toxicity, confounding remains possible. Antidepressant use may be a marker for more severe depression not fully captured by the depression scores.

The Heart and Soul Study [29] was a longitudinal study of the mechanisms underlying the association of depression with CAD prognosis. Statistical adjustment for the use of most antidepressants did not significantly change the association of depressive symptoms with cardiovascular events. However, "other" antidepressants (i.e. not SSRIs or TCAs), reduced the effect size for depressive symptoms on cardiovascular events by 8.8%. The authors suggested two possible explanations: "Other" antidepressants are often prescribed after SSRIs fail. Their presence could be a confounder for another adverse prognostic factor - treatment-resistant depression. Alternatively, many second line antidepressants have noradrenergic activity, which may be cardiotoxic, as discussed below.

As discussed below, data from other longitudinal studies revealed different results: Two trials reported antidepressant safety concerns, and one suggested that antidepressants improve prognosis.

Two longitudinal studies, which showed an association between depression and CAD, did not reproduce these results. The NHANES I study of 7893 study participants without heart disease [167], the LASA (Longitudinal Aging Study Amsterdam) study of 2847 participants with and without cardiac disease [168] reported that antidepressants did not carry an adverse risk independently of depression.

A review of the outcomes of 1834 depressed patients in the ENRICHD trial, suggested that antidepressants might improve 2 year prognosis after an acute coronary event [169]. The relative risk of death/ recurrent MI was significantly lower (RR = 0.66) among patients taking antidepressants compared to those on no antidepressants. Subgroup analysis revealed that, compared to patients on no antidepressants, only patients on SSRIs showed a significant difference in event-free survival (RR= 0.57). No such survival difference was seen in patients on non-SSRI antidepressants.

Noradrenergic Antidepressants

The category of "other antidepressants" in the Heart and Soul trial included medications, such as venlafaxine, mirtazapine, and bupropion, that all affect noradrenergic activity[30].

Hypertension can be a side-effect of antidepressants that inhibit norepinephrine reuptake. High blood pressure is a common risk of venlafaxine [170], but less common in bupropion [171] or duloxetine [170]. Common side effects of mirtazapine include obesity and increased lipids [172].

A further concern involves whether noradrenergic reuptake inhibition increases sympathetic activity. Sympathetic overactivity likely worsens CAD prognosis, given the evidence for its role in atherogenesis [173], its importance in cardiac remodeling [174], and the well-known long term prognostic benefit of Beta-adrenergic blockers [175]. Sympathetic output also increases the risk of arrhythmias [176]

Do antidepressants with noradrenergic activity affect sympathetic activity, and thus, adversely influence prognosis? The pathophysiology is not straightforward. Norepinephrine reuptake inhibition (NRI) does not uniformly increase peripheral sympathetic output, but rather, changes it in complex ways [177]. Indices of sympathetic activity, such as norepinephrine levels or heart rate variability, did not significantly mediate the prognostic effect of depression in the Heart and Soul study [29]. The MIND-IT trial was too underpowered to assess whether mirtazapine affected CAD prognosis.

To our knowledge, there are no longitudinal placebo controlled trials of noradrenergic drugs on depressed CAD patients. However, there is a prospective placebo-controlled study of a 12-week course of bupropion to promote smoking cessation in 248 smokers with acute cardiovascular disease, mostly acute MI or unstable angina [178]. Bupropion was significantly associated with better one year smoking cessation rates (25.0% vs 21.3% placebo, OR = 1.23). There was no significant difference in blood pressure or in non-cardiovascular event rates at 3 and 12 months. Although cardiovascular event rates at 3 and

12 months appeared similar in both groups, a post hoc analysis was completed because some patients in the study group did not actually take bupropion. When comparing participants who took bupropion to those on placebo, cardiovascular event rates were similar within 30 days. However, cardiovascular event rates after 30 days were significantly higher among patients taking bupropion. Even after adjusting for covariates, including coronary risk factors, history of CAD, discharge diagnosis, and smoking status, patients on bupropion had three times more cardiovascular events (rate ratio = 3.12, p = 0.05). The authors questioned the result, commenting that there was no plausible explanation for a higher rate of cardiovascular events taking place over 30 days after bupropion was stopped. However, one might hypothesize that increased sympathetic output from bupropion adversely affected cardiac modeling, which in turn, had long term cardiac consequences.

Without replication of these results, it is not possible to make definitive conclusions, but the study results emphasize the need for caution with noradrenergic drugs, in case they do increase sympathetic output. Particular caution should be exercised to avoid the use of noradrenergic drugs in the presence of arrhythmias, or left ventricular dysfunction. Left ventricular dysfunction, a key adverse prognostic factor, can worsen from pathological cardiac remodeling, promoted by norepinephrine. Beta-blockers may not be able to prevent adverse consequences of noradrenergic drugs. Among patients on beta blockers, with congestive heart failure, mortality correlated with "adrenergic escape" – i.e. norepinephrine levels that were above normal despite beta-blockers [179].

Antidepressants - A Summary and Recommendations

The intervention studies of antidepressants, including the SADHART, MIND-IT, and CREATE trials, were underpowered to address the prognostic effect of antidepressants.

As described above, some studies have shown no relationship between prognosis and antidepressants. The Heart and Soul study reported that only "other" antidepressants – i.e. not SSRIs or TCAs - carried a risk. Nonetheless, several large scale studies, two with tens of thousands of participants, reported adverse medical outcomes associated with antidepressants, including SSRIs, independently of depression. It goes without saying that evidence indicating that antidepressants have no effect, a beneficial effect and an adverse effect on prognosis is ambiguous. Several experts [180-182] have recently recommended that prospective studies are needed to address the question of antidepressant toxicity.

Antidepressants should be prescribed only for clinical necessity, and not with the expectation of improving prognosis. Citalopram and sertraline, the most extensively studied antidepressants in CAD patients, should be considered first line agents. Patients who are depressed within 6 months after an ACS may be more likely to respond to sertraline than to citalopram. Fluoxetine is the next choice, given some evidence of safety. Paroxetine may be the last choice of SSRIs given the lack of data and its anticholinergic effect. Theoretically, paroxetine's stronger anticholinergic activity [183] might adversely change the sympathetic/parasympathetic balance. Tricyclic antidepressants should be avoided.

Noradrenergic drugs should not be prescribed unless SSRIs fail. A decision to give noradrenergic antidepressants to CAD patients should be made with the patient's cardiologist and/or primary provider. Left ventricular dysfunction and a history of arrhythmias likely increase the risk of cardiotoxicity from noradrenergic drugs. Blood pressure should be monitored, particularly in the case of venlafaxine. Patients receiving mirtazapine should additionally be monitored for lipids and weight gain.

Consideration should be given to watchful waiting, psychotherapy, or rehabilitation. Sertraline and citalopram may offer little benefit in first episode depression. Depression that begins after an ACS might be better treated without antidepressants, as it often remits spontaneously. Watchful waiting is a reasonable approach for patients who develop mild-moderate (HAM-D <20) depression after an acute coronary event, whether or not depression is recurrent.

Severe depression at baseline predicted high seven year mortality rates (26%)[92]. When severe, depression improved more with sertraline than placebo. Sertraline did not improve the prognosis of severe depression over placebo. However, the study was underpowered. When severe depression did not improve, patients carried a particularly high seven year mortality rate (32%). In other words, patients who responded to treatment, whether to placebo or sertraline, had better medical outcomes. Thus, it may be worthwhile to treat severe depression with antidepressants, even when depression begins after ACS.

Less caution for the use of antidepressants is needed when depression persists beyond 3 months of an acute coronary event. Patients with persistent/treatment-resistant depression after an MI/unstable angina have a particularly adverse prognosis. Such patients should be considered for the treatment described in the COPES trial, the only intervention which improved prognosis, as discussed above. The COPES intervention is a collaborative stepped approach, emphasizing patient choice and satisfaction. Patients can choose between problem-solving psychotherapy (PST) and/or pharmacotherapy [151]. Follow up with PHQ-9 scores should guide further treatment.

Omega-3 Fatty Acids

Omega-3 fatty acid levels are inversely associated with both depression and an adverse prognosis in CAD [184]. Thus, low omega-3 fatty acid levels have been proposed as an explanation for their link [184].

A large epidemiological study demonstrated an inverse relationship between omega-3 fatty levels and coronary heart disease [185]. The Heart and Soul study reported that omega-3 fatty acids did not significantly mediate the association between depression and adverse CAD prognosis [186]. Nonetheless, considerable evidence has been cited to support omega-3 fatty acids for CAD risk reduction [187], and as a low-risk adjunctive treatment in MDD [188]. Thus, omega-3 fatty acids could be particularly useful in treating concomitant depression and CAD.

In a placebo-controlled trial of patients with CAD, omega-3 fatty acids augmentation of sertraline prevented deterioration of heart rate variability [189]. Low heart rate variability is a predictor of sudden cardiac death. However, in a larger ten week trial of 122 patients, omega-3 fatty acid augmentation of sertraline did not result in better depression or CHD outcomes compared to placebo [190].

It remains to be seen whether further studies reproduce the lack of efficacy. Given the evidence for improved depression from omega-3 fatty acids in the general population, more studies should be done, at least to identify if specific subgroups are responsive to omega-3 fatty acids.

In the meantime, the safety, and possible benefit of omega-3 fatty acids offer a significant advantage. Omega-3 fatty acids should be considered alone or as augmentation treatment for depressed patients with CAD.

Collaborative Care Models Integrating Treatment of Mental and Physical Health

As we described at the beginning of this chapter, the "body as machine" model neglects the importance of the psyche in medical illness. Psychiatry now emphasizes the biological basis of mental illness. However, the treatment of chronic medical illness remains characterized by isolation between providers of mental health and physical health.

An estimated 16-38% of primary care patients have a psychiatric diagnosis. 5-13% of these patients have major depression. As described in this chapter, and by several experts [205-206], co-morbid mental disorders complicate the management and exacerbate the course of chronic physical conditions. Our growing understanding of the role of psychological factors in chronic illness, including CAD, highlights the need for integrated biopsychosocial approach to treatment. Integrating mental health care in primary care practices is hampered by logistical barriers – particularly time pressure for primary care physicians, and low reimbursement for on-site mental health care providers [205-206]. In part, these barriers contribute to the under-diagnosis of major depression, the underuse/ inappropriate use of antidepressants, and the lack of evidence-based psychotherapy in primary care [205].

Systematic reviews/meta-analyses have demonstrated the benefits of collaborative care in depression treatment [207-208]. Collaborative models include the integration of mental health providers, closely supervised by psychiatrists, in primary care practices [205-206]. Nurses can act as care extenders, monitoring outcomes, ensuring patient-provider communication, and coaching patients in self-care. This approach can provide depressed patients with chronic illness (including CAD), superior medical outcomes, mood, quality of life and treatment satisfaction [209]. At this point, strong evidence argues for broad scale implementation of collaborative care.

Future Directions

There has been an upsurge of research in the relationship between depression and CAD. Nonetheless, our understanding of this area is in its early stages.

Defining the role of medications in the prognosis of patients with CAD is an urgent research priority. The study results concerning SSRIs are quite inconsistent. Large scale trials with enough power would clarify questions regarding antidepressant safety. Whether noradrenergic agents can be safely prescribed in patients with CAD also needs to be determined. Further investigation of omega-3 fatty acids would also be valuable. All of the intervention trials should include follow-up echocardiograms to assess whether cardiac remodeling is affected.

Future research could help identify subgroups of depressed patients at high risk for adverse outcomes, and determine which treatments reduce risk. Optimal treatment of the high risk patient subgroup with persistent depression after a coronary event is particularly important.

The Heart and Soul trial was helpful in understanding which variables mediate the prognostic effect of depression on CAD. Further studies on confounders and mediators of the effect of psychosocial factors would be valuable.

Nonpharmacological treatments for depressed CAD patients include psychotherapy, exercise, cardiac rehabilitation and the Ornish intervention. Investigations currently underway include the UPBEAT trial and the READY trial. The UPBEAT study is designed to assess the efficacy of exercise in treating depression in cardiac patients and evaluates the impact of treating depression on important biological markers of cardiovascular risk [193]. The READY study investigates the effect of resilience training, promoting positive emotions, cognitive flexibility, social support, life meaning, and active coping, on mood and cardiac biological markers in the general population [194].

In some patient subgroups, such as those with repressive coping styles, psychotherapy may result in worse outcomes. These patients are more effectively treated with support. Research is needed to match patients with the appropriate form of psychotherapy.

Research into role of the physiological response to stress in the effect of depression on CAD is needed. Sympathetic overactivity has been linked to adverse cardiac remodeling in left ventricular dysfunction. The stress response is known to be associated with sympathetic activation, changes in immune function and increased cortisol [172, 195].

Mindfulness meditation appears to reduce stress, and its physiological consequences. Multiple studies have shown improved quality of life and reductions in cortisol levels [196-199]. There is some evidence for reduced pro-inflammatory cytokines [199], and reduced sympathetic activity [200]. A recent meta-analysis concluded that mindfulness meditation improves depression and anxiety in chronic medical illness [201]. Evidence specific to heart disease is limited to small studies, in which cardiac patients have shown less anxiety [202], depression[203] and CHF symptoms [204] from mindfulness meditation. In a larger study of 154 patients at risk for CAD, lifestyle change, including mindfulness meditation, reduced the Framingham CAD risk score.

These promising findings justify larger scale prospective studies of the benefits of mindfulness meditation. We are looking forward to studies currently underway, such as the HARMONY trial, which will assess the benefit of mindfulness meditation on hypertension.

Summary and Clinical Recommendations

1. Is depression a coronary risk factor?
- There is strong evidence that depression correlates with CAD incidence.
- Less consistent evidence links depression with prognosis of established CAD.

2. What are the proposed mediators of the association between depression and CAD?
- Behavioral smoking, sedentary living, and nonadherence to treatment.
- Biomedical: inflammation, insulin resistance, endothelial function, platelet activation and HRV.

3. Is depression a "true" CAD risk factor, or a confounder?

- It remains to be determined whether association is specific to depression.
- The "true risk factor" may be:
  - Psychosocial: e.g. anxiety, or social support
  - Biomedical: e.g. inflammation, or a genetic basis
- Depression may be the result, rather than the cause, of atherosclerosis.
- *Alternatively*: Relationship may be bidirectional:
  i.e. depression worsens CAD, & atherosclerosis causes vascular depression.
- While future evidence is pending, from a clinical perspective, it seems reasonable to view depression as a likely marker for CAD risk.

4. What role do co-morbid psychosocial factors have in CAD?

- Anxiety and low social support, likely predict adverse medical outcomes.
- Weaker evidence links hostility to CAD.
- The relative prognostic importance of different psychosocial factors has not been determined.
- High social support likely protects against adverse medical outcomes linked to depression.

5. How should a clinician address co-morbid psychological concerns?

- Refer depressed patients for a comprehensive clinical evaluation by providers who can identify and treat co-morbid mental disorders.
- Choose treatments which improve multiple psychological concerns. e.g.:
  - SSRIs can improve depression, anxiety and may reduce aggression.
  - cardiac rehabilitation including psychotherapy, or the Ornish intervention

6. Which symptoms of depression predict prognosis of CAD?

- Affective and somatic symptoms of depression appear most predictive
- Cognitive symptoms, reflecting negative attitudes towards self, may be less predictive.

7. After an acute coronary syndrome (ACS), which characteristics of depression likely predict a high risk for adverse outcomes? What predicts low risk?

High risk subgroups:

- Worsening/new onset of depression months after the ACS
- Recalcitrance to treatment, whether psychotherapy, medication or cardiac rehabilitation
- Persistent depression (evidence is less strong)

Question of increased risk:

- Prognosis *may* be worse in post-MI depression compared to "pre-MI" depression.
- It is unknown if first onset (incident) depression carries a worse prognosis than recurrent depression.

Low risk subgroup
- Transient depression may carry less/ no increased risk.

8. How can providers prevent CAD in depressed patients?
- Educate patients about the following:
  - Depression is associated with a higher risk of CAD.
  - CAD risk factors, i.e. hypertension, high lipids, family history of early CAD, metabolic syndrome/diabetes mellitus, smoking, obesity and physical inactivity
  - how to recognize symptoms of CAD
- Barring health contraindications, encourage exercise for the mood and physical health.
- Antidepressants may reduce the risk of death or MIs in patients without pre-existing CAD, but evidence remains preliminary, and may be confounded by medication adherence.

9. Should providers screen for depression in patients with CAD?
- Yes: Screen for depression soon after an ACS and q 3 months x 1 year.

10. What depression screening instrument should be used in patients with CAD?
- AHA recommends the PHQ-2 depression screen. If PHQ-2 is positive, patients should receive further depression assessment.

11. How should depression in patients with CAD be treated?
- Educate patients about
  - depression as a possible cardiac risk factor
  - possible mediators of the risk e.g. nonadherence, smoking and inactivity
- Identify and address co-morbid concerns e.g. low social support, anxiety, and hostility
- Advise exercise, to improve both CAD and depression, under the guidance of the primary physician or cardiologist.
- Refer to cardiac rehabilitation and/or a mental health provider.
- Watchful waiting for first episode of mild/moderate depression beginning after the ACS.
- Monitor mood closely after an ACS to identify high risk patients with persistent depression.
- Treat depression primarily to enhance quality of life, except for persistent depression.
  - The absence of evidence for prognostic improvement from treatment may relate to underpowered studies, and the high rate of spontaneous remission.
  - Depression treatment may enhance adherence, smoking cessation, and/or exercise
- See below for further answers regarding psychotherapy and medications.

12. How safe is depression treatment in CAD?

A. Psychotherapy
- Psychotherapy is likely to be safe in most patients.
- CBT and IPT are the most studied, but psychodynamic psychotherapy is also reasonable.
- A repressive coping style may predict distress with psychotherapy. Consider support and clinical management instead.
- Among patients with low social support, the addition of IPT to clinical management was inferior to clinical management alone in depression treatment (CREATE trial).

B. Antidepressants
- TCAs should be avoided.
- SSRIs are the safest antidepressants, but evidence for their safety is inconclusive.
- Citalopram or sertraline should be the first choices.
- Because of safety concerns, noradrenergic agents, such as venlafaxine, duloxetine and mirtazapine, should only be considered if SSRIs fail (see below).
- See question 13 re precautions

C. Whatever treatment modality is chosen, monitor patients serially. Switch treatments if patients do not improve after weeks of a fair trial (see question 15).

13. What precautions are needed when prescribing antidepressants to patients with CAD?
- Patients with pre-existing arrhythmias, particularly bradycardia/ AV block:
  - Exercise caution: SSRIs infrequently may cause bradycardia [191].
  - Consult a cardiologist if there are pre-existing arrhythmias, especially bradycardia/AV block
  - Order serial EKGs or EKG monitoring
- If noradrenergic antidepressants are prescribed:
  - Collaborate with the patient's primary physician, or cardiologist.
  - Involve cardiology if there is left ventricular dysfunction/ arrhythmia.
  - Monitor blood pressure, particularly in the case of venlafaxine.
  - Patients on mirtazapine should have lipids and weight monitored.
- Review all concomitant medications and anticipate that levels will rise because all antidepressants inhibit of P450 enzymes [192].

14. Do Omega-3 fatty acids have a role in depression treatment?
- Consider omega-3 fatty acids as augmentation treatment even though the only trial investigating its use in CAD patients showed no benefit.
- Omega-3 fatty acids are a useful antidepressant in the general population
- Omega–3 fatty acids are likely safe, and may benefit cardiac prognosis
- If prescribed, choose a brand tested for mercury and dioxins.

15. How should depression that persists over 3 months after an ACS be treated?

- Depression present months after an ACS likely indicates a high risk whether due to treatment resistance, persistence, or to new onset.
- Address psychological and biomedical cardiac risk factors.
- Refer to cardiac rehabilitation with a behavioral component, or the Ornish intervention
- Strongly consider the COPES intervention, which improved mood and medical prognosis

16. How should post-CABG depression be treated?

- Post-CABG patients have worse medical outcomes when depressed.
- Same recommendations as in question 10 - 12 with the following additions:
- Citalopram has been shown to improve post-CABG depression.
- SSRI safety specific to post-CABG patients is unknown. In general, antidepressants, including SSRIs, may have safety concerns in CAD (see questions 12, 13).
- Aggressive lowering of LDL (60-85 mg/dl) may reduce CAD progression.
- Provide bedside cognitive testing (such as a mini-mental status exam ™) to assess concomitant cognitive deficits, and to rule out delirium in the differential diagnosis.

References

[1] Wagner, R., et al., *Tristan und Isolde.* 2006, Opera d'Oro,: Portland, OR.

[2] Roberts, A., *My Heart My Mother.* 1st [England] ed. 2000, Rottingdean, East Sussex, England: NorthGate Publishers. iv, 265 p.

[3] McMahon, C.E., The psychosomatic approach to heart disease. A study in premodern medicine. *Chest,* 1976. 69(4): p. 531-7.

[4] Damasio, A.R., *Looking for Spinoza : joy, sorrow, and the feeling brain.* 1st ed. 2003, Orlando, Fla.: Harcourt. x, 355 p.

[5] Vivona, J.M., Embodied language in neuroscience and psychoanalysis. *J Am Psychoanal Assoc,* 2009. 57(6): p. 1327-60.

[6] Wulsin, L.R., Is depression a major risk factor for coronary disease? A systematic review of the epidemiologic evidence. *Harv Rev Psychiatry,* 2004. 12(2): p. 79-93.

[7] Rugulies, R., Depression as a predictor for coronary heart disease. a review and meta-analysis. *Am J Prev Med,* 2002. 23(1): p. 51-61.

[8] Frasure-Smith, N. and F. Lesperance, Reflections on depression as a cardiac risk factor. *Psychosom Med,* 2005. 67 Suppl 1: p. S19-25.

[9] Van der Kooy, K., et al., Depression and the risk for cardiovascular diseases: systematic review and meta analysis. *Int J Geriatr Psychiatry,* 2007. 22(7): p. 613-26.

[10] Sorensenf, C., et al., Postmyocardial infarction mortality in relation to depression: a systematic critical review. *Psychother Psychosom,* 2005. 74(2): p. 69-80.

[11] Nicholson, A., H. Kuper, and H. Hemingway, Depression as an aetiologic and prognostic factor in coronary heart disease: a meta-analysis of 6362 events among 146 538 participants in 54 observational studies. *Eur Heart J,* 2006. 27(23): p. 2763-74.

[12] Wang, P.S., et al., Changing profiles of service sectors used for mental health care in the United States. *Am J Psychiatry,* 2006. 163(7): p. 1187-98.

[13] Schulberg, H.C., et al., The 'usual care' of major depression in primary care practice. *Arch Fam Med*, 1997. 6(4): p. 334-9.

[14] Ford, D.E., Optimizing outcomes for patients with depression and chronic medical illnesses. *Am J Med,* 2008. 121(11 Suppl 2): p. S38-44.

[15] Leonard, B.E., The immune system, depression and the action of antidepressants. *Prog Neuropsychopharmacol Biol Psychiatry,* 2001. 25(4): p. 767-80.

[16] Tousoulis, D., et al., Inflammatory and thrombotic mechanisms in coronary atherosclerosis. *Heart,* 2003. 89(9): p. 993-7.

[17] McCaffery, J.M., et al., Common genetic vulnerability to depressive symptoms and coronary artery disease: a review and development of candidate genes related to inflammation and serotonin. *Psychosom Med,* 2006. 68(2): p. 187-200.

[18] Kendler, K.S., et al., Major depression and coronary artery disease in the Swedish twin registry: phenotypic, genetic, and environmental sources of comorbidity. *Arch Gen Psychiatry,* 2009. 66(8): p. 857-63.

[19] Surtees, P.G., et al., Major depression, C-reactive protein, and incident ischemic heart disease in healthy men and women. *Psychosom Med,* 2008. 70(8): p. 850-5.

[20] Vaccarino, V., et al., Depression, inflammation, and incident cardiovascular disease in women with suspected coronary ischemia: the National Heart, Lung, and Blood Institute-sponsored WISE study. *J Am Coll Cardiol,* 2007. 50(21): p. 2044-50.

[21] Davidson, K.W., et al., Relation of inflammation to depression and incident coronary heart disease (from the Canadian Nova Scotia Health Survey [NSHS95] Prospective Population Study). *Am J Cardiol,* 2009. 103(6): p. 755-61.

[22] Stewart, J.C., et al., A prospective evaluation of the directionality of the depression-inflammation relationship. *Brain Behav Immun,* 2009. 23(7): p. 936-44.

[23] Rudisch, B. and C.B. Nemeroff, Epidemiology of comorbid coronary artery disease and depression. *Biol Psychiatry,* 2003. 54(3): p. 227-40.

[24] Alexopoulos, G.S., et al., 'Vascular depression' hypothesis. *Arch Gen Psychiatry,* 1997. 54(10): p. 915-22.

[25] Heart rate variability. Standards of measurement, physiological interpretation, and clinical use. Task Force of the European Society of Cardiology and the North American Society of Pacing and Electrophysiology. *Eur Heart J,* 1996. 17(3): p. 354-81.

[26] Kinder, L.S., et al., Depressive symptomatology and coronary heart disease in Type I diabetes mellitus: a study of possible mechanisms. *Health Psychol,* 2002. 21(6): p. 542-52.

[27] Drago, S., et al., Depression in patients with acute myocardial infarction: influence on autonomic nervous system and prognostic role. Results of a five-year follow-up study. *Int J Cardiol,* 2007. 115(1): p. 46-51.

[28] Jermendy, G., Clinical consequences of cardiovascular autonomic neuropathy in diabetic patients. *Acta Diabetol,* 2003. 40 Suppl 2: p. S370-4.

[29] Whooley, M.A., et al., Depressive symptoms, health behaviors, and risk of cardiovascular events in patients with coronary heart disease. *JAMA,* 2008. 300(20): p. 2379-88.

[30] Stahl, S.M., et al., SNRIs: their pharmacology, clinical efficacy, and tolerability in comparison with other classes of antidepressants. *CNS Spectr,* 2005. 10(9): p. 732-47.

[31] Ladwig, K.H., et al., C-reactive protein, depressed mood, and the prediction of coronary heart disease in initially healthy men: results from the MONICA-KORA Augsburg Cohort Study 1984-1998. *Eur Heart J,* 2005. 26(23): p. 2537-42.

[32] Brummett, B.H., et al., Ratings of positive and depressive emotion as predictors of mortality in coronary patients. *Int J Cardiol,* 2005. 100(2): p. 213-6.

[33] Romanelli, J., et al., The significance of depression in older patients after myocardial infarction. *J Am Geriatr Soc,* 2002. 50(5): p. 817-22.

[34] Gehi, A., et al., Depression and medication adherence in outpatients with coronary heart disease: findings from the Heart and Soul Study. *Arch Intern Med,* 2005. 165(21): p. 2508-13.

[35] Dorn, J., et al., Correlates of compliance in a randomized exercise trial in myocardial infarction patients. *Med Sci Sports Exerc,* 2001. 33(7): p. 1081-9.

[36] Danner, M., et al., Association between depression and elevated C-reactive protein. *Psychosom Med,* 2003. 65(3): p. 347-56.

[37] Empana, J.P., et al., Contributions of depressive mood and circulating inflammatory markers to coronary heart disease in healthy European men: the Prospective Epidemiological Study of Myocardial Infarction (PRIME). *Circulation,* 2005. 111(18)· p. 2299-305.

[38] Winokur, A., et al., Insulin resistance after oral glucose tolerance testing in patients with major depression. *Am J Psychiatry,* 1988. 145(3): p. 325-30.

[39] Wright, J.H., et al., Glucose metabolism in unipolar depression. *Br J Psychiatry,* 1978. 132: p. 386-93.

[40] Hemingway, H., et al., Social and psychosocial influences on inflammatory markers and vascular function in civil servants (the Whitehall II study). *Am J Cardiol,* 2003. 92(8): p. 984-7.

[41] Sherwood, A., et al., Impaired endothelial function in coronary heart disease patients with depressive symptomatology. *J Am Coll Cardiol,* 2005. 46(4): p. 656-9.

[42] Schins, A., et al., Whole blood serotonin and platelet activation in depressed post-myocardial infarction patients. *Life Sci,* 2004. 76(6): p. 637-50.

[43] Whyte, E.M., et al., Influence of serotonin-transporter-linked promoter region polymorphism on platelet activation in geriatric depression. *Am J Psychiatry,* 2001. 158(12): p. 2074-6.

[44] Hughes, J.W., et al., Depression and anxiety symptoms are related to increased 24-hour urinary norepinephrine excretion among healthy middle-aged women. *J Psychosom Res,* 2004. 57(4): p. 353-8.

[45] Otte, C., et al., Depressive symptoms and 24-hour urinary norepinephrine excretion levels in patients with coronary disease: findings from the Heart and Soul Study. *Am J Psychiatry,* 2005. 162(11): p. 2139-45.

[46] Carney, R.M., K.E. Freedland, and R.C. Veith, Depression, the autonomic nervous system, and coronary heart disease. *Psychosom Med,* 2005. 67 Suppl 1: p. S29-33.

[47] Shen, B.J., et al., Anxiety characteristics independently and prospectively predict myocardial infarction in men the unique contribution of anxiety among psychologic factors. *J Am Coll Cardiol,* 2008. 51(2): p. 113-9.

[48] Shemesh, E., et al., Posttraumatic stress, nonadherence, and adverse outcome in survivors of a myocardial infarction. Psychosom Med, 2004. 66(4): p. 521-6.

[49] Dembroski, T.M., et al., Components of hostility as predictors of sudden death and myocardial infarction in the Multiple Risk Factor Intervention Trial. *Psychosom Med,* 1989. 51(5): p. 514-22.

[50] Welin, C., G. Lappas, and L. Wilhelmsen, Independent importance of psychosocial factors for prognosis after myocardial infarction. *J Intern Med,* 2000. 247(6): p. 629-39.

[51] Denollet, J., et al., Personality as independent predictor of long-term mortality in patients with coronary heart disease. *Lancet,* 1996. 347(8999): p. 417-21.

[52] Bankier, B., et al., Association between anxiety and C-reactive protein levels in stable coronary heart disease patients. *Psychosomatics,* 2009. 50(4): p. 347-53.

[53] Narita, K., et al., Interactions among higher trait anxiety, sympathetic activity, and endothelial function in the elderly. *J Psychiatr Res,* 2007. 41(5): p. 418-27.

[54] McGrady, A., et al., Effects of depression and anxiety on adherence to cardiac rehabilitation. *J Cardiopulm Rehabil Prev,* 2009. 29(6): p. 358-64.

[55] Narita, K., et al., The association between anger-related personality trait and cardiac autonomic response abnormalities in elderly subjects. *Eur Arch Psychiatry Clin Neurosci,* 2007. 257(6): p. 325-9.

[56] Goldbacher, E.M. and K.A. Matthews, Are psychological characteristics related to risk of the metabolic syndrome? A review of the literature. *Ann Behav Med,* 2007. 34(3): p. 240-52.

[57] Moynihan, J.A., Mechanisms of stress-induced modulation of immunity. *Brain Behav Immun,* 2003. 17 Suppl 1: p. S11-6.

[58] Lutgendorf, S.K., et al., Effects of acute stress, relaxation, and a neurogenic inflammatory stimulus on interleukin-6 in humans. *Brain Behav Immun,* 2004. 18(1): p. 55-64.

[59] Maes, M., et al., In humans, serum polyunsaturated fatty acid levels predict the response of proinflammatory cytokines to psychologic stress. *Biol Psychiatry,* 2000. 47(10): p. 910-20.

[60] Suls, J. and J. Bunde, Anger, anxiety, and depression as risk factors for cardiovascular disease: the problems and implications of overlapping affective dispositions. *Psychol Bull,* 2005. 131(2): p. 260-300.

[61] Strik, J.J., et al., Comparing symptoms of depression and anxiety as predictors of cardiac events and increased health care consumption after myocardial infarction. *J Am Coll Cardiol,* 2003. 42(10): p. 1801-7.

[62] Ketterer, M.W., et al., Five-year follow-up for adverse outcomes in males with at least minimally positive angiograms: importance of "denial" in assessing psychosocial risk factors. *J Psychosom Res,* 1998. 44(2): p. 241-50.

[63] Stewart, J.C., et al., Negative emotions and 3-year progression of subclinical atherosclerosis. *Arch Gen Psychiatry,* 2007. 64(2): p. 225-33.

[64] Kubzansky, L.D., et al., Shared and unique contributions of anger, anxiety, and depression to coronary heart disease: a prospective study in the normative aging study. *Ann Behav Med,* 2006. 31(1): p. 21-9.

[65] Rutledge, T., et al., Comorbid depression and anxiety symptoms as predictors of cardiovascular events: results from the NHLBI-sponsored Women's Ischemia Syndrome Evaluation (WISE) study. *Psychosom Med,* 2009. 71(9): p. 958-64.

[66] Wang, H.X., et al., Depressive symptoms, social isolation, and progression of coronary artery atherosclerosis: the Stockholm Female Coronary Angiography Study. *Psychother Psychosom,* 2006. 75(2): p. 96-102.

[67] Frasure-Smith, N., et al., Social support, depression, and mortality during the first year after myocardial infarction. *Circulation,* 2000. 101(16): p. 1919-24.

[68] Dickens, C.M., et al., Lack of a close confidant, but not depression, predicts further cardiac events after myocardial infarction. *Heart,* 2004. 90(5): p. 518-22.

[69] Effect of the antiarrhythmic agent moricizine on survival after myocardial infarction. The Cardiac Arrhythmia Suppression Trial II Investigators. *N Engl J Med,* 1992. 327(4): p. 227-33.

[70] Berkman, L.F., et al., Effects of treating depression and low perceived social support on clinical events after myocardial infarction: the Enhancing Recovery in Coronary Heart Disease Patients (ENRICHD) Randomized Trial. *Jama,* 2003. 289(23): p. 3106-16.

[71] Horsten, M., et al., Depressive symptoms and lack of social integration in relation to prognosis of CHD in middle-aged women. The Stockholm Female Coronary Risk Study. *Eur Heart J*, 2000. 21(13): p. 1072-80.

[72] Lett, H.S., et al., Social support and prognosis in patients at increased psychosocial risk recovering from myocardial infarction. *Health Psychol*, 2007. 26(4): p. 418-27.

[73] Berkman, L.F., L. Leo-Summers, and R.I. Horwitz, Emotional support and survival after myocardial infarction. A prospective, population-based study of the elderly. *Ann Intern Med*, 1992. 117(12): p. 1003-9.

[74] Lichtman, J.H., et al., Depression and coronary heart disease: recommendations for screening, referral, and treatment: a science advisory from the American Heart Association Prevention Committee of the Council on Cardiovascular Nursing, Council on Clinical Cardiology, Council on Epidemiology and Prevention, and Interdisciplinary Council on Quality of Care and Outcomes Research: endorsed by the American Psychiatric Association. *Circulation*, 2008. 118(17): p. 1768-75.

[75] Gorman, J.M. and J.M. Kent, SSRIs and SNRIs: broad spectrum of efficacy beyond major depression. *J Clin Psychiatry*, 1999. 60 Suppl 4: p. 33-8; discussion 39.

[76] Hoffman, E.J. and S.J. Mathew, Anxiety disorders: a comprehensive review of pharmacotherapies. *Mt Sinai J Med*, 2008. 75(3): p. 248-62.

[77] Fuller, R.W., The influence of fluoxetine on aggressive behavior. *Neuropsychopharmacology*, 1996. 14(2): p. 77-81.

[78] Thombs, B.D., et al., Probit structural equation regression model: general depressive symptoms predicted post-myocardial infarction mortality after controlling for somatic symptoms of depression. *J Clin Epidemiol*, 2008. 61(8): p. 832-9.

[79] Barefoot, J.C., et al., Depressive symptoms and survival of patients with coronary artery disease. *Psychosom Med*, 2000. 62(6): p. 790-5.

[80] Joiner, T.E., Jr., et al., Hopelessness depression as a distinct dimension of depressive symptoms among clinical and non-clinical samples. *Behav Res Ther*, 2001. 39(5): p. 523-36.

[81] McKenzie, D.P., et al., Pessimism, worthlessness, anhedonia, and thoughts of death identify DSM-IV major depression in hospitalized, medically ill patients. *Psychosomatics*, 2010. 51(4): p. 302-11.

[82] Leroy, M., G. Loas, and F. Perez-Diaz, Anhedonia as predictor of clinical events after acute coronary syndromes: a 3-year prospective study. *Compr Psychiatry*, 2010. 51(1): p. 8-14.

[83] Everson, S.A., et al., Hopelessness and risk of mortality and incidence of myocardial infarction and cancer. Psychosom Med, 1996. 58(2): p. 113-21.

[84] Frasure-Smith, N. and F. Lesperance, Depression and other psychological risks following myocardial infarction. *Arch Gen Psychiatry*, 2003. 60(6): p. 627-36.

[85] Hoen, P.W., et al., Differential associations between specific depressive symptoms and cardiovascular prognosis in patients with stable coronary heart disease. *J Am Coll Cardiol*, 2010. 56(11): p. 838-44.

[86] Linke, S.E., et al., Depressive symptom dimensions and cardiovascular prognosis among women with suspected myocardial ischemia: A report from the National Heart, Lung, and Blood Institute-sponsored Women's Ischemia Syndrome Evaluation. *Arch Gen Psychiatry*, 2009. 66(5): p. 499-507.

[87] de Jonge, P., et al., Symptom dimensions of depression following myocardial infarction and their relationship with somatic health status and cardiovascular prognosis. *Am J Psychiatry*, 2006. 163(1): p. 138-44.

[88] Martens, E.J., et al., Symptom dimensions of post-myocardial infarction depression, disease severity and cardiac prognosis. *Psychol Med*, 2010. 40(5): p. 807-14.

[89] de Jonge, P., D. Mangano, and M.A. Whooley, Differential association of cognitive and somatic depressive symptoms with heart rate variability in patients with stable coronary heart disease: findings from the Heart and Soul Study. *Psychosom Med,* 2007. 69(8): p. 735-9.

[90] Glassman, A.H., et al., Onset of major depression associated with acute coronary syndromes: relationship of onset, major depressive disorder history, and episode severity to sertraline benefit. *Arch Gen Psychiatry,* 2006. 63(3): p. 283-8.

[91] Lesperance, F., et al., Effects of citalopram and interpersonal psychotherapy on depression in patients with coronary artery disease: the Canadian Cardiac Randomized Evaluation of Antidepressant and Psychotherapy Efficacy (CREATE) trial. *JAMA,* 2007. 297(4): p. 367-79.

[92] Glassman, A.H., J.T. Bigger, Jr., and M. Gaffney, Psychiatric characteristics associated with long-term mortality among 361 patients having an acute coronary syndrome and major depression: seven-year follow-up of SADHART participants. *Arch Gen Psychiatry,* 2009. 66(9): p. 1022-9.

[93] Dickens, C., et al., Depression is a risk factor for mortality after myocardial infarction: fact or artifact? *J Am Coll Cardiol,* 2007. 49(18): p. 1834-40.

[94] Parker, G., et al., Specificity of depression following an acute coronary syndrome to an adverse outcome extends over five years. *Psychiatry Res,* 2010.

[95] de Jonge, P., et al., Only incident depressive episodes after myocardial infarction are associated with new cardiovascular events. *J Am Coll Cardiol,* 2006. 48(11): p. 2204-8.

[96] Carney, R.M., et al., History of depression and survival after acute myocardial infarction. *Psychosom Med,* 2009. 71(3): p. 253-9.

[97] Grace, S.L., et al., Effect of depression on five-year mortality after an acute coronary syndrome. *Am J Cardiol,* 2005. 96(9): p. 1179-85.

[98] Lesperance, F., N. Frasure-Smith, and M. Talajic, Major depression before and after myocardial infarction: its nature and consequences. *Psychosom Med,* 1996. 58(2): p. 99-110.

[99] Kaptein, K.I., et al., Course of depressive symptoms after myocardial infarction and cardiac prognosis: a latent class analysis. Psychosom Med, 2006. 68(5): p. 662-8.

[100] de Jonge, P., et al., Nonresponse to treatment for depression following myocardial infarction: association with subsequent cardiac events. *Am J Psychiatry,* 2007. 164(9): p. 1371-8.

[101] Lesperance, F., et al., Five-year risk of cardiac mortality in relation to initial severity and one-year changes in depression symptoms after myocardial infarction. *Circulation,* 2002. 105(9): p. 1049-53.

[102] Carney, R.M., et al., Depression and late mortality after myocardial infarction in the Enhancing Recovery in Coronary Heart Disease (ENRICHD) study. *Psychosom Med,* 2004. 66(4): p. 466-74.

[103] Milani, R.V. and C.J. Lavie, Impact of cardiac rehabilitation on depression and its associated mortality. *Am J Med,* 2007. 120(9): p. 799-806.

[104] Carney, R.M. and K.E. Freedland, Treatment-resistant depression and mortality after acute coronary syndrome. *Am J Psychiatry,* 2009. 166(4): p. 410-7.

[105] AAFP guideline for the detection and management of post-myocardial infarction depression. *Ann Fam Med,* 2009. 7(1): p. 71-9.

[106] Ziegelstein, R.C., et al., Routine screening for depression in patients with coronary heart disease never mind. *J Am Coll Cardiol,* 2009. 54(10): p. 886-90.

[107] Thombs, B.D., R.C. Ziegelstein, and M.A. Whooley, Optimizing detection of major depression among patients with coronary artery disease using the patient health

questionnaire: data from the heart and soul study. *J Gen Intern Med,* 2008. 23(12): p. 2014-7.

[108] Stafford, L., M. Berk, and H.J. Jackson, Validity of the Hospital Anxiety and Depression Scale and Patient Health Questionnaire-9 to screen for depression in patients with coronary artery disease. *Gen Hosp Psychiatry,* 2007. 29(5): p. 417-24.

[109] Thombs, B.D., et al., Performance characteristics of depression screening instruments in survivors of acute myocardial infarction: review of the evidence. *Psychosomatics,* 2007. 48(3): p. 185-94.

[110] Balady, G.J., et al., Core components of cardiac rehabilitation/secondary prevention programs: 2007 update: a scientific statement from the American Heart Association Exercise, Cardiac Rehabilitation, and Prevention Committee, the Council on Clinical Cardiology; the Councils on Cardiovascular Nursing, Epidemiology and Prevention, and Nutrition, Physical Activity, and Metabolism; and the American Association of Cardiovascular and Pulmonary Rehabilitation. *Circulation,* 2007. 115(20): p. 2675-82.

[111] Beckie, T.M., J.W. Beckstead, and M.W. Groer, The influence of cardiac rehabilitation on inflammation and metabolic syndrome in women with coronary heart disease. *J Cardiovasc Nurs,* 2010. 25(1): p. 52-60.

[112] Artham, S.M., C.J. Lavie, and R.V. Milani, Cardiac rehabilitation programs markedly improve high-risk profiles in coronary patients with high psychological distress. *South Med J,* 2008. 101(3): p. 262-7.

[113] Appels, A., et al., Effects of treating exhaustion in angioplasty patients on new coronary events: results of the randomized Exhaustion Intervention Trial (EXIT). *Psychosom Med,* 2005. 67(2): p. 217-23.

[114] Appels, A., et al., Effects of a behavioural intervention on quality of life and related variables in angioplasty patients: results of the EXhaustion Intervention Trial. *J Psychosom Res,* 2006. 61(1): p. 1-7; discussion 9-10.

[115] Sebregts, E.H., et al., Psychological effects of a short behavior modification program in patients with acute myocardial infarction or coronary artery bypass grafting. A randomized controlled trial. *J Psychosom Res,* 2005. 58(5): p. 417-24.

[116] Jolliffe, J.A., et al., Exercise-based rehabilitation for coronary heart disease. *Cochrane Database Syst Rev,* 2001(1): p. CD001800.

[117] Vizza, J., et al., Improvement in psychosocial functioning during an intensive cardiovascular lifestyle modification program. *J Cardiopulm Rehabil Prev,* 2007. 27(6): p. 376-83; quiz 384-5.

[118] Ornish, D., et al., Intensive lifestyle changes for reversal of coronary heart disease. *JAMA,* 1998. 280(23): p. 2001-7.

[119] Pischke, C.R., et al., Long-term effects of lifestyle changes on well-being and cardiac variables among coronary heart disease patients. *Health Psychol,* 2008. 27(5): p. 584-92.

[120] Daubenmier, J.J., et al., The contribution of changes in diet, exercise, and stress management to changes in coronary risk in women and men in the multisite cardiac lifestyle intervention program. *Ann Behav Med,* 2007. 33(1): p. 57-68.

[121] Thompson, P.D., et al., Exercise and physical activity in the prevention and treatment of atherosclerotic cardiovascular disease: a statement from the Council on Clinical Cardiology (Subcommittee on Exercise, Rehabilitation, and Prevention) and the Council on Nutrition, Physical Activity, and Metabolism (Subcommittee on Physical Activity). *Circulation,* 2003. 107(24): p. 3109-16.

[122] Fraker, T.D., Jr., et al., 2007 chronic angina focused update of the ACC/AHA 2002 Guidelines for the management of patients with chronic stable angina: a report of the American College of Cardiology/American Heart Association Task Force on Practice

Guidelines Writing Group to develop the focused update of the 2002 Guidelines for the management of patients with chronic stable angina. *Circulation,* 2007. 116(23): p. 2762-72.

[123] Babyak, M., et al., Exercise treatment for major depression: maintenance of therapeutic benefit at 10 months. *Psychosom Med,* 2000. 62(5): p. 633-8.

[124] Group, P.A.G.W., 2008 Physical Activity Guidelines for Americans. *US Department of Health and Human Services,* 2008.

[125] Mead, G.E., et al., Exercise for depression. *Cochrane Database Syst Rev,* 2009(3): p. CD004366.

[126] Scherrer, J.F., et al., Antidepressant drug compliance: reduced risk of MI and mortality in depressed patients. *Am J Med,* 2011. 124(4): p. 318-24.

[127] Blumenthal, J.A., et al., Exercise, depression, and mortality after myocardial infarction in the ENRICHD trial. *Med Sci Sports Exerc,* 2004. 36(5): p. 746-55.

[128] Burg, M.M., et al., Presurgical depression predicts medical morbidity 6 months after coronary artery bypass graft surgery. *Psychosom Med,* 2003. 65(1): p. 111-8.

[129] Peterson, J.C., et al., New postoperative depressive symptoms and long-term cardiac outcomes after coronary artery bypass surgery. *Am J Geriatr Psychiatry,* 2002. 10(2): p. 192-8.

[130] Connerney, I., et al., Relation between depression after coronary artery bypass surgery and 12-month outcome: a prospective study. Lancet, 2001. 358(9295): p. 1766-71.

[131] Connerney, I., et al., Depression is associated with increased mortality 10 years after coronary artery bypass surgery. *Psychosom Med,* 2010. 72(9): p. 874-81.

[132] Rowland, L.P., T.A. Pedley, and W. Kneass, Merritt's neurology. 12th ed. 2010, *Philadelphia: Wolters Kluwer Lippincott Williams & Wilkins.* xxi, 1172 p.

[133] Newman, M.F., et al., Longitudinal assessment of neurocognitive function after coronary-artery bypass surgery. *N Engl J Med,* 2001. 344(6): p. 395-402.

[134] Gottesman, R.F., et al., Delirium after coronary artery bypass graft surgery and late mortality. *Ann Neurol,* 2010. 67(3): p. 338-44.

[135] Serebruany, V.L., Selective serotonin reuptake inhibitors and increased bleeding risk: are we missing something? *Am J Med,* 2006. 119(2): p. 113-6.

[136] Movig, K.L., et al., Relationship of serotonergic antidepressants and need for blood transfusion in orthopedic surgical patients. *Arch Intern Med,* 2003. 163(19): p. 2354-8.

[137] Andreasen, J.J., et al., Effect of selective serotonin reuptake inhibitors on requirement for allogeneic red blood cell transfusion following coronary artery bypass surgery. *Am J Cardiovasc Drugs,* 2006. 6(4): p. 243-50.

[138] Wellenius, G.A., et al., Depressive symptoms and the risk of atherosclerotic progression among patients with coronary artery bypass grafts. *Circulation,* 2008. 117(18): p. 2313-9.

[139] Rollman, B.L., et al., Telephone-delivered collaborative care for treating post-CABG depression: a randomized controlled trial. *JAMA,* 2009. 302(19): p. 2095-103.

[140] Burton, R. and H. Jackson, The anatomy of melancholy. *New York Review Books classics.* 2001, New York: New York Review of Books. xxx, 523, 312, 547 p.

[141] Frasure-Smith, N., et al., Randomised trial of home-based psychosocial nursing intervention for patients recovering from myocardial infarction. *Lancet,* 1997. 350(9076): p. 473-9.

[142] Frasure-Smith, N., et al., Long-term survival differences among low-anxious, high-anxious and repressive copers enrolled in the Montreal heart attack readjustment trial. *Psychosom Med,* 2002. 64(4): p. 571-9.

[143] Cossette, S., N. Frasure-Smith, and F. Lesperance, Clinical implications of a reduction in psychological distress on cardiac prognosis in patients participating in a psychosocial intervention program. *Psychosom Med,* 2001. 63(2): p. 257-66.

[144] Denollet, J., et al., Clinical events in coronary patients who report low distress: adverse effect of repressive coping. *Health Psychol,* 2008. 27(3): p. 302-8.

[145] Shaw, R.E., et al., The impact of denial and repressive style on information gain and rehabilitation outcomes in myocardial infarction patients. *Psychosom Med,* 1985. 47(3): p. 262-73.

[146] Myers, L.B., The importance of the repressive coping style: findings from 30 years of research. *Anxiety Stress Coping,* 2010. 23(1): p. 3-17.

[147] Saab, P.G., et al., The impact of cognitive behavioral group training on event-free survival in patients with myocardial infarction: the ENRICHD experience. *J Psychosom Res,* 2009. 67(1): p. 45-56.

[148] Sotsky, S.M., et al., Patient predictors of response to psychotherapy and pharmacotherapy: findings in the NIMH Treatment of Depression Collaborative Research Program. *Am J Psychiatry,* 1991. 148(8): p. 997-1008.

[149] Burg, M.M., et al., Treating persistent depressive symptoms in post-ACS patients: the project COPES phase-I randomized controlled trial. *Contemp Clin Trials,* 2008. 29(2): p. 231-40.

[150] Unutzer, J., et al., Collaborative care management of late-life depression in the primary care setting: a randomized controlled trial. *JAMA,* 2002. 288(22): p. 2836-45.

[151] Davidson, K.W., et al., Enhanced depression care for patients with acute coronary syndrome and persistent depressive symptoms: coronary psychosocial evaluation studies randomized controlled trial. *Arch Intern Med,* 2010. 170(7): p. 600-8.

[152] Roose, S.P., et al., Comparison of paroxetine and nortriptyline in depressed patients with ischemic heart disease. *JAMA,* 1998. 279(4): p. 287-91.

[153] Habra, M.E., et al., First episode of major depressive disorder and vascular factors in coronary artery disease patients: Baseline characteristics and response to antidepressant treatment in the CREATE trial. *J Psychosom Res,* 2010. 69(2): p. 133-41.

[154] Glassman, A.H., et al., Sertraline treatment of major depression in patients with acute MI or unstable angina. *JAMA,* 2002. 288(6): p. 701-9.

[155] Strik, J.J., et al., Efficacy and safety of fluoxetine in the treatment of patients with major depression after first myocardial infarction: findings from a double-blind, placebo-controlled trial. *Psychosom Med,* 2000. 62(6): p. 783-9.

[156] Honig, A., et al., Treatment of post-myocardial infarction depressive disorder: a randomized, placebo-controlled trial with mirtazapine. *Psychosom Med,* 2007. 69(7): p. 606-13.

[157] Stevenson, B.E., The home book of verse, American and English, 1580-1912. 1912, New York,: H. Holt and company. lxxv, 3742 p.

[158] Glassman, A.H., Cardiovascular effects of antidepressant drugs: updated. *J Clin Psychiatry,* 1998. 59 Suppl 15: p. 13-8.

[159] Rivelli, S. and W. Jiang, Depression and ischemic heart disease: what have we learned from clinical trials? *Curr Opin Cardiol,* 2007. 22(4): p. 286-91.

[160] Jiang, W. and J.R. Davidson, Antidepressant therapy in patients with ischemic heart disease. *Am Heart J,* 2005. 150(5): p. 871-81.

[161] Roose, S.P. and M. Miyazaki, Pharmacologic treatment of depression in patients with heart disease. *Psychosom Med,* 2005. 67 Suppl 1: p. S54-7.

[162] Ovsiew, F. and R.L. Munich, *Principles of inpatient psychiatry.* 2009, Philadelphia: Lippincott Williams and Wilkins. xiv, 383 p.

[163] Gaudron, P., et al., Progressive left ventricular dysfunction and remodeling after myocardial infarction. Potential mechanisms and early predictors. *Circulation,* 1993. 87(3): p. 755-63.

[164] Whang, W., et al., Depression and risk of sudden cardiac death and coronary heart disease in women: results from the Nurses' Health Study. *J Am Coll Cardiol,* 2009. 53(11): p. 950-8.

[165] Krantz, D.S., et al., Psychotropic medication use and risk of adverse cardiovascular events in women with suspected coronary artery disease: outcomes from the Women's Ischemia Syndrome Evaluation (WISE) study. *Heart,* 2009. 95(23): p. 1901-6.

[166] Smoller, J.W., et al., Antidepressant use and risk of incident cardiovascular morbidity and mortality among postmenopausal women in the Women's Health Initiative study. *Arch Intern Med,* 2009. 169(22): p. 2128-39.

[167] Ferketich, A.K., et al., Depression as an antecedent to heart disease among women and men in the NHANES I study. National Health and Nutrition Examination Survey. *Arch Intern Med,* 2000. 160(9): p. 1261-8.

[168] Penninx, B.W., et al., Depression and cardiac mortality: results from a community-based longitudinal study. *Arch Gen Psychiatry,* 2001. 58(3): p. 221-7.

[169] Taylor, C.B., et al., Effects of antidepressant medication on morbidity and mortality in depressed patients after myocardial infarction. *Arch Gen Psychiatry,* 2005. 62(7): p. 792-8.

[170] Michael E Thase, M., *Kaplan & Sadock's comprehensive textbook of psychiatry.* 9th ed, ed. B.J. Sadock, et al. Vol. II. 2009, Philadelphia: Wolters Kluwer Health/Lippincott Williams & Wilkins. 2 v. (lix, 4520, I-138 p.).

[171] Charles DeBattista D.M.H., M.D. and A.F.S. M.D., Kaplan & Sadock's comprehensive textbook of psychiatry. 9th ed, ed. B.J. Sadock, et al. Vol. II. 2009, Philadelphia: Wolters Kluwer Health/Lippincott Williams & Wilkins. 2 v. (lix, 4520, I-138 p.).

[172] Sadock, B.J., et al., Kaplan & Sadock's comprehensive textbook of psychiatry. 9th ed. 2009, Philadelphia: Wolters Kluwer/Lippincott Williams & Wilkins. 2 v. (li, 4520, I-138 p.), [16] p. of plates.

[173] Julius, S., Corcoran Lecture. Sympathetic hyperactivity and coronary risk in hypertension. *Hypertension,* 1993. 21(6 Pt 2): p. 886-93.

[174] Sabbah, H.N., Biologic rationale for the use of beta-blockers in the treatment of heart failure. *Heart Fail Rev,* 2004. 9(2): p. 91-7.

[175] Kendall, M.J., Clinical trial data on the cardioprotective effects of beta-blockade. Basic Res Cardiol, 2000. 95 Suppl 1: p. I25-30.

[176] Hjalmarson, A., Effects of beta blockade on sudden cardiac death during acute myocardial infarction and the postinfarction period. *Am J Cardiol,* 1997. 80(9B): p. 35J-39J.

[177] Mayer, A.F., et al., Influences of norepinephrine transporter function on the distribution of sympathetic activity in humans. *Hypertension,* 2006. 48(1): p. 120-6.

[178] Rigotti, N.A., et al., Bupropion for smokers hospitalized with acute cardiovascular disease. *Am J Med,* 2006. 119(12): p. 1080-7.

[179] Frankenstein, L., et al., Prevalence and prognostic significance of adrenergic escape during chronic beta-blocker therapy in chronic heart failure. Eur J Heart Fail, 2009. 11(2): p. 178-84.

[180] Narayan, S.M. and M.B. Stein, Do depression or antidepressants increase cardiovascular mortality? The absence of proof might be more important than the proof of absence. *J Am Coll Cardiol,* 2009. 53(11): p. 959-61.

[181] O'Connor, C. and M. Fiuzat, Antidepressant Use, Depression, and Poor Cardiovascular Outcomes: The Chicken or the Egg?: Comment on "Antidepressant Use and Risk of

Incident Cardiovascular Morbidity and Mortality Among Postmenopausal Women in the Women's Health Initiative Study". *Arch Intern Med,* 2009. 169(22): p. 2140-1.

[182] Jolly, K. and M.J. Langman, Psychotropic medication: curing illness or creating problems? *Heart,* 2009. 95(23): p. 1893-4.

[183] Gunasekara, N.S., S. Noble, and P. Benfield, Paroxetine. An update of its pharmacology and therapeutic use in depression and a review of its use in other disorders. *Drugs,* 1998. 55(1): p. 85-120.

[184] Parker, G., et al., Omega-3 fatty acids and mood disorders. *Am J Psychiatry,* 2006. 163(6): p. 969-78.

[185] Dolecek, T.A., Epidemiological evidence of relationships between dietary polyunsaturated fatty acids and mortality in the multiple risk factor intervention trial. *Proc Soc Exp Biol Med,* 1992. 200(2): p. 177-82.

[186] Ali, S., et al., Association between omega-3 fatty acids and depressive symptoms among patients with established coronary artery disease: data from the Heart and Soul Study. *Psychother Psychosom,* 2009. 78(2): p. 125-7.

[187] Harper, C.R. and T.A. Jacobson, The fats of life: the role of omega-3 fatty acids in the prevention of coronary heart disease. Arch Intern Med, 2001. 161(18): p. 2185-92.

[188] Freeman, M.P., et al., Complementary and alternative medicine in major depressive disorder: the American Psychiatric Association Task Force report. J Clin Psychiatry, 2010. 71(6): p. 669-81.

[189] Carney, R.M., et al., Effect of omega-3 fatty acids on heart rate variability in depressed patients with coronary heart disease. Psychosom Med, 2010. 72(8): p. 748-54.

[190] Carney, R.M., et al., Omega-3 augmentation of sertraline in treatment of depression in patients with coronary heart disease: a randomized controlled trial. *JAMA,* 2009. 302(15): p. 1651-7.

[191] Goldberg, R.J., Selective serotonin reuptake inhibitors: infrequent medical adverse effects. *Arch Fam Med,* 1998. 7(1): p. 78-84.

[192] Goodman, L.S., et al., Goodman & Gilman's the pharmacological basis of therapeutics. 11th ed. 2006, New York: McGraw-Hill. xxiii, 2021 p.

[193] Blumenthal, J.A., et al., Understanding prognostic benefits of exercise and antidepressant therapy for persons with depression and heart disease: the UPBEAT study--rationale, design, and methodological issues. *Clin Trials,* 2007. 4(5): p. 548-59.

[194] Burton, N.W., K.I. Pakenham, and W.J. Brown, Feasibility and effectiveness of psychosocial resilience training: a pilot study of the READY program. *Psychol Health Med,* 2010. 15(3): p. 266-77.

[195] Cacioppo, J.T., et al., Autonomic, neuroendocrine, and immune responses to psychological stress: the reactivity hypothesis. *Ann N Y Acad Sci,* 1998. 840: p. 664-73.

[196] Klatt, M.D., J. Buckworth, and W.B. Malarkey, Effects of low-dose mindfulness-based stress reduction (MBSR-ld) on working adults. *Health Educ Behav,* 2009. 36(3): p. 601-14.

[197] Witek-Janusek, L., et al., Effect of mindfulness based stress reduction on immune function, quality of life and coping in women newly diagnosed with early stage breast cancer. *Brain Behav Immun,* 2008. 22(6): p. 969-81.

[198] Tang, Y.Y., et al., Short-term meditation training improves attention and self-regulation. Proc Natl Acad Sci U S A, 2007. 104(43): p. 17152-6.

[199] Carlson, L.E., et al., One year pre-post intervention follow-up of psychological, immune, endocrine and blood pressure outcomes of mindfulness-based stress reduction (MBSR) in breast and prostate cancer outpatients. Brain Behav Immun, 2007. 21(8): p. 1038-49.

[200] Takahashi, T., et al., Changes in EEG and autonomic nervous activity during meditation and their association with personality traits. *Int J Psychophysiol,* 2005. 55(2): p. 199-207.

[201] Bohlmeijer, E., et al., The effects of mindfulness-based stress reduction therapy on mental health of adults with a chronic medical disease: a meta-analysis. *J Psychosom Res,* 2010. 68(6): p. 539-44.

[202] Zeidan, F., et al., Effects of brief and sham mindfulness meditation on mood and cardiovascular variables. *J Altern Complement Med,* 2010. 16(8): p. 867-73.

[203] Olivo, E.L., et al., Feasibility and effectiveness of a brief meditation-based stress management intervention for patients diagnosed with or at risk for coronary heart disease: a pilot study. *Psychol Health Med,* 2009. 14(5): p. 513-23.

[204] Sullivan, M.J., et al., The Support, Education, and Research in Chronic Heart Failure Study (SEARCH): a mindfulness-based psychoeducational intervention improves depression and clinical symptoms in patients with chronic heart failure. *Am Heart J,* 2009. 157(1): p. 84-90.

[205] Katon, W.J., The Institute of Medicine "Chasm" report: implications for depression collaborative care models. *Gen Hosp Psychiatry,* 2003. 25(4): p. 222-9.

[206] Meyer, F., J. Peteet, and R. Joseph, Models of care for co-occurring mental and medical disorders. *Harv Rev Psychiatry*, 2009. 17(6): p. 353-60.

[207] Bower, P., et al., Collaborative care for depression in primary care. Making sense of a complex intervention: systematic review and meta-regression. *Br J Psychiatry,* 2006. 189: p. 484-93.

[208] Gilbody, S., et al., Collaborative care for depression: a cumulative meta-analysis and review of longer-term outcomes. *Arch Intern Med,* 2006. 166(21): p. 2314-21.

[209] Katon, W.J., et al., Collaborative care for patients with depression and chronic illnesses. *N Engl J Med,* 2010. 363(27): p. 2611-20.

In: Current Advances in Cardiovascular Risk. Volume 2   ISBN: 978-1-62081-746-9
Editor: Sandeep Ajoy Saha   © 2012 Nova Science Publishers, Inc.

Chapter XXII

Cardiovascular Risk Factors and Their Management in Bipolar Disorder (BD) and Schizophrenic Spectrum Illness (SSI)

James L. Megna[1], Mariela Rojas[1], Shilpa Sachdeva[1],
Robert Nastasi[1], Umar A. Siddiqui[1],
Thomas L. Schwartz[1] and Roger S. McIntyre[2]*

[1]Psychiatry Department, SUNY Upstate Medical University.
Syracuse, NY, US
[2]Psychiatry Dept. University of Toronto University Health Network.
Toronto, Canada

Abstract

Introduction: Cardiovascular risk factors are quite prevalent in the general population, but they are especially so in patients with serious and persistent mental illness [SPMI] (BD and SSI). This contributes significantly to the morbidity and mortality of the group.

Methods: An extensive literature search was conducted with the following keywords: obesity, hypertension, diabetes mellitus type II, dyslipidemias, metabolic syndrome, atypical antipsychotics, mood stabilizers, antidepressants, and SPMI (BD and SSI).

Results: The rates of obesity, hypertension, diabetes mellitus type II, dyslipidemias and metabolic syndrome are almost twice as high in individuals with BD and SSI compared with individuals from the general population. This contributes to the more than doubled risk of mortality from cardiovascular disease in the SPMI population. There is some evidence that obesity is the core problem in this group of patients, such that hypertension, dyslipidemias, DM type II and metabolic syndrome will ultimately develop

* Corresponding Author: Dr James L. Megna Psychiatry Department, SUNY Upstate Medical University. 750 East Adams Street, Syracuse, NY13210, USA. TEL: 315 464-3100 ; FAX: 315 464-3163, Email: megnaj@upstate.edu.

as a result. However, direct effects of psychotropic medications (i.e., not via weight gain) on glucose metabolism have been observed. There are both non-pharmacologic and pharmacologic factors that contribute to the problem of increased cardiovascular risk. Examples of non-pharmacologic factors include biologic (certain receptors[5HT2C, H1], genetic polymorphisms, baseline insulin resistance) and non-biologic factors (e.g.,life-style [activity level, smoking, food choices], health system factors, childhood trauma, diminished concern over body weight). Pharmacologic factors include atypical antipsychotics, mood stabilizers, and antidepressants. A number of interventions has been attempted to reduce the development of cardiovascular risk factors. Monitoring strategies such as checking baseline lipid profiles and serum glucose have produced very small effects, predominately because of under-usage by psychiatrists. However, evidence-based weight reduction strategies, both pharmacologic and non-pharmacologic, have produced effect sizes into the moderate range with non-pharmacologic interventions showing a slight superiority. Unfortunately, the interventions studied were not of long duration, and it is not clear if the weight reductions were maintained after study completion. In addition, an unanswered question is when to begin such weight loss intervention strategies (as primary or secondary treatments). Based upon the extant literature we recommend the following approach for minimizing cardiovascular risk factors: checking family history and past medical history, judicious prescribing of weight increasing medications, checking vital signs, lipid profile, EKG, waist circumference and body weight (at baseline and at regular intervals thereafter). Unfortunately, there are no good long term data on the effects of these interventions on the incidence of developing cardiovascular risk factors, as well as the effect on mortality for patients with BD and SSI.

Conclusion: While there have been some successes in reducing the development of cardiovascular risk factors, at least in the short term, there is a great need for longer term follow-up studies to assess the impact of recommended interventions on cardiovascular risk factor development, quality of life, and mortality.

Introduction

Cardiovascular risk factors are prevalent and increasing in the general population. This is especially so in individuals with serious and persistent mental illness (SPMI) and contributes significantly to the morbidity and mortality of this group [1].

Patients with schizophrenia are known to have a 20% shorter life expectancy (age 61 yrs) than that of the general U.S. population. Individuals with bipolar disorder as well as individuals with schizophrenia, incur an increase in health service utilization and public assistance. [2] Medical conditions such as hyperlipidemia, hypertension, obesity, and diabetes mellitus are factors that contribute to shortened life expectancy and greater demand of medical resources; more recently, this constellation of medical illnesses has been qualified as metabolic syndrome. [3-5] Cardiovascular disease is the leading cause of premature deaths in patients with chronic mental illness (schizophrenia and bipolar disorder), [6]accounting for 50-75% of deaths in this patient population, twice as high as that of the general population. [7].

Obesity rates (BMI >30) in the U.S. are estimated at 30%. [8] Individuals with bipolar (Type I)disorder and schizophrenia are found to have rates of 32% and 42%, respectively. [9, 10]More specifically, schizophrenia and bipolar patients are shown to have an increase in visceral fat when compared to control patients. [5, 9, 11] The accumulation of visceral fat is associated with an increased risk for insulin resistance, type 2 diabetes mellitus, and metabolic syndrome. [12] Ryan et al. report that schizophrenia and bipolar disorder may be independent risk factors for developing diabetes mellitus [13].

The lifetime risk of developing diabetes for people born in the United States after 2000 is estimated at 32.8% for men and 38.5% for women, with current rates of detected diabetes at 6.9%. [14] While there is a paucity of recent studies forecasting trends in patients with psychiatric illness, at present, detected rates are as high as 15% for patients with bipolar disorder and schizophrenia. [15, 16].

Hypertension (30%) and hyperlipidemia (28%) are found more commonly in the chronically mental ill patient population than the general U.S. population. [17] Elevations of cholesterol and triglyceride levels are associated with ischemic heart disease, coronary artery disease and myocardial infarction. [18] Cerebrovascular accidents (CVA) are found to be more common in the bipolar patient population than the general U.S. population (4.8%). [15].

Metabolic syndrome, characterized by three or more of the following: abdominal obesity, elevated triglycerides, lower plasma levels of high density lipoprotein –cholesterol (HDL), elevated blood pressure, and elevated fasting plasma glucose is estimated at 25% of the United States population. [19] The rate of metabolic syndrome in schizophrenia and bipolar patients is 40.9% and 30%, respectively. [20, 21].

Contributing Factors

Mechanisms accounting for the risk of metabolic syndrome and its individual components, and for cardiovascular disease (CVD) risk, in patients with SPMI are multifactorial and can be classified as non-pharmacologic and pharmacologic. The first category comprises biologic and non-biologic factors, such as those related to the psychiatric disease itself and to life style often attributed to SPMI patients. Health-related behaviors, pathophysiological changes, access and content of medical care can all influence the onset or worsening in the example of coronary heart disease [22]. Psychotropic medications can also interact with these non-pharmacologic factors but can also directly induce metabolic disturbances and increase the cardiovascular risk in this group of patients. [23] The information that follows will attempt to simplify what is known about these complex interactions.

Non-Pharmacologic

It is hypothesized that patients with SPMI have baseline metabolic disturbances that might be related to the psychiatric diagnosis itself and are present even before starting treatment. Indeed, there is evidence supporting this from studies including cohorts of neuroleptic-naïve or first episode schizophrenia patients (and, in some, their family members). Fewer studies have been completed with bipolar disorder patients during the first manic episode [24] However, sample sizes and methodological difficulties limit the power and reliability of some of these studies. Schizophrenia had been clearly associated with diabetes and abnormal glucose metabolism before the neuroleptic era [25-27], although, at the time, problems with diagnosis, small study sample size and other methodological problems, make it difficult to draw definitive conclusions. Taken together, the findings suggest that interactions among environmental, lifestyle, genetics, or disease-related factors could account, at least in part, for the metabolic abnormalities observed in patients with SPMI. The issue of weight gain and metabolic disorder clearly began before the invention of the atypical antipsychotic class of medications.

In one particular study, patients with newly diagnosed, non-affective psychosis who were antipsychotic-naïve (n=50) were compared with matched controls (n=50) for 2 hours glucose tolerance testing. Fasting concentrations of adiponectin, interleukin-6 and C-reactive protein were also assessed, since these are considered markers associated with an increased risk of diabetes. The authors found a significant difference in 2h serum glucose between the two groups, with mean concentrations of 111 mg/dl (s.d.=35.2) in the psychosis group and 82 mg/dl (s.d.=19.3) in the control group (p<0.001). This impaired glucose tolerance and/or diabetes was present in 16% of the psychosis group and in 0% of the control group (p=0.003). Also significantly different was the percentage of people with abnormal interleukin-6 (23% vs 8% in the psychosis and control group, respectively; p=0.012), but no differences were found in the levels of C-reactive protein or adiponectin. The differences could not be attributed to confounding factors, including BMI, gender, age, psychotropic medications, cortisol concentration, socioeconomic status, smoking, aerobic conditioning, or drugs that affect glucose tolerance. The results suggest an association between schizophrenia and diabetes that is not dependent on medication. [28]

In a smaller study, mean insulin sensitivity index was 42% lower in a cohort of nine schizophrenia patients (7 drug naïve and 2 out of antipsychotic treatment for more than a year) compared to nine matched controls (p=0.026), suggesting baseline insulin resistance and susceptibility to type 2 diabetes inherent to schizophrenia. Furthermore, the patient group not only displayed insulin resistance but also a failed compensation in insulin secretion needed to maintain glucose disposal in the setting of their reduced insulin sensitivity. Adiponectin levels were also studied and there was no significant difference between the two groups [29]. In a cohort of drug-naïve schizophrenia subjects (n=99) affected with first-episode psychosis (FEP), patients had higher fasting 2-hour plasma glucose levels, compared with matched healthy control subjects (p=0.002). [30] Another study found that neuroleptic naïve schizophrenia patients (n=44), compared to matched controls, had significantly higher mean plasma insulin levels that were independent of hypercortisolemia (p=0.039), significantly higher insulin resistance scores (p=0.039), and significantly lower levels of insulin-like growth factor-1 (IGF-1) (p=0.026) , an essential factor for optimal insulin sensitivity, suggesting that deficient IGF-1 might underlie baseline insulin resistance in schizophrenia. [31] Hepatic insulin resistance was also linked to schizophrenia in a smaller study of a cohort of seven neuroleptic-naïve schizophrenia and schizoaffective disordered patients who were FEP. It was found that they had a significantly greater endogenous glucose production during a hyperinsulinemic-euglycemic clamp procedure compared to matched controls (p=0.02). The hepatic insulin resistance could not be attributed to an increased visceral fat mass or differences in plasma free fatty acids (FFAs), plasma adiponectin, glucoregulatory hormones, or plasma retinol-binding protein 4 concentrations. [32] Another large study detected that drug-naïve patients with FEP (n=166) had a significantly elevated incidence of type 2 diabetes (p=0.007) compared to matched healthy controls even though controls had a significantly higher body mass index (p<0.05) and plasma LDL cholesterol levels (p=0.01). [33].

Studies have also been completed investigating the first-degree relatives of schizophrenia patients. One of these studies evaluated differences in a glucose tolerance test between first-degree non-affected siblings of schizophrenia patients (n=6) and matched controls (n=12). Although the sample sizes were small, they did find a significantly increased (p<0.03) two hour postprandial mean glucose concentration in the sibling group (100.5 mg/dl, s.d. 27.7) compared to the control group (78 mg/dl, s.d.12.3) and the differences could not be attributed to confounding factors. The authors suggested the presence of shared familial risk factors between schizophrenia and diabetes, but recommended confirmation with larger samples. [34] Another study compared the results of the oral glucose tolerance test among 38 non-obese drug-naïve first episode schizophrenia patients, 44 non-obese first degree unaffected relatives, and 38 matched controls, finding an impaired glucose tolerance in 10.5% of patients, 18.2% of relatives, and none of the controls (p<0.001). Both patients and relatives had significantly higher levels of insulin in fasting (p<0.01) and at two hours postprandial (p<0.001), and had significantly higher scores of insulin resistance (p<0.05) compared with control subjects. These differences were independent of BMI, saturated and unsaturated fat intake, fiber intake, exercise level, or cortisol levels. These findings again point to a possible shared environmental or genetic predisposition to impaired glucose tolerance in the absence of pharmacological management. [35] Finally, a cross sectional study of patients with bipolar disorder, psychotropic-naïve subjects (n=70) were compared to 114 who were previously treated via medication. No significant differences were found in metabolic parameters of BMI, fasting plasma glucose (including patients on anti-diabetic medication) or cholesterol abnormality (including those on a cholesterol lowering agent. [36].

There are also studies suggesting a genetic overlap among diabetes, schizophrenia, and bipolar disorder. Genetic linkage studies have identified multiple chromosomal regions associated with both schizophrenia and diabetes type 2. [26] It is hypothesized that these two diseases might share a DNA sequence in putative susceptibility genes that may play a role in two different pathological pathways simultaneously, causing various phenotypic products, one associated with the psychopathology of schizophrenia and the other with glucose metabolism alterations, increasing the risks of both diseases in a carrier. A total of 37 common genes in the two diseases were reported in a systemic review discussing approaches and methods of identifying genetic loci that contribute to the comorbidity between schizophrenia and type 2 diabetes. [37] Furthermore, the gene cluster of tyrosine hydroxylase/insulin/insulin-like growth factor II (TH/INS/IGF-II) located on chromosome 11p has been linked as a susceptibility locus for diabetes mellitus and there are studies reporting an association of tyrosine hydroxylase markers with bipolar disorder as well [38] Similarly, there appears to be a link among migraine headaches, obesity and bipolar disorder. Genetic association studies are beginning to reveal this link where vulnerabilities may lie and the level of the serotonin transporter or with certain inflammatory cytokines. [39-41].

Biological factors that contribute to weight gain include serotonin (5-HT2C and 5-HT1A) and histamine (H1) receptors. [42] The interaction between dopamine and serotonin/histamine neurotransmission may affect the regulation of appetite, whereby dopamine is believed to mediate the primary rewarding properties of natural stimuli, such as food intake, in the brain. [43-45] Thus, manipulation of the dopamine system has an influence on the desire for food e.g., D2 receptor antagonism in the hypothalamus increases food intake and central dopamine dysfunction is linked to increased feeding behavior and obesity. [43] Indeed, dopaminergic deficits have been found in both mood disorders and obesity[44] , leading to a "reward deficiency syndrome" in mood disorders, in which low intrinsic dopamine activity in brain reward mechanisms is compensated for by the development of a variety of reinforcing behaviors, such as increased feeding. [43] Antagonistic action at the serotonin 5-HT2C receptor and agonist action at the 5-HT1A receptor increase appetite [42, 45, 46] as does histamine antagonism [46, 47]. The latter and action at the alpha-1 adrenergic receptor [47] also have sedative effects, leading some investigators to speculate that sedation may induce weight gain because of reduced mobility [47], making physical activity problematic. [45] Also of importance is the cholinergic system. Blockade of the muscarinic acetylcholine receptor can produce dryness of mouth, stimulating liquid intake and eventually greater consumption of calorie laden drinks. Adrenergic receptors are also implicated in food intake regulation through the role of noradrenaline as a hypothalamic neurotransmitter. Interestingly, it has been noted that alpha-1 and alpha-2 adrenoreceptors have opposing effects on food intake. [48, 49].

Bipolar disorder has been associated with an increased risk of hypertension and has higher systolic blood pressures when experiencing manic episodes. [38, 43] Depressive episodes are present more often than manic episodes in the disease course of the majority of patients with bipolar disorder. A 5-year study has shown an association between depressive symptoms and hypertension incidence that was present after adjustment for other hypertension risk factors in a cohort of relatively young individuals with high scores on the Centre for Epidemiological Studies Depression (CES-D) scale ($p \leq 0.01$), but also significant ($p \leq 0.05$) for those with intermediate depressive symptoms. [50] Depressed mood has also been positively associated with higher levels of systolic blood pressure ($p = 0.037$) and diastolic blood pressure ($p = 0.030$) in 24-hour monitoring of fifteen subjects over seven days. [51] Unfortunately, depressive symptoms are associated with poor BP control in hypertensive patients and may allow for further development of complications of hypertension, including stroke and cardiovascular-related mortality. [52].

One of the proposed physiological mechanisms explaining the relationship between depression and blood pressure is the observation of increased sympathetic nerve activity and poor vagal control in depressed patients. It has been suggested that depressed patients have a maximal neural sympathetic activity according to studies of heart rate during orthostasis and exercise, as well as decreased parasympathetic activity as indicated by diminished heart rate variability. [52] There is also evidence of an increased sympathetic tone in manic episodes compared with controls and a lower heart rate variability in euthymic patients with bipolar disorder, as well, compared to normal controls. [38] This may be related to increased levels of norepinephrine and its major central nervous system metabolite, 3-methoxy-4-hydroxyphenylglycol (MHPG) in cerebrospinal fluid, plasma and urine.

Another theory supporting the aforementioned association is a relative failure in the regulation of the neurotransmitter systems in patients with affective disorders, rather than simple increases or decreases in activity. The consequence of this dysregulation would be a disturbance in the individual affective responsiveness to stimuli, either external or internal. It is known that stressful stimuli increase noradrenergic activity, and, according to this theory, in the presence of affective disorders, this arousal would not be dampened by feedback mechanisms. [52] Indeed, the excessive regularity in heart rate manifested by tight control of normal cardiac fluctuations may be explained by a tightened cortical control that has been reset to withstand stressful changes to mood stability, and to dampen the changes associated with fluctuating mood. [38] Another suggested mechanism that could explain the relationship between depression and hypertension is a shared genetic vulnerability, but results of studies thus far have been controversial. [52].

Bipolar disorder has been associated with an increased risk of diabetes, independent of the effects of BMI and psychotropic medication use. Furthermore, impaired glucose tolerance and insulin resistance are found more frequently in bipolar disorder patients compared to the general population, and might be found as commonly as in schizophrenia, a disease that has been identified as an independent risk factor for diabetes by diabetes associations. [38, 43] Among populations in the United States with low educational attainment, it has been shown that depressive symptoms are a risk factor for the development of diabetes. [53] There is an increased incidence and prevalence of diabetes in schizophrenia and bipolar disorder that seems to be multifactorial. An increase in risk factors for diabetes accounts for part of this, including family history of diabetes, obesity and physical inactivity. Metabolic derangements and alterations in cytokines and stress hormones can also mediate the risk of diabetes in patients with mood disorders. [16] Lastly, bipolar disorder has been associated with an increased risk of dyslipidemia. [43].

The causes of metabolic syndrome are not fully understood, but visceral adiposity and insulin resistance seem to play a central role. [27] Schizophrenia patients are known to have greater visceral adiposity than healthy individuals. [25, 54] Studies of patients with bipolar disorder have shown an increased frequency of overweight and obesity compared to that of healthy controls, with a predominance of central distribution of the excess fat. This visceral fat increases the risk of elevated blood pressure, diabetes and derangements in glucose, dyslipidemia, and cardiovascular disease. [38, 43] Therefore, metabolic syndrome is often more common in bipolar patients than those in the general population. [55] This type of metabolic finding has been replicated internationally as well.

Individuals with metabolic syndrome have approximately a 3-fold increased risk of developing diabetes, and several separate studies found they have double the risk for CVD. This strongly indicates that the higher risk for developing CVD in persons with schizophrenia and bipolar disorder may be attributed to a certain extent by the presence of metabolic syndrome. [53].

Cortisol dysregulation may be a contributing factor in the association between the disorders of bipolar and schizophrenia and abdominal obesity, insulin resistance, dyslipidemia, metabolic syndrome, and increased cardiovascular risk as well. It has been shown that schizophrenia, and both first episode and relapses in mood disorders, are often associated with, or preceded by psychosocial stressors. This stress response is commonly associated with hyperactivity of the HPA. [5, 38] This can produce alterations of metabolism [56], both in the depressed and manic phases of bipolar disorder patients. A cross-sectional study found nearly equal levels of CVD risk factors in bipolar disorder (n=110) and schizophrenia (n=163) patients, with both groups having almost double the prevalence of CVD risk factors when compared to 15186 matched healthy individuals. The only significant differences between both diseases were the presence of a lower HDL level in women with schizophrenia (p<0.001) and higher systolic blood pressure in bipolar disorder patients.

Even in remission bipolar patients display HPA dysfunction, suggesting that this is a trait abnormality of the illness. The mechanisms accounting for increased risk of metabolic syndrome and CVD during chronic hypercortisolemia include insulin resistance, increased levels of leptin (a satiety hormone), obesity, deposition of body fat, increased visceral fat, and formation of atherosclerotic plaques in the coronary. [43].

Hyperactivation of the HPA axis and insulin resistance in the central nervous system are also linked with increased tone of the sympathetic nervous system, which produces an increase in blood pressure as noted previously. This has also been displayed in obesity and might partially account for the shared symptoms between bipolar disorder and metabolic syndrome. [38].

Another proposed mechanism for the relation of bipolar disorder and schizophrenia with metabolic syndrome and CVD is an immune mediated. This theory proposes mediation by adipokines, such as leptin, resistin, adiponectin and vistafin, which are highly active and lead to local and generalized inflammation by release of cytokines like tumor necrosis factor-alpha (TNF-alpha), interleukin-6 (IL-6), monocyte chemoattractant protein 1 (MCP-1) and IL-1. They also might influence vascular function by the modulation of vascular nitric oxide, and might also influence insulin [57].

Some inflammatory factors, like interleukin-6 and C-reactive protein, have been associated with depression, bipolar disorder [38, 58], and schizophrenia. These studies have found that the intensity of manic symptoms may be associated with C-reactive protein levels. A cross-sectional study evaluated the role of adipokines (adiponectine and leptin) in development of metabolic syndrome and its components in patients with paranoid schizophrenia (n=138) compared to 138 matched individuals. Patients in the schizophrenia group with metabolic syndrome had higher serum leptin levels than patients in the control group that had metabolic syndrome. Moreover, in both groups serum leptin levels positively and independently correlated with the HOMA index, which is a method to quantify insulin resistance, and in the schizophrenia group only, with triglycerides concentration. The authors suggest that metabolic syndrome can be a result of hyperleptinemia and/or leptin resistance in these cases [59].

Interleukin-6 is released from adipocyte tissue and leptin induces its upregulation by white blood cells. Interleukin-6 induces hepatic release of C-reactive protein which is an independent risk factor for CVD. [58] Interleukin-6 is also a potent stimulator of corticotropin-releasing hormone, leading to hyperactivity of the HPA axis with resultant hypercortisolemia. Elevated levels of C-reactive protein (relative risk 15.7) and interleukin-6 (relative risk 7.5) have also been found to be predictors of the development of diabetes in healthy women, after adjustment for potential confounding variables , and CRP is associated not only with insulin resistance, but also with obesity and the other components of the metabolic syndrome. Furthermore, metabolic syndrome has been defined as a chronic inflammatory state. In both bipolar disorder and schizophrenia, a specific alteration of endothelium inflammatory reactions is shared. [58] A cross-sectional study evaluated differences in CRP levels in patients with schizophrenia (n=63) and euthymic bipolar disorder (n=60), and the presence of metabolic syndrome. There was a significantly elevated proportion of bipolar patients with high CRP in comparison with schizophrenia patients (33% vs 22%, respectively, p=0.041), but no statistically significant differences in mean CRP values were found between the groups. There was an association in the total sample between high CRP and the prevalence of metabolic syndrome (p=0.031), with a more than two fold increase in the risk for having metabolic syndrome when CRP was high [58].

Bipolar disorder symptoms, either depressive or manic, can sometimes be associated with thyroid dysfunction, including hypothyroidism, which is linked to cardiovascular disease and dyslipidemia. However, it is not clear if the thyroid dysfunction is secondary to lithium use or independent of it in certain cases. Depressive symptoms have also been found to be associated with an increased risk for incidence and recurrence of coronary artery disease, decreased quality of life and all-cause mortality in patients with pre-existent heart disease.

The risk attributable to the effect of depressive symptoms is independent of other known prognostic factors for coronary artery disease. This association was found to be moderate and mediated by economic, behavioral, physiologic and iatrogenic factors [60] Heightened susceptibility to platelet activation may be a mechanism underlying the increased risk of ischemic heart and cerebrovascular disease and/or mortality after myocardial infarction in depression. This is suggested by evidence of significantly greater platelet reactivity following serotonin stimulation in patients with hypertension with higher scores on depression rating scales compared to those with lower depression scores[52], and findings in depressed patients of platelet activity up to 40% greater than controls and similar to patients with large-vessel atherosclerotic disease. Furthermore, there is an up-regulation of 5HT2a receptors in medication-free patients with bipolar disorder and a further increased 5HT2A receptor density in suicidal patients and in those treated with lithium. [38] Components of hemostasis other than platelet activity: like blood coagulation, anticoagulation and fibrinolysis, involved in the development and prognosis of CVD, seem to be involved in the mechanism as well. Lastly, it has been suggested that there may be a common vascular element in the etiology between late-onset mania and CVD, but not for earlier onset bipolar disorder [53].

Life style factors also contribute to the metabolic disturbances seen in people with SPMI. This group of patients is more likely to have poor diet, smoke cigarettes, use illegal drugs, and are less likely to exercise regularly [16]. [45] Cigarette smoking increases insulin resistance, carrying with it a decrease in glucose tolerance and a predisposition to future hyperinsulinemia. [61] The unhealthy lifestyle choices combined with a delayed diagnosis and treatment of hypertension, dyslipidemia, and prediabetic states are the main nonbiological factors accounting for the increased risk of cardiovascular disease in patients with severe mental illness [26].

In bipolar disorder, many variables play a role in the onset and maintenance of metabolic derangements. Unhealthy eating habit behavior and higher physical inactivity increase the rate of obesity and metabolic syndrome in this population. [38, 48, 56] Dysfunctional eating behavior and habits reported in bipolar disorder include increased total energy intake, total daily sucrose intake, percentage of energy from carbohydrates, total fluid intake and intake of sweetened drinks. Binge eating and other eating disorders are frequently comorbid in patients with bipolar disorder. Indeed, there is particular overlap in the prevalence of Bipolar II disorder and bulimia nervosa. [43,62,63].

Lower basal metabolic rates have been found in patients with bipolar disorder compared to individuals without mood disorders with a reduction in spent energy. [48] Nicotine dependence in bipolar disorder, which is a major risk factor for cardiovascular disease and has been found to impair insulin action increasing the risk for metabolic syndrome, has a higher prevalence compared with that of the general population. Alcohol and substance abuse have also been found to be similarly higher in patients with bipolar disorder which is also associated with the likelihood of developing metabolic syndrome. [43] Lastly, atypical depressive episodes can be observed in bipolar disorder, during which patients present with hypersomnia, carbohydrate hyperphagia, and psychomotor retardation, [64] all of which can contribute to increased weight. Accordingly, there has been speculation about an overlap between emotional dysregulation and abnormal eating behaviors, interfering specifically with hunger and feeding mechanisms, which then lead to obesity and metabolic disturbances in bipolar disorder patients [56, 62, 63].

Schizophrenic patients have also been found to have a sedentary lifestyle, [37, 65] in part due to recurrent hospitalizations and negative symptoms, such as social withdrawal and psychomotor retardation. Also, patient exercise is inadequate and their diet is unhealthy, with high intake of fat and sugar and low intake of fiber [66], fruits and vegetables [67], in part due to a limited access to lower calorie and higher nutrient foods. [10] They also display a high prevalence of smoking [50, 65, 67], higher than the rates reported in the general population and in many cigarette use is heavy. [68].

Certain environmental factors have been found, in some studies, to be common to schizophrenia and obesity or glucose metabolism derangements, such a lower educational achievement, poverty, prenatal and perinatal exposures to famine, and low levels of Vitamin D during childhood. [37] Childhood adversity has been associated, in cross-sectional and longitudinal studies, with overweight/obesity, derangements in glucose metabolism, and incidence of CVD. Adversity is also very frequent in patients with mood disorder and is considered a vulnerability factor for illness onset, recurrence, co-morbidity, and chronicity. Based on these facts, a cross-sectional study sought to determine whether a reported history of childhood adversity has a role in the association between mood disorders and metabolic syndrome and its components. Results suggested that childhood adversity is associated with components of the metabolic syndrome in individuals with mood disorders. Childhood adversity was assessed retrospectively with the Klein Trauma and Abuse-Neglect self-report scale in 373 patients with MDD, bipolar disorder 1, bipolar disorder 2, and mood disorder NOS. There was no significant difference in the rate of metabolic syndrome in patients with and without a history of any childhood adversity nor the specific types of childhood adversity evaluated in the scale. However, when each component of the metabolic syndrome was assessed, systolic blood pressure was significantly higher in patients with a history of physical abuse, parental loss, or any trauma, and diastolic blood pressure was significantly higher in patients reporting any type of adversity during childhood. Also, HDL cholesterol levels were lower in subjects with a history of loss and of any trauma. Lower glucose levels were found in patients with a history of parental loss and sexual abuse. Amongst subjects with a history of sexual abuse, a significant proportion met criteria for obesity. After adjustment for potential confounders, systolic blood pressure remained significantly higher in subjects with parental loss, as did lower glucose levels amongst subjects with a history of sexual abuse. When different diagnoses were compared, patients with BD but not MDD who reported a history of parental loss had significantly higher systolic blood pressure, but this difference became insignificant after adjustment for confounders. The overall duration of any adversity was not associated with metabolic syndrome or its components. The authors discuss potential mechanisms explaining this association, including persistent behavioral alterations, modulation of neuroendocrine and immunological systems, and permanent changes in neuroanatomical architecture, based on results from animal and human studies (McIntyre et al childhood adversity). [69].

Additional factors that have been associated with weight gain in patients with SPMI include age and gender, [42, 70, 71], lower basal BMI [72], lower bodyweight before initiation of drug treatment [73, 74], rapid initial weight gain [74], decreased cigarette smoking activity [73], and socioeconomic status [42].

A survey completed by outpatients with schizophrenia and affective disorders showed that people with SPMI are less physically active overall than individuals in the general population (49% vs 22% in the 2005-2006 NHANES sample). A lack of social contacts in the past month and female gender were factors found to be associated with the aforementioned outcome [75].

Similar results were obtained in another survey including 234 patients with psychotic or affective disorders attending community mental health services in Australia and exhibiting chronic psychiatric symptoms. The investigators inquired on a wide range of cardiovascular risk factors and compared the results with those obtained from the Risk Factor Prevalence Study and from the National Health Survey. The results showed that mentally ill patients were 5 times more likely to smoke, twice as likely to start smoking and four times less likely to be ex-smokers. The odds ratios in the patient group for overweight and obesity were >1 (1.3 and 7.8, respectively). Patients with mental illness were also 2 times more likely to have abstained from alcohol during the previous 2 weeks, but were 4 times more likely to have used harmful levels of alcohol (5 or more glasses a day in women or 7 or more glasses a day in men). The authors proposed that this characteristic made it less likely for the patient group to gain the protective benefits of consuming daily, small amounts of alcohol. They were also more likely to add salt to their food. There was no difference between the groups in blood pressure readings and in the number of patients that didn't exercise during the two weeks before the survey. [50].

In another questionnaire, chronic psychotic inpatients accurately perceived their obesity status but their level of concern didn't correlate with body mass index, and the obese were resistant to engaging in dieting as a remedy [76]. In another cross-sectional study of outpatient schizophrenic subjects using a questionnaire, a high proportion had insight about their unhealthy lifestyles [67].

Cardiovascular risk factors in schizophrenia patients include non-modifiable ones, such as sex, family history, personal history, and age, as well as modifiable ones such as obesity (relative risk [RR] 1.5-2), smoking (RR 2-3), inactivity, diabetes (RR 3), hypertension (RR 2-3), and dyslipidemia (RR ≤5) compared to the general population [16, 53]. Studies have examined some of these risk factors to see if their contribution to cardiovascular-related mortality in the general population can be extrapolated to the schizophrenia population. It has been found that cardiac-related deaths in schizophrenia are 12-fold higher in young smokers compared to non smokers. Another study showed that diabetes is an important risk factor for cardiac-related death in schizophrenia. Low physical activity showed higher hazard ratios than smoking for heart disease mortality in schizophrenia patients. Surprisingly, another study including 22,817 patients with schizophrenia showed that hyperlipidemia was protective for cardiovascular related mortality. That same study demonstrated that both diabetes and hypertension increased cardiac mortality risk in schizophrenia patients [68]. Cardiovascular risk factors in bipolar disorder have not been studied as widely as in schizophrenia, but there is evidence showing an increase (1-5 fold RR) in the modifiable risk factors of obesity (RR 1-2), smoking (RR 2-3), diabetes (RR 1.5-2), hypertension (RR 2-3) and dyslipidemia (≤3) compared with the general population [16].

The underrecognition of medical problems in people with SPMI is worrisome because it decreases the chances for them to seek healthcare when they need it [43, 53], and it has been reported that they have a limited access to appropriate primary care screening or treatment [37]. Also, the combination of having to cope with a chronic illness that may require lifelong medication, with a lack of educational attainment and employment problems, may all impact obtaining effective medical care. This is one of the reasons why patients with SPMI have a general health that is poorer than that of controls in the general population and have more comorbidities like obesity and metabolic syndrome [53], with higher risks of complications from poorly controlled illnesses secondary to their lack of concern and poor lifestyle. As reviewed above, patients with schizophrenia and bipolar disorder are more prone to present with the cluster of risk factors for CVD, including diabetes mellitus, overweight or obesity, and substance abuse (including high rates of cigarette smoking) [53].

These problems are complicated by non-adherence with medical treatment in patients with SPMI, which increases the frequency of uncontrolled diseases and, therefore, increases the risk of cardiovascular complications and might explain, in part, the increased mortality in this population. Some have pointed out that older patients with psychotic disorders might be at risk of non adherence due to their increased likelihood of being prescribed medications for concomitant medical disorder and of having more complex medical regimens, cognitive and sensory deficits, plus the well known lack of insight of patients with schizophrenia that might be extended to medical illnesses as well (Dolder et al). A study assessed medication adherence of 76 middle-age and older Veterans Affairs outpatients with schizophrenia or other psychotic disorders on an oral antipsychotic in addition to an oral medication for hypertension, hyperlipidemia, or diabetes during a 12 month period by review of medication fill records. Non-adherence rates were found to be equally problematic for both antipsychotic and non-psychiatric medications in these middle-age and older patients, with the 12-month mean compliance fill rates ranging from 52% to 64% [77]. However, another study did not replicate these findings in patients with schizophrenia and diabetes mellitus taking an oral hypoglycemic (n=11,454) compared to diabetics without a diagnosis of schizophrenia on an oral hypoglycemic (n=10,560). They found that poor adherence was less prevalent in the schizophrenia group (43%) compared to the non schizophrenia group (52%, p<0.001) [78]. Bipolar patients exhibit high rates of non-adherence with prescribed treatments, both pharmacological and psychosocial for their psychiatric condition (Kim B et al).

Some hypothesize that the cognitive impairment associated with schizophrenia may affect functions considered essential for effective self-care in type 2 diabetes like attentiveness, learning, and motivation [66]. A cross-sectional study assessed the levels of glycemic control in 38 outpatients with schizophrenia and diabetes in Tokyo and the influence of the severity of the psychiatric illness on diabetes self-care and glycemic control. It found the average HbA1c in the group was 7.65%, and 73% of the patients had an HbA1c >6.5%. There was no significant association between the score in the Brief Psychiatry Rating Scale (BPRS) and the level of HbA1c. However, some of the diabetes knowledge and self-care behaviors were significantly lower in the high BPRS score group, including exercise, bathing frequency, number of dietary guidance items, and Diabetes Knowledge Test scores [66].

Finally, it has been shown that patients with schizophrenia rarely receive appropriate treatment for hypertension, dyslipidemia and diabetes mellitus. A cross-sectional study using the VA's National Psychosis Registry, and the VA External Peer Review Program's national random sample of chart reviews for the assessment of quality of care for CVD-related conditions, assessed if patients with serious mental illness compared with a control group of patients without mental illness received care following guidelines for hypertension (n=24,016), hyperlipidemia (n=46,430), and diabetes (n=10,943). After adjustments for confounding factors, results showed that patients with SPMI were 42% less likely to be assessed for CVD risk factors, notably screening for hyperlipidemia (OR=0.58, p<0.001). They were also less likely to receive recommended follow up for diabetes, notably foot exam

(OR=0.68, p<0.001), retinal exam (OR=0.65, p<0.001), or renal testing (OR=0.64, p<0.001). Also, a higher percentage of patients in the SPMI group had a HbA1c>9 or one not recorded compared to the no psychiatry diagnosis group (19.1% vs 14%, respectively, p<0.001). The results remained unchanged after controlling for race, interaction between race and diagnosis, and comorbidity. Finally, there were no significant differences for quality of care of hypertension among the groups [79]. When a physical healthcare need is diagnosed in this group of patients, treatment is less intensive than in the general population [68]. For example, in those with established cardiovascular disease less intensive treatment for their cardiac condition is received and they are less likely to undergo invasive cardiac procedures or to receive guideline-consistent treatment for a cardiovascular event [65]. Medical illnesses in patients with bipolar disorder also have been reported to be undetected and inadequately treated [43].

Pharmacologic

Antidepressants (ATDs)

It is speculated that the variable effects of different antidepressants are due to their dissimilar actions on monoaminase signaling [60, 80]. Potentiation of noradrenergic neurotransmission may be a mechanism by which antidepressants increase BP [52]. They also exert different effects on serotoninergic, dopaminergic, noradrenergic, histaminergic and cholinergic systems [80]. Another hypothesis is that central serotoninergic neurotransmission may play an essential role in BP regulation. Serotonin reuptake blockade could trigger a cascade of changes in central serotonin neurotransmission that results in an enhancement of autonomic tone [52]. Monoamines interact with neuropeptides and hormones to control satiety mechanisms and eating behaviors [80].The propensity for weight gain with ATD's may also be influenced by this symptom constellation, which will dictate the antidepressant chosen. Each class and type of ATD exerts different effects on aspects of the metabolic syndrome [60].

Postulated mechanisms include altered appetite and effects on weight; habitual inactivity caused by side effects such as sedation and somnolence; dietary composition changes; altered insulin receptor sensitivity; altered glucose transporter effects; anticholinergic activity; neuropeptides/adipokines (like leptin and insulin resistance); cortisol dysregulation (and other contraregulatory hormones); increased hepatic lipid biosynthesis and decreased peripheral lipid utilization; central/peripheral monoaminergic receptor modulation; activation of proinflammatory networks (i.e. cytokines) [60].

In addition, the contribution of ATDs to changes in body weight is difficult to ascertain because disease associated features of depression, like alterations in appetite, energy level, and physical activity, significantly impact weight. Individual variables, such as sex, premorbid weight and age, as well as genetic susceptibility, likely all play a role in the induced weight changes [80].

Serotonin exerts control on the ratio of carbohydrate, [23, 80] and protein ingestion, and SSRIs are expected to cause a weight reduction. However, each antidepressant from this group has variable selectivity and pharmacologic action, and each interacts in a different way with dopaminergic activity [80]. It has been proposed that the multiple serotonergic activities of SSRIs play a role in weight gain, one of which is an affinity for serotonin 5-HT2C receptors [23, 53]. As mentioned above, research has implicated these receptors as having a role in the regulation of appetite [53]. It is possible that the increase in serotonin levels downregulates 5-HTC2c receptors, mimicking the 5HT2c blockade by antipsychotics (see below) [23].

Fluoxetine (FXT) has a favorable effect on insulin sensitivity and glucose metabolism in both diabetic and mood disorder populations [60]. It may have a beneficial effect on lipid fraction in mixed populations as well, including non-depressed, diabetic individuals [60]. It has shown to be weight neutral in most studies, with minimal weight loss in fewer studies [60]. Fluoxetine has a high level of noradrenergic and dopaminergic action [80].

Paroxetine (PXT) has been associated with glucose control impairment [60]. Increases in LDL-chol, HDL-chol, and TG levels have been documented, which may normalize after discontinuation of treatment [60]. It also causes clinically significant weight gain [38, 60] (≥7% from baseline) [60]. In a metaanalysis it showed marginal weight loss during acute treatment and weight gain over medium and long periods, particularly after 8 months of treatment [80]. This medication has the greatest affinity for cholinergic receptors amongst the SSRIs [80].

Other SSRIs (non FXT or PXT) don't predictably affect glucose levels [60] and seem to have favorable effects on glycemic control and insulin resistance [43]. SSRIs other than PXT have no clinically significant effects on lipids [60] SSRIs in general are considered "weight neutral" in chronic administration, except for paroxetine [38, 60], with favorable effects on food intake [43]. Fluvoxamine in most studies shows weight neutrality, with minimal weight loss in fewer studies. Both citalopram and escitalopram are more selective for serotonin reuptake inhibition [80]. SSRIs in general are considered to have neutral effects on blood pressure, with reports of hypotension and hypertension documented [60].

SNRIs in general have been demonstrated to cause a dose-dependent elevation in systolic and diastolic blood pressures and sustained diastolic hypertension in a small number of studies. They are expected to have stronger anorexigenic effects compared to SSRIs due to their combined serotonin and norepinephrine reuptake inhibition [80]. This hypothesis was not confirmed in a metaanalysis [80], and they are considered weight neutral [60].

Venlafaxine doesn't consistently demonstrate a detrimental effect on glucose metabolism. [60]. It causes dose- and duration-dependent increases in LDL-chol, HDL-chol and TG levels [60]. In a meta-anlaysis, sustained hypertension (defined as a resting diastolic BP value ≥90 mm Hg plus a ≥10 mm Hg rise above baseline diastolic BP for at least 3 consecutive clinical visits) was observed in 4.8% of patients treated with venlafaxine and 2.1% of those receiving placebo. The largest increases (13.2%) occurred at doses ≥300 mg daily [52].

Desvenlafaxine has shown increases in blood glucose levels in short-term registration trials. It has also demonstrated increases in total cholesterol, LDL-chol, HDL chol, and TG levels [60].

Duloxetine may increase fasting blood glucose levels in some populations (i.e. diabetic peripheral neuropathy patients) [60].

As for SNRA's, mirtazapine causes variable effects on carbohydrate craving and causes significant weight gain, both in acute and maintenance treatment [60, 80]. It enhances noradrenergic and serotoninergic neurotransmission due to its antagonism of central α2-adrenergic autoreceptors and heteroreceptors as well to its postsynaptic blockade of 5HT2 and 5HT3 receptors. Blockade of α2 adrenoceptors, along with affinity for histamine H1 receptors, and low affinity for dopaminergic D1 and D2 receptors, may explain the induced weight gain [80]. Its use is associated with an increase in glucose levels, and significant increases in serum TG and LDL-chol levels, with no consistent effect on HDL-chol and minimal effects on BP. There are reports of orthostatic hypotension [60].

Nefazodone and trazodone don't affect glucose metabolism, serum lipids or weight. They also cause minimal effects on blood pressure, with reports of orthostatic hypotension [60].

TCA's in general increase TGs and have a variable effect on HDL-chol and LDL-chol. Imipramine specifically increases the total cholesterol/HDL ratio. TCA's in general are not associated with hypertension and they actually cause orthostatic hypotension [60] except for desimpramine, a potent norepinephrine reuptake inhibitor, which has been reported to increase blood pressure, with the mechanism being a regional increase of cardiac noradrenergic activity [52]. Sustained hypertension was observed in 4.7% of the patients treated with imipramine and 2.1% of those receiving placebo in a metaanalysis [52]. TCA use increases caloric intake, probably related to carbohydrate craving, with clinically significant weight gain [60, 80], and TCAs may be more likely to cause weight gain than all antidepressants other than mirtazapine [38, 43]. Amitryptiline treatment is associated with increased severity of weight gain when compared to treatment with imipramine, [60], both in acute and maintenance treatment [80]. It is the most potent weight gain inducer among all the TCAs and has high affinity for alpha-adrenergic, histaminergic, and cholinergic receptors. Imipramine also has anticholinergic and antimuscarinic effects, but it too is a strong inhibitor of the reuptake of norepinephrine and has some affinity for D1 and D2 receptors, which could explain the difference when compared with amitryptiline. Tertiary TCA's are not known to cause changes in glucose levels in the absence of weight gain, while secondary TCAs are associated with increases in plasma glucose [60] and insulin resistance [43].

It is well recognized that MAOI's are associated with hypertensive crises when co-administered with agents altering the monoamine system or with tyramine containing foods [60]. High levels of unmetabolized tyramine or sympathomimetics trigger norepinephrine release from peripheral sympathetic neurons [52] MAOI's facilitate glucose disposal but cause significant weight gain [38, 60] and, in general, may be more likely to cause weight gain than all antidepressants other than mirtazapine, [38, 43] except for moclobemide, which is considered weight neutral with both short- and long-term use and has no effect on glucose metabolism. This last agent has no clinically significant effect on lipids [60].

Bupropion has no significant effect on glucose metabolism or lipids. There are reports of hypertension with its use, but a RCT evaluating vasopressor actions demonstrated neutral and/or minimal effects on BP measurements.

It is less likely to cause weight gain [38], and there is increasing evidence of weight loss with its use [60]. In a recent meta-analysis SSRIs, SNRIs, bupropion and moclobemide were associated with weight loss to various extents in the acute period, but, over maintenance, only bupropion maintained a significant effect on weight [80].

This antidepressant selectively inhibits dopamine and, to a lesser extent, norepinephrine reuptake. It has no action on postsynaptic histamine, β-adrenergic, or acetylcholine receptors. In fact, recently the combination product of bupropion-naltrexone was evaluated to promote weight loss in non-psychiatric patients.

Some studies have shown up to 5-10% of initial weight loss on the combination product when compared with placebo. Although weight loss was notable, it was not felt to be effective enough to gather a full regulatory approval. [81].

A meta-analysis showed only slight effects on weight for the majority of antidepressants, with few exceptions: amytriptiline, mirtazapine, paroxetine (which significantly increased weight), and bupropion (which significantly decreased weight) [80].

The study included patients in monotherapy with antidepressants at doses no lower than the minimal therapeutic dose for at least 4 weeks. It assessed the effects divided in acute (4-12 weeks), and maintenance treatment (at 4-7 months and at ≥8 months). However, it excuded patients with obesity and eating disorders, and the former are encountered frequently in clinical practice.

Mood Stabilizers

Studies in bipolar disorder have found a positive correlation between BMI and both the number and the specific types of weight gain-inducing medications with which patients are treated [43].

Lithium use causes significant weight gain [38, 43, 57] in up to 60% of patients, [38] reported as 13% at 1 year vs 7% with placebo, [43] with an estimated range of 4.5 to 15.6 kg over 2 years [38]. This increase in weight has been associated with carbohydrate craving [23, 38, 57], increased appetite [38, 43] secondary in part to appetite-stimulation in the hypothalamus, [43] fluid retention, altered carbohydrate and fat metabolism, hypothyroidism, [23, 38], and increased dry mouth [23] and thirst with consumption of high-calorie beverages [43] [23]. Lithium may be associated with lower total cholesterol levels [57]. It has an insulin-like effect on carbohydrate metabolism and increases glucose absorption into adipocytes.

Valproic acid use is also associated with significant weight gain [38, 43], with up to 71% of patients gaining more than 4 kg, and reported ranges of weight gain between 0.9 and 14 kg [82] in 21% at 1 year compared to 7% with placebo. This seems to be a consequence of impaired fatty acid metabolism [43], [23], increased thirst and consumption of high-calorie beverages, and appetite-stimulation through a direct effect on the hypothalamus [43], and increase in serum leptin levels [23]. It also may cause insulin resistance, hyperlipidemia, impaired glucose tolerance, and hyperinsulinemia [38] though data on hyperlipidemia is mixed depending on patient populations studied [83, 84].

In general, anticonvulsant mood stabilizers may decrease lipid levels [57].

The association with weight gain and metabolic syndrome components is lower for carbamazepine (CBZ), [38] which is associated with stable weight in a 6-month, open-label study [43]. However, other studies report weight gains of up to 15 kg [82]. Even lower is the risk for lamotrigine [38], in which use as monotherapy for bipolar disorder at 1 year has been reported as having a weight neutral effect in one retrospective study [43] and reported changes in weight ranging from a 2 kg weight loss to a 0.6 kg weight gain [82].

In a small (n=98) cross-sectional study of the prevalence of metabolic syndrome in bipolar patients from the a VA Medical Center Bipolar Clinic, subjects taking carbamazepine were less likely to have metabolic syndrome compared to those on lamotrigine, divalproex, lithium, and gabapentin, although the sample size for each drug was small. The authors argued that these results were produced by carbamazepine's ability to induce a long-term increase in HDL and total cholesterol (observed to remain for 1-5 years), while its induced increase of LDL cholesterol and triglycerides seemed to be transient during the first year of treatment. Importantly, the increase in HDL might eliminate one criterion for metabolic syndrome [64]. Also, CBZ is a potent inducer of the hepatic isozyme CYP3A4 which can then reduce levels of concurrently prescribed medications that might cause derangements in the components of the metabolic syndrome [64].

Atypical Antipsychotics

Atypical antipsychotics have been associated with a higher prevalence of obesity [75]. Clinical trials show a variability by antipsychotic agent in mean weight gain and in the incidence of clinically significant weight gain, with greater than placebo-level effects on weight reported for all currently available agents in the U.S. [54]. The effects range from minimal to significant [38].

In short-term studies, a definite rank order of weight-gain potential among atypical antipsychotics has been demonstrated: clozapine has the highest risk of weight gain followed by olanzapine [53, 85], [38], [43]. SGAs induce weight gain by blockade of H1 and 5HT2C receptors, which enhances appetite [26]. Clozapine and olanzapine have the greatest affinity for both receptors [42, 46, 53], and the combined blockade of H1 and 5HT2C receptors has been especially associated with weight gain, sometimes profound [42, 46]. They both have high affinity for M1 receptors [53] [23], and this effect, as explained above, can cause dry mouth stimulating the intake of high calorie liquids. The descending order continues with quetiapine and risperidone [85], [53], [38],[43], at least in short-term studies; in long-term studies, however, quetiapine appears to produce more weight gain [85] although other authors mention that quetiapine and risperidone do not differ substantially in their effect on body weight [46]. Risperidone has lesser yet substantial 5HT2C antagonism activity with low affinity for H1 receptors and, thereby (presumably), produces less weight gain [85], [53]). Quetiapine, however, has high affinity for H1 receptors but is a weak antagonist of the 5HT2C receptor ([86], which places it at about the same level of associated weight gain as that of risperidone, yet lower than that of clozapine and olanzapine. Amisulpride, aripiprazole and ziprasidone seem to have the lowest risk for weight gain ([85], [53] [38], [43]. Ziprazidone is a potent agonist at 5HT1a receptors and is a potent 5HT2C receptor antagonist. It is also a synaptic reuptake inhibitor of serotonin ([42], [23, 53] and noradrenaline [23, 53] with very low affinity for H1 receptors [86]. Aripiprazole is a partial D2 agonist [53] with moderate affinity for the histamine receptor [42], agonism or partial agonism at some forms of the 5HT2c receptor, partial 5HT1a agonism [42] and antagonism at 5HT2a receptors [53]. Its affinity for the H1 receptor is low [86]. The mixed receptor activity profile of these agents likely contributes to their lowered weight gain potential. It is mentioned that both ziprasidone and aripiprazole can even have a protective effect against weight gain [53]. A meta-analysis, including 81 studies on body weight changes after 10 weeks of treatment, supported these findings. The mean weight change for the different first generation antipsychotics (FGAs) and second generation antipsychotics (SGAs) included was 4.45 kg for clozapine and 4.15 kg for olanzapine; thioridazine, sertindole, chlorpromazine, and risperidone were considered to induce moderate weight gain (from 3.19 kg to 2.10 kg), and haloperidol, aripiprazole, fluphenazine, and ziprasidone were associated with low or very low weight gain (from 1.08 kg to 0.04 kg) ([10]. In the Comparison of Atypicals in First-Episode Psychosis double blind study, the percentages of patients gainig more than 7% of their baseline body weight after 52 weeks of treatment were 80% for olanzapine, 57.6% for risperidone, and 50% for quetiapine [87]. Another prospective, observational study, including almost 5000 patients with schizophrenia, the Intercontinental Schizophrenia Outpatients Health Outcome study, showed a weight gain after 12 months of treatment of 3.4 kg for olanzapine, 2.2 kg with haloperidol and risperidone, and 1.9 kg for quetiapine [88]. In the CATIE study, 1493 chronic schizophrenic patients were treated for up to 18 months, and the average weight gain was 4.3 kg for olanzapine, 0.5 kg for quetiapine, and 0.36 kg for risperidone. For ziprasidone, the mean weight change was a loss of 0.73 kg and for perphenazine it was a loss of 0.91 kg [10]. Since aripiprazole has been approved as adjunctive treatment for depression, reports have emerged on increased weight gain potential when it is prescribed with serotoninergic antidepressants [82].

Newer FDA-approved antipsychotics for schizophrenia include asenapine, lurasidone, iloperidone, and paliperidone. Iloperidone has shown mild to moderate weight gain (1.5-2.1 kg), comparable to that caused by risperidone. Paliperidone, over both the short and long term (52 weeks), has shown no significant weight gain. Lurasidone, in short-term, placebo-controlled pooled data, shows a mean weight gain of 0.75 kg, compared to 0.26 kg with placebo. Asenapine over the first three weeks of treatment showed a 0.9 kg weight gain, and over 52 weeks was considered to cause negligible weight gain [82]. The differences in molecular structure of the SGA agents may be, in part, responsible for the differences in associated weight gain. Structural differences may result in slightly dissimilar interactions and combinations of neurotransmitter receptor blocking that may explain the different propensities to cause weight gain [53]. Also, patient-specific factors such as genetic vulnerability, sex, age, BMI, weight before starting antipsychotic treatment, type of psychiatric disorder, and individual lifestyle may also play a role in the differences ([85].

In a study of weight change during treatment of acute mania in an inpatient hospital setting, patients on any kind of atypical antipsychotic showed greater weight gain than those on typicals or without antipsychotics [36]. In another study of acutely hospitalized patients, individuals on atypical antipsychotics also gained more weight [73].

In some cases, weight gain may occur via indirect effects on glucose and lipid levels. Olanzapine and clozapine have the greatest impact on increasing blood glucose and lipids [89] independent of adiposity [42]. However, there exists a complex relationship among adiposity, blood glucose, and serum lipid levels in relation to antipsychotic treatment [42].

Associated with increased weight gain is an increased risk for type 2 diabetes [38]. The weight gain seen with antipsychotics may produce a state of overweight or obesity [53] or a change in body fat distribution [43]. Such changes, particularly abdominal obesity, are a risk factor for the development of insulin resistance [53], [43], which in turn is thought to be a precursor of type 2 diabetes. Patients taking aripiprazole and ziprasidone, therefore, have a greatly reduced risk for the development of diabetes compared to other SGAs. Also, it has been found that after 1 year of treatment, patients taking risperidone had approximately half the risk of development or worsening of metabolic syndrome than those on olanzapine [53]. In the CATIE study, olanzapine was associated with higher increases in HbA1c compared to all other antipsychotics. Clozapine and olanzapine carry the greatest risk for diabetes [65]. Using the Food and Drug Administration (FDA) adverse events database, the risk of diabetes mellitus was increased for olanzapine, risperidone, clozapine and quetiapine, whereas a decreased risk was found for haloperidol, aripiprazole [90] and ziprasidone [65].

Overall, the rank order for development or worsening of diabetes with antipsychotics support the hypothesis that weight gain is playing a role [27]. Blockade of the H1 and 5HT2C receptors increases body weight, and weight from fatty tissue, resulting in insulin resistance [49]. However, some patients on SGAs develop diabetes in the absence of weight gain or obesity, and the effect size from different second generation antipsychotics on weight doesn't always correlate with the extent of disturbance in glucose metabolism, [26] which suggests that weight gain and obesity are not the only mechanisms accounting for diabetes onset or worsening in this population. This is also supported by the fact that diabetes can resolve after discontinuation of the antipsychotic without any weight loss, and often recurs rapidly if the medication is started again.

A direct mechanism, independent of weight changes, is thought to be a metabolic one, including a direct effect on insulin-sensitive target tissues [43]. A decrease in insulin-sensitive transporters or an inability to stimulate the recruitment of glucose transporters from microsomes to the plasma membrane are hypothesized [57]. Such alterations could result in hyperglycemia, with a homeostatic increase in insulin release, followed by insulin resistance secondary to prolonged hyperinsulinemia [53]. An elevation of serum free fatty acids can also cause insulin resistance [57]. Blockade of the 5-HT1a receptor may directly decrease insulin secretion and α-1 adrenergic receptor activity may directly increase blood glucose [49]. Also, the blockade of muscarinic 3 receptors at the level of the pancreatic beta cells decreases insulin secretion [26]. Studies show that low concentrations of clozapine and olanzapine can markedly and selectively impair cholinergic-stimulated insulin secretion by blocking muscarinic M2 receptors [27]. Olanzapine in a canine study caused preferential deposition of energy into adipose tissue and induced hepatic insulin resistance [43].

Some cases of new-onset diabetes, associated with acute pancreatitis, were seen with the use of olanzapine and clozapine. Interestingly, hyperinsulinemia rather than failure of insulin release were observed in those cases, indicating a complex etiology rather than simple chemical damage to the pancreas, which would reflect an indirect action caused by atypical antipsychotic (AAP)-induced hyperlipidemia [53]. Furthermore, in patients developing diabetic ketoacidosis with AAPs, the derangement is reversible after discontinuation of the medication, supporting a complex pathophysiology, including a functional defect rather than destruction of pancreatic β-cells [27].

Another putative mechanism for the increased risk of diabetes type 2 with AAPs is an effect of these medications on the level of adiponectin, a hormone derived from adipocytes that moderates lipid and carbohydrate metabolism [37]. In a study in male rats, olanzapine increased the levels of adiponectin without causing significant changes in insulin, glucose or leptin, and without causing hyperphagia. As mentioned before, this molecule causes release of many inflammatory factors that have been linked with metabolic syndrome and CVD.

Lipid profiles are also often negatively altered by atypical antipsychotics [38]. Prospective studies have shown an increase in LDL cholesterol and a decrease in HDL cholesterol associated with the use of antipsychotics. There is also a marked effect on triglycerides that differs among these medications [16]. Similar to the observation for weight gain and glucose derangements, patients taking olanzapine have an increased chance of developing hyperlipidemia compared with patients who have been given conventional antipsychotic agents or for those who have not received therapy [53], and the risk of hyperlipidemia appears to be higher for patients under treatment with clozapine and olanzapine, particularly the younger patients [65]. In the CATIE study, olanzapine was associated with significantly greater increases in serum levels of cholesterol and triglyceride compared to the other medications. In that study, ziprasidone and risperidone were the only SGAs linked with reductions in cholesterol and triglycerides. There is growing evidence suggesting that newer SGAs (aripiprazole and ziprasidone) are associated with little or no dyslipidemia; in contrast, risperidone and quetiapine appear to have "intermediate" effects on lipids (Casey), however, in other studies risperidone's relative risk for hyperlipidemia is considered low [27].

The mechanisms accounting for antipsychotic-induced dyslipidemia have been less studied compared with those related to weight gain and diabetes. As with diabetes, weight gain can be in some cases the culprit of new onset dyslipidemia with SGAs, but, in other cases, dyslipidemia occurs without any weight gain, and the effect size of various SGAs on weight doesn't always correlate with the extent of disturbance in lipid metabolism [26]. Particularly, olanzapine and quetiapine have been noted to cause extreme elevations in triglyceride levels without causing weight gain [53]. The development of glucose intolerance could be involved in the effects of antipsychotics on lipid levels because insulin resistance is associated with an abnormal physiology of serum lipids [27], but some patients develop hyperlipidemia without showing glucose intolerance. Interferences with leptin have also been mentioned as a direct mechanism, although it is not clear if the changes in leptin are a cause or a consequence of the changes in lipids associated with antipsychotics [57].

In general, antipsychotics have not shown to cause or to worsen hypertension, except for clozapine, which appears to be associated with an increased risk of hypertension in a small number of patients [57].

The increased risk of developing metabolic syndrome with AP medications is in part related to their potential to induce weight gain and glucose intolerance. However, in up to 25% of cases of metabolic syndrome with AP treatment, no weight gain, or increased abdominal adiposity, was present, suggesting again a direct link between the antipsychotic agent and the development of metabolic abnormalities [27].

Since SGA's have been approved for the treatment of bipolar disorder, there has been an increasing interest in knowing if there is a difference in the degree and appearance of metabolic changes according to the diagnosis, and in the effect of the combined use of mood stabilizers with atypical antipsychotics, since such combinations may result in additional risk for obesity and associated metabolic abnormalities [36, 55]. This was specifically noted when combined olanzapine and divalproex was compared to monotherapy and statistical increases in weight and blood sugars were noted [91].

A cross-sectional study suggested a shared susceptibility to antipsychotic-related metabolic dysregulations, not primarily related to the psychiatric diagnoses of schizophrenia or bipolar disorder, nor to the concomitant mood stabilizer treatment. The investigators assessed the prevalence rates of metabolic syndrome and coronary heart disease in 74 bipolar disorder patients compared to 111 matched schizophrenia patients treated with SGAs at the time of presentation for admission, with or without mood stabilizers. Patients were randomly selected from 1420 consecutive admissions into a psychiatric tertiary care hospital. The results showed essentially identical increases in rates of metabolic syndrome and cardiovascular risk parameters in patients with bipolar disorder (43.2%) and schizophrenia (45.9%) with second generation antipsychotics and, interestingly, a lack of effects of co-treatment with mood stabilizers on these outcomes [92].

A cross-sectional study from medical records of patients with bipolar disorder attending a clinic in Korea examined the prevalence of metabolic syndrome in those receiving medications for their diagnosis (including antipsychotics other than clozapine and mood stabilizers) for 90 days or more compared to that of matched, healthy individuals. 15.1% of the patient sample were on antipsychotics only and 11.8% on mood stabilizers only, while 73% were on a combined regimen. The prevalence of metabolic syndrome in the patient group was 27%, which was significantly higher than that in the control group (OR 2.44). No significant difference was found in the number of patients diagnosed with metabolic syndrome according to the three groups of treatments: antipsychotic only, mood stabilizer only or combined regimen. Patients on clozapine were excluded from the study, which might cause an underestimation of the prevalence of metabolic syndrome in the patient group and in the antipsychotic-only group [93].

Another smaller, cross-sectional study with non-random assignment of bipolar patients to treatment showed a metabolic rate significantly higher in patients treated with SGAs only (54.5%), compared to those treated with mood stabilizers only (24.2%) or those receiving generation SGAs along with mood stabilizer treatment (23.7%), with no significant difference between the last two groups [94]. Other studies, however, have found that combinations of atypical antipsychotics and mood stabilizers may result in additional risks for obesity and associated metabolic abnormalities in bipolar patients [36].

Lastly, in a cross-sectional chart review evaluating the effect of SGAs on components of the metabolic syndrome in 277 patients with bipolar disorder, no significant association was found between medication use and any specific component of the metabolic syndrome or the metabolic syndrome itself. However, a trend toward higher burden of cardiovascular risk factors was observed among the SGAs associated with weight gain (clozapine, risperidone, olanzapine, or quetiapine) since 67% of the patients on those medications showed metabolic syndrome compared to 42% not taking these medications ($p < 0.062$) [95].

Management Interventions

The key to preventing significant drug-related weight gain and treating obesity if it occurs is early intervention. Patients should always be told about weight gain as a potential adverse effect before they begin treatment and their weight should be monitored as long as they continue taking the drugs that we know may increase weight. Ideally, a diet and exercise plan should be initiated with the patient to prevent or treat weight gain before medically significant weight gain occurs [96]. The management of overweight and obesity in patients with Bipolar Disorder and Schizophrenic Spectrum illness has included non-pharmacologic as well as pharmacologic interventions which are primarily directed at the metabolic/weight gain effects of antipsychotic medications [97].

Non-Pharmacological Weight Reduction Strategies

Diet, exercise and cognitive behavior therapy (behavioral modification) are the principal non-pharmacological means of promoting (and maintaining) weight loss. Diet and exercise produce maximum benefit, but require considerable commitment and motivation on the part of the patient. This is often difficult or impossible in the mentally ill. A successful weight loss program is one which can produce a loss of 0.5–1% of the patient's initial body weight per week, a rate of loss considered safe and acceptable [98].

Weight gain because of psychotropics can result from eating too many high-fat, high-calorie foods, although in some cases it may be related to a metabolic abnormality in appetite control.

Simple use of 'portion control' behaviors can teach patients to eat less at every meal without the complexity of counting fat versus carbohydrate calories and does not require the willpower to follow a bland low salt, low fat, low sugar diet. [99] Thus, the first step in losing weight is to restrict the number of high-fat and high-calorie foods in the form of oils and sweets, while increasing the proportions of fruits, vegetables and fiber in the diet by following an ad libitum (patients eat freely, provided they stay within the physician-recommended calorie limits) diet, which is portion controlled and incorporates healthy meals and snack-replacement foods. If this low-fat diet fails, then one can switch to a low-calorie or very-low-calorie diet, which provides a quick initial weight loss. Many patients benefit from the structured approach to weight loss provided by commercial weight loss programs, but the likelihood of regaining the weight on discontinuation of the program is high.

Exercise, especially aerobic, is often least addressed but is one of the most important components of weight maintenance and appetite control. Walking at least 40 min /day produces maximal benefit, but requires considerable commitment and motivation on the part of the patient. [100] However, it has also been shown that walking for only 30 min, three times a week, can be of some benefit. Other than having both physiologic and psychological benefits, it helps in inhibiting food intake, and hence, promoting a sense of self control as well. Exercise, as we know, reduces the risk of medical problems, like heart disease and increases insulin sensitivity in subjects with insulin resistance (as occurs in cases of obesity and diabetes). [101,102].

Cognitive-Behavioral Therapy

Besides diet and exercise, behavior modification techniques involve changing eating habits through identifying the eating or related lifestyle behavior that need to be modified, setting specific goals, modifying determinants of the behavior that need to be changed and reinforcing the desired behaviors.

Through cognitive therapy patients can achieve satisfaction with body image and acceptance of modest weight loss.

Behavior modification programs are offered in groups or individual sessions under the guidance of a professional or a trained lay person. They usually lead to gradual changes in behavior which is more consistent. The effects of cognitive-behavioral therapy on weight gain due to psychotropics was studied in six schizophrenia patients (mean age 37.3 years). It was seen that the mean BMI (kg /m2) decreased from 29.6 in the pretreatment group to 25.1 in the post-treatment group when these techniques were employed [104] They also reported that behavior modification alone can generate a weight loss of 0.5–0.7 kg per week [103].

Pharmacological Weight Reduction Strategies

As mentioned above, informed consent, active monitoring of weight and early intervention (or even prophylaxis with diet and exercise) are the first treatment options. Current clinical practice suggests that anti-obesity drugs are appropriate only when non-pharmacologic approaches have failed or as an adjunct to them; they should not be used as primary therapy for obesity. In general, drug treatment for obesity should be reserved for patients with a BMI greater than 30 or a BMI of 27 with other risk factors like diabetes, stroke or cardiovascular disease. Risks and benefits should be evaluated for each anti-obesity agent and discussed with the patient. Sometimes, prior to trying an anti-obesity medication, one may choose to switch the current psychotropic medication to one with the same indication but less weight gain potential.

Risks and benefits should be evaluated and the decision to resort to antiobesity medication in a population already treated with psychotropic drugs should be made in conjunction with the patient and possibly his/her general physician. The goal of pharmacotherapy is to lose 5–10% of one's baseline weight over 3–6 months. Failure to achieve the initial goal is an indication to stop the medication. However, a plateau in weight loss after 6–9 months is expected and is not cause for stopping the drug. If successful, drug treatment may be continued indefinitely and both the physician and patient must understand and accept the intention to treat long-term.

Drugs that reduce caloric intake, commonly known as anorectic agents or appetite suppressants, do so by decreasing appetite or increasing satiety. They are classified as centrally acting sympathomimetic agents or serotonergic agents. Sympathomimetic agents include phendimetrazine, phentermine, mazindol, diethylpropion (all of which are schedule III and IV controlled substances), amphetamine and related compounds, and phenylpropanolamine. Of the serotonergic agents, fenfluramine and dexfenfluramine were withdrawn from the market in September 1997 over concerns about valvular heart disease. [104] Because of their high potential for abuse, amphetamines are generally not recommended for treating obesity [105].

Sibutramine, a weight loss agent affecting both serotonin and norepinephrine reuptake ,was an effective and well-tolerated adjunct to behavior modification for weight loss in patients with schizophrenia and schizoaffective disorder being treated with olanzapine.[106] However, sibutramine was removed from the US market in October 2010 because of data indicating an increased risk of heart attack and stroke.

Metformin

Short-term studies have suggested that the effects of metformin on body weight and body mass index may be mediated in part by reductions in food intake [107] [108] [109] [110] Metformin has been shown to reduce the rates of weight gain and body fat accumulation in non-diabetic adults. [107] Klein et al. (2006) found that metformin therapy is safe and effective in decreasing weight gain and impaired insulin sensitivity, as well as abnormal glucose metabolism resulting from the treatment with olanzapine in children and adolescents. [111] A recent randomized placebo-controlled study attempted to explore the effectiveness of metformin in preventing antipsychotic-induced weight gain in first-episode schizophrenia patients. It was found to be safe and effective in attenuating olanzapine-induced weight gain and insulin resistance in this group. Good adherence to this type of preventive intervention was seen, as well. [112].

Orlistat is a synthetic inhibitor of gastrointestinal lipases [113]. This results in decreased fat-absorption and increased fat excretion which is dose-dependent. The recommended starting dose is 120 mg PO three times a day but a 60-mg pill (Brand name: Alli) is available for over-the-counter purchase. Several studies have demonstrated significant weight-loss with orlistat compared to placebo in the general population. [114] [115] [116] Common side effects of orlistat include diarrhea, flatulence, dyspepsia and abdominal pain, [117] although some cases of severe liver injury have also been identified. [118] In a randomized, double-blind, placebo-controlled trial, adult patients who were receiving stable clozapine or olanzapine regimens who were not compliant with non-pharmacologic programs or hypocaloric diet were given orlistat. [119] The authors concluded that the effect of orlistat in overweight/obese clozapine-or olanzapine-treated patients is modest and may only be seen in men. Similar results were found in a study from Finland [120]. Interestingly, in this study, patients who did not respond to orlistat within the first 16 weeks did not benefit from continuation treatment.

Topiramate

Preliminary findings suggest that topiramate may serve as a dual purpose agent in the treatment of obese patients with affective disorders. In a 10-week, randomized, double-blind, placebo-controlled study 43 women who had been treated with olanzapine, and had gained weight as a side effect ,weight loss was observed and was significantly more pronounced in the topiramate-treated group . It was seen to be a safe and effective agent in the treatment of weight gain that occurred during olanzapine treatment. A positive effect on health-related quality of life, the patients' actual state of health, and psychological impairments was also observed. [121].

Additionally, topiramate add-on studies for bipolar disorder have shown 33–55% of patients losing weight. (10–15 lbs)[122] [123] Side-effects of fatigue, cognitive dulling, ataxia, glaucoma, oligohydrosis and acidosis are reported at a dose of 100–400 mg/ d.

Rimonabant

Rimonabant, an endocannabinoid receptor (subtype 1) blocker, was developed as a result of observations on the appetite stimulation associated with recreational cannabis use. The drug has a range of both central and metabolic peripheral effects and had also been investigated for smoking cessation. [124] Rimonabant is of interest in schizophrenia also because of evidence from animal and human studies that abnormalities in the endocannabinoid system may play a role in the etiology or expression of schizophrenia [125].

A study showed that rimonabant reduced body weight and waist circumference as compared to placebo ($P < .001$)in the non-diabetic sub group [126]. The most commonly experienced adverse events were gastrointestinal disorders, mood alterations with depressive symptoms, anxiety, dizziness, nausea, and upper respiratory tract infections [127]. A randomized double blind pilot study with rimonabant on weight loss in schizophrenia found that it was safe and well tolerated. In fact, significant improvement in anxiety/depression and hostility factors in the rimonabant group was observed compared with the placebo group. Because of the small sample size a significant effect on BMI was not found [128].

Bupropion

Although bupropion is not approved for weight loss, it has been used *off-label* and is currently under evaluation as combination therapy with naltrexone, a μ-opioid receptor antagonist and zonisamide, a GABA receptor activator. Bupropion is an antidepressant which inhibits reuptake of dopamine (DA) and noradrenaline (NA) resulting in a loss of appetite and decreased food intake [129] and modest weight loss in obese people. [130] [131] [132] [133] The efficacy of bupropion as a sustained release (SR) formulation was demonstrated at 48 weeks in obese patients [134].

Naltrexone

Administration of naloxone to rats results in a significant reduction in short-term food intake by blocking β-endorphin, a find which initially demonstrated the role of opioid receptors in eating behavior. [134]. Naltrexone is a high affinity , long-acting opioid receptor antagonist which was originally produced for the treatment of opioid and alcohol dependence and was also noted to decrease food intake, and led to weight loss in former narcotic addicts. In randomized controlled trials, naltrexone has not consistently demonstrated statistically significant weight loss in obese and lean subjects [135] [136] [137].

Naltrexone, at a dose of 50 mg/d, has been shown to decrease weight by reversing the observed hunger and craving for sweet and fatty foods caused by tricyclic antidepressants and lithium. It does this, possibly, by decreasing food ingestion especially of highly palatable foods. Subjects reported decreased pleasantness ratings of palatable foodstuffs and also diminished subjective feelings of hunger. No adverse effects of opioid antagonism were seen regarding depressive symptoms.

Bupropion Combinations

The use of the combination of bupropion and naltrexone is still under investigation. Since naltrexone blocks β-endorphin mediated pro-opiomelanocortin (POMC) autoinhibition to sustain α-MSH release, while bupropion activates POMC neurons and enhances the release of the anorexiant neuropeptide α-MSH in the hypothalamus ,bupropion has been combined with naltrexone.[138][139] Significant improvements in depressive symptoms in addition to weight loss and improved control of eating in overweight and obese women, with major depression, were observed in an open-label 24-week study that used naltrexone 32 mg SR/bupropion-SR 360 mg. [140] The combination of bupropion with the epilepsy agent zonisamide has been evaluated in three Phase II trials. [141,142] The mechanism of action for zonisamide has not been fully characterised, however it has demonstrated biphasic DA and 5HT activity. [143] The role of bupropion, naltrexone, and [141] zonisamide, as well as their various combinations, in the management of overweight and obesity in the SPMI is yet to be determined. However, the aforementioned study results are encouraging.

Bariatric Surgery

In patients with morbid obesity who fail to maintain weight loss through behavioral programs, or in those for whom the weight loss achieved through behavioral programs is insufficient to improve obesity-related comorbidities, bariatric surgery is a treatment option. Bariatric surgery is the most effective treatment for morbid obesity. In contrast to the modest and often temporary effect of behavioral weight loss programs, bariatric surgery results in profound, sustained weight loss, resolution or improvement of obesity-associated comorbidities, and improved quality of life [144]. More data are required before the proper role of this intervention is understood, however.

Screening and Monitoring

Straker et al. indicated that the presence of abdominal obesity was most sensitive (92.0%), while fasting glucose >110 mg/dl was most specific (95.2%) in correctly identifying the presence of metabolic syndrome. Further, combining the two had 100% sensitivity. It was concluded that the measurement of both abdominal obesity and fasting blood glucose is a simple, cost-effective screening test to detect patients on antipsychotic medications at high risk for future cardiovascular morbidity [145]. Due to the known association between central adiposity and insulin resistance in adults and children ,it was mandated by the International Diabetes Federation Metabolic Syndrome diagnostic scheme that waist circumference must be 1 of at least 3 of 5 criteria met [146] [147]. The results of a recent study by Jin et al (2010) indicated several common clinical and laboratory markers, waist circumference, triglyceride: HDL ratio, and body mass index, as the optimal predictors of metabolic syndrome, and that the use of all three measures combined increased specificity to 97% but achieved a sensitivity of only 50% .Most easily available in psychiatric settings is the BMI. Consequently, the presence of its elevation during a course of treatment should prompt investigation of the other markers, especially fasting lipid and glucose levels.[148] According to the Consensus Guidelines on Metabolic Monitoring all patients receiving an atypical antipsychotic medication should have fasting blood glucose as well as a lipid profile determined at baseline and after 12 weeks of treatment. [149].

Our suggestions would include taking an extensive family history, past medical history and also judicious prescribing of medications to patients with SSI and BD. As discussed above, measuring baseline body weight and subsequent monitoring becomes important on initiation of an antipsychotic. Further monitoring of the lipid profile, blood pressure, blood glucose, EKG, and waist circumference should become an integral part of clinical practice for patients on antipsychotic medications. Collateral contact with the involved primary care doctor should also regularly take place. An example of clinical application of these suggestions is as follows: a patient with SPMI who has a personal and/or first-degree family history of obesity, diabetes, hyperlipidemia, or hypertension would be best served (metabolically) by being prescribed an antipsychotic agent associated with less weight gain (e.g., ziprazdone, aripipirzole). However, if there is no such history the choice of antipsychotic agent can be made from among a greater number of options (influenced, of course, by clinical need). Nevertheless, if more than 5% of baseline body weight is gained, or hyperglycemia or dyslipidemia develops, switching to a drug associated with lower weight gain must be seriously considered.

It has been shown by many data sets that guidelines alone do not lead to an adequate level of monitoring of and interventions for cardiometabolic risk factors among patients with SPMI. Furthermore, the effect on weight gain of monitoring alone has not been robust [150, 151]. It thus becomes important for mental health providers, patients, and their families to be educated and also to make medical monitoring and management an integral part of treating individuals with SPMI. [92] The goal is that, through regular screening, manifest metabolic comorbidities can be prevented or, at least, decreased in drug related weight gain via implementation of early interventions.

Thus far, effect sizes for pharmacologic and non-pharmacologic weight reduction strategies have been in the small to medium range, with the latter displaying a slight superiority. As indicated above, monitoring has produced even smaller effects. Furthermore, the retention of accrued weight loss has not been followed in longer term studies. Accordingly, effects on the incidence of CVD risk factors/metabolic syndrome and mortality are unknown. This remains a challenge for future investigations which need to be adequately powered and of sufficient duration, and which focus on weight loss retention strategies [150,151]. Nevertheless, there is cause for optimism as the mechanisms involved in CVD risk production are becoming better understood, which portends the development of more targeted and effective interventions for SPMI patients [152].

Conclusion

This chapter attempted to review many facets of weight gain and metabolic disorder as it relates to schizophrenia and bipolar disorder. Epidemiology, etiology and treatment options were discussed. It appears that bipolar and schizophrenia patients may be at risk greater than the general population for developing these clinical conditions regardless of medications used. This may be due to genetic and familial loading towards these medical conditions, or due to the fact that patients with severe and persistent mental illness seek care less often and often obtain substandard care as well. Clearly, a majority of psychotropic medications may induce obesity, hypertension, hyperlipdemia, and hyperglucosemia all of which lend themselves to greater cardiovascular risk and shortened life span. Clinicians should take into account the patient's diagnosis, history of adequate healthcare utilization, family history of metabolic disorder, and medication compliance prior to prescribing psychotropics. The greater the current and potential risk a bipolar or schizophrenia patient has after undergoing this clinical evaluation and process, then use of more metabolically friendly psychotropics, where indicated and possible, should be utilized. Psychiatrists who prescribe medications known to increase metabolic risks should become adept at detecting initial signs and symptoms of metabolic disorder and should be quick to refer or treat impending iatrogenic metabolic complications resultant to their prescribing. This suggests that psychiatric prescribers must become aware of treatment guidelines for hypertension, diabetes, and hyperlipidemia often utilized in the realm of primary care. Prescribers should be able to detect these pending medical complications as a standard of care and be willing to treat these aggressively themselves, or refer to appropriate clinicians after initial detection. Metabolic illness has been discussed and reported in the medical literature for over a decade and, slowly, the standard of care is changing where psychiatric practitioners are being held accountable in regards to developing this new skill set. Finally, much of the focus of increased metabolic risk and illness has centered around the increasing use of the (atypical) second generation antipsychotics. Clinicians must be aware that many psychotropics outside of this class of medications will clearly cause weight gain. Where there is weight gain, metabolic illness also likely will exist. It is prudent for clinicians to consider monitoring any type of psychotropic with known weight gain potential and to routinely evaluate these patients as if they were taking a metabolically unfriendly atypical antipsychotic. The same practices and principles outlined in this chapter should apply to them.

References

[1]   Newman SC, Bland RC. Mortality in a cohort of patients with schizophrenia: a record linkage study. *Canadian Journal of Psychiatry.* 1991;36:239-45.

[2]   Judd LL, Akiskal HS. The prevalence and disability of bipolar spectrum disorders in the US population:a reanalysis of the ECA database taking into account subthreshold cases. *Journal of Affective Disorders.* 2003;73(1-2):123-31.

[3]   Must A, Spaers J, Cockley EH ea. The disease burden associated with overweight and obesity. *Journal of the American Medical Association.* 1999;282:1523-59.

[4]   Osborn DP, Nazareth I, King M. Risk for coronary artery disease in people with severe mental illness:corss-sectional comparative study in primary care. *British Journal of Psychiatry.* 2006;188(3):271-77.

[5]   Thakore JH, Mann JN, Vlahos L. Increased visceral fat distribution in drug-naive and drug free patients with schizophrenia. *International Journal of Obesity Related Metabolic Disorders.* 2002;26:137-41.

[6]   Hennekens CH. Increasing global burden of cardiovascular disease in general populations and in patients with schizophrenia. *Journal Of Clinical Psychiatry.* 2007;68:4-7.

[7]   Hennekens CH, Hennekens AR, Hollar D ea. Schizophrenia and increased risks of cardiovascular disease. *American Heart Journal.* 2005;150(6):1115-21.

[8]   Flegal KM, Carroll MD, Ogden CL ea. Prevelance and trends in obesity among US adults. *Journal of the American Medical Association.* 2002;288:1723-27.

[9]   Fagiolini A, Frank A, Houck PR. Prevalence of obesity and weight change during treatment in patients with bipolar I disorder. *Journal Of Clinical Psychiatry.* 2002;63:528-33.

[10]   Allison DB, Fontaine KR, Heo M ea. The distribution of body mass index among individuals witha nd without schizophrenia. *Journal Of Clinical Psychiatry.* 1999;60(215-20).

[11]   McIntyre RS, Konarski JZ, Wilkins K ea. Obesity in bipolar disorder and major depressive disorder:results from a national community survey on mental health and well being. *Canadian Journal of Psychiatry*. 2006;51:274-80.

[12]   Citrome L, Blonde L, Damatarca C. Metabolic issues in patients with severe mental illness. *Southern Medical Journal*. 2005;98(7):714-20.

[13]   Ryan MC, Collins P, Thakore JH. Impaired fasting glucose tolerance in first episode, drug naive patients with schizophrenia. *American Journal of Psychiatry*. 2003;160:284-9.

[14]   Narayan KM, Boyle JP, Thompson TJ ea. Lifetime risk for diabetes mellitus in the United States. *Journal of the American Medical Association*. 2003(290):1884-90.

[15]   McIntyre RS, Soczynska JK, Beyer JL ea. Medical comorbidity in bipolar disorder:reprioritizing unmet needs. *Current Opinion in Psychiatry*. 2007;20:406-16.

[16]   DeHert M, Schreurs V, Vancampfort D ea. Metabolic syndrome in people with schizophrenia:a review. *World Psychiatry*. 2009;8:15-22.

[17]   Sokai J, Messias E, Dickerson FB ea. Comorbidity of medical illnesses among adults with serious mental illness who are receiving community psychiatric services. *Journal of Nervous and Mental Disorders*. 2004;192(421-7).

[18]   Kannel WB, Castelli WP, Gordon T, McNamara PM. Serum cholesterol, lipoproteins, and the risk of coronary artery disease. *Annals of Internal Medicine*. 1971;74:1-12.

[19]   Ford ES, Giles WH, Dietz WH. Prevalence of the metabolic syndrome among US adults: findings from the third national halth and nutrition examination survey. *Journal of the American Medical Association*. 2002;287(356-59).

[20]   McEvoy JP, Meyer JM, Goff DC ea. Prevalence of the metabolic syndrome in patients with schizophrenia:baseline results from the Clinical Antipsychotic Trial of Intervention Effectiveness (CATIE) schizophrenia trial and comparison with national estimates from NHANES III. *Schizophrenia Research*. 2005;80:19-32.

[21]   Krishnan KR. Psychiatric and medical comorbidities of bipolar disorder. *Psychosomatic Medicine*. 2005;67:1-8.

[22]   Davidson S, Judd F, Jolley D, Hocking B, Thompson S, Hyland B. Cardiovascular risk factors for people with mental illness. Australian and *New Zealand Journal of Psychiatry* 2001;35:196-202.

[23]   Schwartz TL, Virk S, Nihalani N ea, . Psychiatric Medication Induced Obesity: An Etiologic Review. *Obesity Reviews*. 2004;5:167-70.

[24]   Meyer JM, Stahl SM. The metabolic syndrome and schizophrenia. *Acta Psychiatrica Scandinavica*. 2008;119(1):4-14.

[25]   Thakore JH. Metabolic disturbance in first episode schizophrenia. *British Journal of Psychiatry*. 2004;184(47suppl):s76-s9.

[26]   Pramyothin P, Khaodhiar L. Metabolic syndrome with the atypical antipsychotics. . *Current opinion in endocrinology, diabetes and obesity*. 2010;17:460-66.

[27]   Monteleone P, Martiadis V, Maj M. Management of schizophrenia with obesity, metabolic, and endocrinological disorders. *Psychiatric Clinics of North America*. 2009;32:775-94.

[28]   Fernandez-Egea E, Bernardo M, Donner T, Conget I, Parellada E, Justicia A, et al. Metabolic profile of antipsychotic-naïve individuals with non-affective psychosis. *British Journal of Psychiatry*. 2009;194:434-8.

[29] Cohn TA, Remington G, Zipursky RB, Azad A, Connolly P, Wolever TM. Resistance and Adiponectin Levels in Drug-Free Patients With Schizophrenia: A Preliminary Report. *Canadian Journal of Psychiatry*. 2006;51(6):382-6.

[30] Saddicha S, Manjunatha N, Ameen S, Akhtar S. Diabetes and schizophrenia – effect of disease or drug? Results from a randomized, double-blind, controlled prospective study in first-episode schizophrenia. *Acta Psychiatrica Scandinava*. 2008;117:342-7.

[31] Venkatasubramanian G, Chittiprol S, Neelakantachar N, Naveen MN, Thirthall J, Gangadhar BN, et al. Insulin and Insulin-Like Growth Factor-1 Abnormalities in Antipsychotic-Naïve Schizophren. *American Journal of Psychiatry*. 2007;164(10):1557-60.

[32] van Nimwegen LJ, Storosum JG, Blumer RM, Allick G, Venema HW, de Haan L, et al. Hepatic Insulin Resistance in Antipsychotic Naive Schizophrenic Patients: Stable Isotope Studies of Glucose Metabolism. *Clinical Endocrinology and Metabolism*. 2008;93(2):572-7.

[33] Verma SK, Subramaniam M, Liew A, Poon LY. Metabolic risk factors in drug-naïve patients with first-episode psychosis. *Journal Of Clinical Psychiatry*. 2009;70(7):997-1000.

[34] Fernandez-Egea E, Bernardo M, Parellada E, Justicia A, Garcia-Rizo C, Esmatjes E, et al. Glucose abnormalities in the siblings of people with schizophrenia. *Schizophrenia Research*. 2008;103:110-3.

[35] Spelman LM, Walsh PI, Sharifi N, Collins P, Thakore JH. Impaired glucose tolerance in first-episode drug-naïve patients with schizophrenia. *Diabetes Medicine*. 2007;24:481-5.

[36] Kim B, Kim SJ, Son JI, Joo YH. Weight change in the acute treatment of bipolar I disorder: a naturalistic observational study of psychiatric inpatients. *Journal of Affective Disorders*. 2008;105(1-3):45-52.

[37] Lin PI, Shuldiner AR. Rethinking the genetic basis for comorbidity of schizophrenia and type 2 diabetes. *Schizophrenia Research*. 2010;123:234-43.

[38] Taylor V, MacQueen G. Associations between bipolar disorder and metabolic syndrome: a review. *Journal Of Clinical Psychiatry*. 2006;67:1034-41.

[39] Bond DS, Roth J, Nash JM, Wing RR. Migraine and obesity: epidemiology, possible mechanisms and the potential role of weight loss treatment. *Obesity Reviews* 2011;12:362-71.

[40] Oedegaard KJ, TA G, Johansson S, Jacobsen KK, Halmoy A, Fasmer OB, et al. A genome-wide association study of bipolar disorder and comorbid migraine. *Genes, Brain, and Behavior*. 2010;9(7):673-80.

[41] Ortiz A, Cervantes P, Zlotnik G, van de Velde C, Slaney C, GarnhAm. J., et al. Cross-prevalence of migraine and bipolar disorder. *Bipolar Disorders*. 2010;12(3):397-403.

[42] Rege S. Antipsychotic induced weight gain in schizophrenia: mechanisms and management. *Austraila and New Zealand Journal of Psychiatry*. 2008;42(5):369-81.

[43] Fagiolini A C, Soreca I, Chang J. Bipolar disorder and the metabolic syndrome. Causal factors, psychiatric outcomes and economic burden. *CNS Drugs*. 2008;22(8):655-69.

[44] Soczynska JK, Kennedy SH, Woldeyohannes HO, Liauw SS, Alsuwaidan M, Yim CY, et al. Mood disorders and obesity: understanding inflammation as a pathophysiological nexus. *Neuromolecular Medicine*.

[45] Jones M, Jones A. The effect of antipsychotic medication on metabolic syndrome. *Acta Psychiatrica Scandanava.* 2008;118(1):4-12.

[46] Stahl SM, Mignon L, Meyer JM. Which comes first: atypical treatment or cardiometabolic risk? *Acta Psychiatrica Scandanava.* 2009;119(3):171-9.

[47] Nasrallah HA. Atypical antipsychotic-induced metabolic side effects : insights from receptor-binding profiles. *Molecular Psychiatry.* 2008;13:7-35.

[48] Torrent C, Amann B, Sánchez-Moreno J, Colom F, Reinares M, Comes M, et al. Weight gain in bipolar disorder: pharmacological treatment as a contributing factor. *Acta Psychiatrica Scandanava.* 2008;118(1):4-18.

[49] Matsui-Sakata A, Ohtani H, Sawada Y. Receptor occupancy-based analysis of the contributions of various receptors to antipsychotics-induced weight gain and diabetes mellitus. *Drug Metabolism and Pharmacokinetics.* 2005;20(5):368-78.

[50] Davidson K, Jonas BS, Dixon KE, Markovitz JH. Do depression symptoms predict early hypertension incidence in young adults in the CARDIA Study? *Archives of Internal Medicine.* 2000;160:1495-500.

[51] Shinagawa M, Otsuka K, Murakami S, Kubo Y, Cornelissen G, Matsubayashi K, et al. Seven-day (24-h) ambulatory blood pressure monitoring, self-reported depression and quality of life scores. Blood *Pressure Monitoring.* 2002;7(1):69-76.

[52] Scalco AZ, Scalco MZ, Azul JBS, Lotufo Neto F. Hypertension and depression. *Clinics.* 2005;60(3).

[53] Casey DE. Metabolic issues and cardiovascular disease in patients with psychiatric disorders. *American Journal of Medicine.* 2005;118(Suppl 2):15s-22s.

[54] Tschoner A, Engl J, Laimer M, Kaser S, Rettenbacher M, Fleischhacker WW, et al. Metabolic side effects of antipsychotic medication. *International Journal of Clinical Practice.* 2007;61(8):1356-70.

[55] McIntyre RS, Danilewitz M, Liauw SS, Kemp DE, Nguyen HT, Kahn LS, et al. Bipolar disorder and metabolic syndrome: an international perspective. *J. Affect Disord.* 2010;126(13):366-87.

[56] Birkenaes AB, Opjordsmoen S, Brunborg C, Engh JA, Jonsdottir H, Ringen PA, et al. The level of cardiovascular risk factors in bipolar disorder equals that of schizophrenia: A comparative study. *Journal Of Clinical Psychiatry.* 2007;68:917-23.

[57] De Leon J, Diaz FJ. Planning for the optimal design of studies to personalize antipsychotic prescriptions in the post-CATIE era: The clinical and pharmacoepidemiological data suggest that pursuing the pharmacogenetics of metabolic syndrome complications (hypertension, diabetes mellitus and hyperlipidemia) may be a reasonable strategy. *Schizophrneia Research* 2007;96:185-97.

[58] Vuksan-Cusa B, Sagud M, Jakovljevic M. C-Reactive protein and metabolic syndrome in patients with bipolar disorder compared to patients with schizophrenia. *Psychiatria Danubia* 2010;22(2):275-77.

[59] Rotar O, Tanyansky D, Martynikhin I, Konradi A, Sokolian N, Denisenko A, et al. Prevalence of metabolic syndrome and serum levels of adipokines in patients with schizophrenia. *Journal of hypertension. Journal of Hypertension.* 2010;38(eSuppl A):e136.

[60] McIntyre RS, Park KY, Law CWY, Sultan F, Adams A, Lourenco MT, et al. The association between conventional antidepressants and the metabolic syndrome.A review of the evidence and clinical implications. *CNS Drugs. 2010*;24(9):741-53.

[61] Bergman RN, Ader M. Atypical antipsychotics and glucose homeostasis. *Journal Of Clinical Psychiatry*. 2005;66(4):504-14.

[62] McElroy SL, Kotwal R, Keck PE Jr, Akiskal HS. Comorbidity of bipolar and eating disorders: distinct or related disorders with shared dysregulations?. *J. Affect Disord*. 2005;86(2-3):107-27.

[63] McElroy SL, Frye MA, Hellemann G, Altshuler L, Leverich GS, Suppes T, et al. Prevalence and correlates of eating disorders in 875 patients with bipolar disorder. *Journal of Affective Disorders*. 2011;128(3):191-98.

[64] Cardenas J, Frye M, Marusak SL, Levander EM, Chirichigno JW, Lewis S, et al. Modal subcomponents of metabolic syndrome in patients with bipolar disorder. *Journal of Affective Disorders*. 2008;106:97-108.

[65] Raedler TJ. Cardiovascular aspects of antipsychotics. *Current Opinion in Psychiatry*. 2010;23:574-81.

[66] Ogawa M, Miyamoto, Kawakami N. Factors associated with glycemic control and diabetes self-care among outpatients with schizophrenia and type 2 diabetes. *Archives of Psychiatric Nursing*. 2011;25(1):63-73.

[67] Heald AH, Sein K, Anderson SG, Pendlebury J, Guy M, Narayan V, et al. Diet, exercise and metabolic syndrome in schizophrenia: a cross-sectional study. *Diabetes Medicine*. 2009;24(Suppl 1):116.

[68] Wildgust HJ, Hodgson R, Beary M. The paradox of premature mortality in schizophrenia: new research questions. Journal of *Psychopharmacology*. 2010;24(11):9-15.

[69] McIntyre RS, Soczynska J, Liauw S, Woldeyohannes H, Brietzke E, Nathanson J, et al. The association between childhood adversity and components of metabolic syndrome in adults with mood disorders: results from the international mood disorders collaborative project. 2010.

[70] Lane HY, Liu YC, Huang CL, Chang YC, Wu PL, Lu CT, et al. Risperidone-related weight gain: genetic and nongenetic predictors. *Journal of Clinical Psychopharmacology*. 2006;26(2):128-34.

[71] Aichhorn W, Whitworth AB, Weiss EM, Marksteiner J. Second-generation antipsychotics: is there evidence for sex differences in pharmacokinetic and adverse effect profiles? *Drug Safety*. 2006;29(7):587-89.

[72] Saddichha S, Ameen S, Akhtar S. Predictors of antipsychotic-induced weight gain in first-episode psychosis: conclusions from a randomized, double-blind, controlled prospective study of olanzapine, risperidone, and haloperidol. *Journal of Clinical Psychopharmacology*. 2008; 28(1):27-31.

[73] Megna JL, Raj Kunwar A, Wade MJ. A retrospective study of weight changes and the contributing factors in short term adult psychiatric inpatients. *Annals of Clinical Psychiatry*. 2006;18(3):163-7.

[74] Haddad P. Weight change with atypical antipsychotics in the treatment of schizophrenia. *Journal of Psychopharmacology*. 2005;19(6 Suppl):16-27.

[75] Daumit GL, Goldberg RW, Anthony C, Dickerson F, Brown CH, Kreyenbuhl J, et al. Physical activity patterns in adults with severe mental illness. *Journal of Nervous and Mental Disorders*. 2005;193(10):641-6.

[76] Meyer JM. Awareness of obesity and weight issues among chronically mentally ill inpatients: a pilot study. *Ann. Clin. Psychiatry*. 2002 Mar;14(1):39-45.

[77] Dolder CR, Lacro JP, Jeste DV. Adherence to antipsychotic and nonpsychiatric medications in middle-aged and older patients with psychotic disorders. *Psychosomatic Medicine* 2003;65 156-62.

[78] Kreyenbuhl J, Dixon LB, McCarthy JF, Soliman S, Ignacio RV, Valenstein M. Does adherence to medications for type 2 diabetes differ between individuals with vs without schizophrenia?. *Schizophrenia Bulletin* 2010;36(2):428-35.

[79] Kilbourne A, Welsh D, McCarthy JF, Post EP, Blow FC. Quality of care for cardiovascular disease-related conditions in patients with and without mental disorders. *J. Gen. Intern. Med.* 2008;23(10):1628-33.

[80] Serretti A, Mandelli L. Antidepressants and body weight: a comprehensive review and meta-analysis. Journal of Clinical Psychiatry *Journal of Clinical Psychiatry* 2010;71(10):1259-72.

[81] Greenway FL, Fujioka K, Plodkowski RA, Mudaliar S, Guttadauria M, Erickson J, et al. Effect of naltrexone plus bupropion on weight loss in overweight and obese adults (COR-I): a multicentre, randomised, double-blind, placebo-controlled, phase 3 trial. *Lancet.* 2010;376(9741).

[82] Nihalani N, Schwartz TL, Siddiqui UA, Megna JL. Obesity and Psychotropics. *Journal of obesity.* 2011.

[83] Verrotti A, Domizio S, Angelozzi B, Sabatino G, Morgese G, Chiarelli F. Changes in serum lipids and lipoproteins in epileptic children treated with anticonvulsants. *Journal of Paediatrics and Child Health.* 1997;33:242-5.

[84] Pita-Calandre E, Rodriguez-Lopez C M, Cano M D, Pena-Bernal M. Serum lipids, lipoproteins, and apolipoproteins in adult epileptics treated with carbamazepine, valproic acid, or phenytoin. *Revista de Neurologia.* 1998;27:785-9.

[85] Gentile S. Long-term treatment with atypical antipsychotics and the risk of weight gain : a literature analysis. *Drug Saf.* 2006;29(4):303-19.

[86] Henderson DC. Schizophrenia and comorbid metabolic disorders. *Journal of Clinical Psychiatry.* 2005;66(6):11-20.

[87] Lieberman J, McEvoy JP, Perkins D ea. Comparison of atypicals in first episode psychosis: a randomized, 52-week comparison of olanzapine, quetiapine and risperidone *Eur. Neuropsychopharmacol.* 2005;15(3):525.

[88] Dossenbach M, Arango-Davila C, Silva IH ea. Response and relapse in patients with schizophrenia treated with olanzapine, risperidone, quetiapine or haloperidol: 12-month follow-up of the Intercontinental Schizophrenia Outpatient Health Outcomes (IC-SOHO) Study. *Clin. Psychiatry* 2005;66:1021–30.

[89] Starrenburg FC, Bogers JP. How can antipsychotics cause Diabetes Mellitus? Insights based on receptor-binding profiles, humoral factors and transporter proteins. *European Psychiatry.* 2009;24(3):164-70.

[90] Blonde L, Kan HJ, Gutterman EM, L'Italien GJ, Kim MS, Hanssens L, et al. Predicted risk of diabetes and coronary heart disease in patients with schizophrenia. *Journal of Clinical Psychiatry.* 2008;69(5):741-8.

[91] Houston JP, Tohen M, Degenhardt EK, Jamal HH, Liu LL, Ketter TA. Olanzapine-divalproex combination versus divalproex monotherapy in the treatment of bipolar mixed episodes: a double-blind, placebo-controlled study. *Journal of Clinical Psychiatry* 2009;70:1540-7.

[92] Correll CU, Frederickson AM, Kane JM, Manu P. Equally increased risk for metabolic syndrome in patients with bipolar disorder and schizophrenia treated with second-generation antipsychotics. *Bipolar Disorders* 2008;10:788-97.

[93] Lee NY, Kim SH, Cho B, Lee YJ, Chang JS, Kang UG, et al. Patients taking medications for bipolar disorder are more prone to metabolic syndrome than Korea's general population. *Progress in neuro-psychopharmacology and biological psychiatry* 2010;34:1243-9.

[94] Yumru M, Savas HA, Kurt E et al. Atypical antipsychotics related metabolic sindrome in bipolar patients. *J. Affect. Disord.* 2007;98:247-52.

[95] Fiedorowicz JG, Palagummi NM, Forman-Hoffman VL, Miller DD, Haynes WG. Elevated prevalence of obesity, metabolic syndrome, and cardiovascular risk factors in bipolar disorder. *Annals of clinical psychiatry.* 2008;20(3):131-7.

[96] Weiss D. How to help your patients lose weight: current therapy for obesity. *Cleve Clin. J. Med.* 2000;67(10):739, 43-6, 49-54.

[97] Mauri M, Castrogiovanni S, Simoncini M, Iovieno N, Miniati M, Rossi A, et al. Effects of an educational intervention on weight gain in patients treated with antipsychotic. *J. Clin. Psychopharmacol.* 2006;26(5):462-6.

[98] Thomas PR. Weighing the Options: Criteria for Evaluating Weight Management Programs/Committee to Develop Criteria for Evaluating the Outcomes of Approaches to Prevent and ·Treat Obesity,Food and Nutrition Board, Institute of Medicine. Washington DC: National Academy Press; 1995.

[99] Hannum SM, Carson L, Evans EM, Canene KA, Petr EL, Bui L, et al. Use of portion-controlled entrees enhances weight loss in women. *Obes. Res.* 2004;12(3):538-46.

[100] Greenburg I, Chan S, Blackburn GL. Nonpharmacologic and pharmacologic management of weight gain. *J. Clin. Psychiatry* 1999;60:31-7.

[101] Kelley DE, Goodpaster BH. Effects of physical activity on insulin action and glucose tolerance in obesity. *Med. Sci. Sports Exerc* 1999;31:S619–S23.

[102] Pajonk FG, Wobrock T, Gruber O, Scherk H, Berner D, Kaizl I, et al. Hippocampal Plasticity in Response to Exercise in Schizophrenia. *Arch. Gen. Psychiatry.* 2010;67(2):133-43.

[103] Umbricht D, Flury H, Bridler R. Cognitive Behavior Therapy for weight gain. *Am. J. Psychiatry* 2001;158:971–2.

[104] Connolly HM, Crary JL, McGoon MD, Hensrud DD, Edwards BS, Edwards WD, et al. Valvular heart disease associated with fenfluramine-phentermine. *N. Engl. J. Med.* 1997;227:581–8.

[105] Bray GA. Use and abuse of appetite suppressant drugs in the treatment of obesity. *Ann. Intern. Med.* 1993;119:707–13.

[106] Henderson DC, Copeland PM, Daley TB, Borba CP, Cather C, Nguyen DD, Louie PM, Evins AE, Freudenreich O, Hayden D, Goff DC. A Double-Blind, Placebo-Controlled Trial of Sibutramine for Olanzapine-Associated Weight Gain. *Am. J. Psychiatry* 2005;162:954-62.

[107] Fontbonne A, Charles MA, Juhan-Vague I. The effect of metformin on the metabolic abnormalities associated with upper-body fat distribution. *Diabetes Care* 1996;19:920–6.

[108] Paolisso G, Amatao L, Eccellente R. Effect of metformin on food intake in obese subjects. . *Eur J. Clin. Invest* 1998;28:441–6.

[109] Nestler JE, Beer NA, Jakubowicz DJ, Beer RM. Effects of a reduction in circulating insulin by metformin on serum dehydroepiandrosterone sulfate in nondiabetic men. *J. Clin. Endocrinol. Metab.* 1994;78:549–54.

[110] Glueck CJ, Fontaine RN, Wang P, Subbiah MT, Weber K, Illig E, et al. Metformin reduces weight, centripetal obesity, insulin, leptin, and low-density lipoprotein cholesterol in nondiabetic, morbidly obese subjects with body mass index greater than 30. *Metabolism* 2001;50:856–61.

[111] Klein DJ, Cottingham EM, Sorter M, Barton BA, Morrison JA. A randomized, double-blind, placebo-controlled trial of metformin treatment of weight gain associated with initiation of atypical antipsychotic therapy in children and adolescents. *Am. J. Psychiatry* 2006;163:2072–9.

[112] Ren-Rong Wu, Jing-Ping Zhao, Xiao-Feng Guo, Yi-Qun He, Mao-Sheng Fang, Wen-Bin Guo, et al. Metformin Addition Attenuates Olanzapine-Induced Weight Gain in Drug-Naive First-Episode Schizophrenia Patients.A Double-Blind, Placebo-Controlled Study *Am. J. Psychiatry* 2008;165:352-8.

[113] Guerciolini R. Mode of action of orlistat. *Int. J. Obes. Relat. Metab. Disord* 1997;21:S12–S3.

[114] Franz MJ, VanWormer JJ, Crain AL ea. Weight-loss outcomes: a systematic review and meta-analysis of weight-loss clinical trials with a minimum 1-year follow-up. *Journal of the American Dietetic Association.* 2007;107(10):1755–67.

[115] O'Meara S, Riemsma R, Shirran L, Mather L, Ter Riet G. A systematic review of the clinical effectiveness of orlistat used for the management of obesity. *Obesity Reviews.* 2004;5(1):51-68.

[116] Sjöström L, Rissanen A, Andersen T ea. Randomised placebo-controlled trial of orlistat for weight loss and prevention of weight regain in obese patients.European Multicentre Orlistat Study Group. *Lancet* 1998;352:167.

[117] Hollander PA, Elbein SC, Hirsch IB ea. Role of orlistat in the treatment of obese patients with type 2 diabetes. A 1-year randomized double-blind study. *Diabetes Care.* 1998;21:1288.

[118] FDA, Communication DS. Completed safety review of Xenical/Alli (orlistat) and severe liver injury; 2010.

[119] Joffe G, Takala P, Tchoukhine E, Hakko H, Raidma M, Putkonen H, et al. Orlistat in clozapine- or olanzapine-treated patients with overweight or obesity. *J. Clin. Psychiatry.* 2008;69(5):706-11

[120] Tchoukhine E, Takala P, Hakko H, Raidma M, Putkonen H, Räsänen P, et al. Orlistat in clozapine- or olanzapine-treated patients with overweight or obesity: a 16-week open-label extension phase and both phases of a randomized controlled trial. *J. Clin. Psychiatry.* 2011;72(3):326-30.

[121] Nickel MK, Nickel C, Muehlbacher M, Leiberich PK, Kaplan P, Lahmann C, et al. Influence of topiramate on olanzapine-related adiposity in women: a random, double-blind, placebo-controlled study. *J. Clin. Psychopharmacol.* 2005;25(3):211-7.

[122] Ghaemi SN, Manwani SG, Katzow JJ, Ko JY, Goodwin FK. Topiramate treatment of bipolar spectrum disorders: a retrospective chart review. *Ann. Clin. Psychiatry* 2001;13:185–9.

[123] Vieta E, Torrent C, Garcia-Ribas G, Gilabert A, Garcia-Pares G, Rodriguez A, et al. Use of topiramate in treatment-resistant bipolar spectrum disorders. *J. Clin. Psychopharmacol.* 2002;22:431–5.

[124] Cahill K, Ussher M. Cannabinoid type 1 receptor antagonists (rimonabant) for smoking cessation. *Cochrane Database of Systematic Reviews* 2007;4.

[125] Fernandez-Espejo E, Viveros MP, Nunez L ea. Role of cannabis and endocannabinoids in the genesis of schizophrenia. *Psychopharmacology* (Berl). 2009;206(4):531-49.

[126] Van Gaal L, Pi-Sunyer X, Després JP, McCarthy C, Scheen A. Efficacy and safety of rimonabant for improvement of multiple cardiometabolic risk factors in overweight/obese patients: pooled 1-year data from the Rimonabant in Obesity (RIO) program. *Diabetes care.* 2008;31(2):S229–40.

[127] Galve-Roperh I, Palazuelos J, Aguado T ea. The endocannabinoid system and the regulation of neural development: potential implications in psychiatric disorders. *Eur. Arch. Psychiatry Clin. Neurosci.* 2009;259(7):371-82.

[128] Kelly DL, Gorelick DA, Conley RR, Boggs DL , Linthicum J, Liu F , et al. Effects of the Cannabinoid-1 Receptor Antagonist Rimonabant on Psychiatric Symptoms in Overweight People With Schizophrenia: A Randomized, Double-Blind, Pilot Study. *Journal of Clinical Psychopharmacology.* 2011;31(1):86-91.

[129] Plodkowski RA, Nguyen Q, Sundaram U, Nguyen L, Chau DL, St Jeor S. Bupropion and naltrexone: a review of their use individually and in combination for the treatment of obesity. *Expert Opinion on Pharmacotherapy.* 2009;10(6):1069–81.

[130] Anderson JW, Greenway FL, Fujioka K, Gadde KM, McKenney J, O'Neil PM. Bupropion SR enhances weight loss: a 48-week double-blind, placebo-controlled trial. *Obesity Research.* 2002;10(7):633–41.

[131] Croft H, Houser T, Leadbetter R, Jamerson B. Effect of bupropion SR on weight in the long-term treatment of depression. *Obesity Research.* 2000;8(1):10.

[132] Gadde KM, Parker CB, Maner LG ea. Bupropion for weight loss: an investigation of efficacy and tolerability in overweight and obese women. *Obesity Research.* 2001;9(9):544–51.

[133] Li Z, Maglione M, Tu W ea. Meta-analysis: pharmacologic treatment of obesity. *Annals of Internal Medicine.* 2005;142(7):532–46.

[134] Holtzman SG. Suppression of appetitive behavior in the rat by naloxone: lack of effect of prior morphine dependence. *Life Sciences.* 1979;24(3):219–26.

[135] Bertino M, Beauchamp GK, Engelman K. Naltrexone, an opioid blocker, alters taste perception and nutrient intake in humans. . *American Journal of Physiology.* 1991;261(1):R59–R63.

[136] Atkinson RL, Berke LK, Drake CR. Effects of long-term therapy with naltrexone on body weight in obesity. *Clinical Pharmacology and Therapeutics.* 1985;38(4):419–22.

[137] Spiegel TA, Stunkard AJ, Shrager EE. Effect of Naltrexone on food intake, hunger, and satiety in obese men. *Physiology and Behavior.* 1987;40(2).

[138] Cone RD. Anatomy and regulation of the central melanocortin system. *Nature Neuroscience.* 2005;8(5):571–8.

[139] Grossman HC, Hadjimarkou MM, Silva RM ea. Interrelationships between mu opiod and melanocortin receptors in mediating food intake in rats. *Brain Research.* 2003;991:240-4.

[140] Mcelroy SL, Guerdjikova AI, Rosen A, Kim DD, Landbloom R, Dunayevich E. An open-label study evaluating the naltrexone SR/bupropion SR combination therapy in overweight or obese subjects with major depression. *American Diabetes Association 70th Scientific Meeting*. 2010.

[141] Gadde KM, Yonish GM, Foust MS, Wagner HR II. Combination therapy of zonisamide and bupropion for weight reduction in obese women: a preliminary, randomized,open-label study. *Journal of Clinical Psychiatry*. 2007;68(8):1226–9.

[142] Greenway F, Anderson J, Atkinson R et al. Bupropion and zonisamide for the treatment of obesity *Obesity Research*. 2006;14.

[143] Gadde KM, Franciscy DM, Wagner HR 2nd, Krishnan KR. *JAMA*. 2003;289(14):1820–5.

[144] Ahmed AT, Blair TR, McIntyre RS. Surgical treatment of morbid obesity among patients with bipolar disorder: a research agenda. *Adv. Ther.* 2011;28(5):389-400.

[145] Straker D, Correll CU, Kramer-Ginsberg E, Abdulhamid N, Koshy F, Rubens E, Saint-Vil R, Kane JM, Manu P. Cost-Effective Screening for the Metabolic Syndrome in Patients Treated With Second-Generation Antipsychotic Medications *Am. J. Psychiatry*. 2005;162(6).

[146] Wahrenberg H, Hertel K, Leijonhufvud BM ea. Use of waist circumference to predict insulin resistance: retrospective study. 2005;330:1363–4.

[147] Hirschler V, Maccallini G, Calcagno M ea. Waist circumference identifies primary school children with metabolic syndrome abnormalities. *Diabetes Technol Ther.* 2007;9(2):149–57.

[148] Jin H, Meyer J, Mudaliar S, Henry R, Khandrika S, Glorioso DK, Kraemer H, Jeste D. Use of Clinical Markers to Identify Metabolic Syndrome in Antipsychotic-Treated Patients *J. Clin. Psychiatry* 2010;71(10):1273–8.

[149] Association. ADAaAP. *J. Clin. Psychiatry* 2004;65:267-72.

[150] Megna JL, Schwartz TL, Siddiqui UA, Herrera Rojas M. Obesity in adults with serious and persistent mental illness: a review of postulated mechanisms and current interventions. *Ann. Clin. Psychiatry.* 2011;23(2):131-40.

[151] Dixon L, Perkins D, Calmes C. Guideline watch (september 2009) Practice guideline for treatment of patients with Schizophrenia. Second ed. Arlington: *American Psychiatric Publishing* Inc.; 2009.

[152] Schwartz TL,Nihalani N, Virk S, Jindal S, Chilton M. Psychiatric medication-induced obesity:treatment options. *Obesity reviews* 2004:233–8.

In: Current Advances in Cardiovascular Risk. Volume 2   ISBN: 978-1-62081-746-9
Editor: Sandeep Ajoy Saha   © 2012 Nova Science Publishers, Inc.

Chapter XXIII

Management of Cardiovascular Risk in African-American Patients

Tochukwu M. Okwuosa[*] *and Kim A. Williams*
Wayne State University School of Medicine, Detroit, MI, US

Abstract

Compared with any other race/ethnic group in the United States, African-Americans have the highest incidence of CHD and heart failure – with an earlier age of onset. They also exhibit the highest overall prevalence of hypertension, LVH, stroke and heart failure; as well as the highest rate of out-of-hospital coronary death, and mortality from hypertension, heart failure, stroke and sudden cardiac death. The high rate of CVD and CHD observed in African-Americans appears to be out of proportion to risk burden. As such, different mechanisms for CHD and CVD have been suggested in this group.

Some observed differences in pathophysiology of CVD in African-Americans compared with any other race/ethnicity within the US include higher salt-sensitivity, and more microvascular disease/endothelial dysfunction as a contributor to CHD. For those with CAD, stabilization of coronary plaque through fibrosis and calcification appears to be less common in this population.

This could explain the higher rate of coronary-related deaths in African-Americans, despite an observed lower rate of obstructive CAD. In African-Americans, the mechanism of heart failure – which is more common in this race compared with any other race in the U.S. – appears to be more often a function of hypertension and LVH, rather than CAD as observed in non-African-Americans. These differences in pathophysiology have therapeutic implications for different aspects of CVD in African-American patients, such as heart failure and even blood pressure control.

Given the higher prevalence of obesity in African-Americans, efforts aimed at weight reduction in this population, as well as obesity prevention in African-American children – through education on diet and exercise – could translate into immense risk factor modification, and reduced overall CVD incidence and prevalence in African-

[*] Corresponding Author: Tochukwu E. M. Okwuosa, D.O., FACC, Assistant Professor of Medicine and Cardiology, Wayne State University School of Medicine, Harper University Hospital, 3990 John R – 4 Hudson, Detroit, MI 48201, Telephone: 313.966.0273 or 773.354.1497, Fax: 313.745.8643, Email: tokwuosa@gmail.com.

Americans. Some genetic polymorphisms have been linked to mechanisms of different aspects of CVD in African-Americans and are discussed here, along with the role of proteomics, ribomics, metabolomics, lipomics and pharmacogenomics in future prevention of CVD.

Abbreviations

ACE	Angiotensin Converting Enzyme
A-Heft	African-American Heart Failure Trial
ALLHAT	Antihypertensive and Lipid-Lowering Treatment to Prevent Heart Attack Trial
ALLHAT-LLT	ALLHAT Lipid-Lowering Trial
ARB	Angiotensin Receptor Blocker
ARIC	Atherosclerotic Risk in Communities
BMI	Body Mass Index
CABG	Coronary Artery Bypass Grafting
CAC	Coronary Artery Calcium
CAD	Coronary Artery Disease
CARDIA	Coronary Artery Risk Development In young Adults
CCB	Calcium-Channel Blocker
CDC	Center for Disease Control and Prevention
CHD	Coronary Heart Disease
CHF	Congestive Heart Failure
CHS	Cardiovascular Health Study
CIMT	Carotid Intima-Medial Thickness
CVD	Cardiovascular Disease
CRP	C-Reactive Protein
CRT	Cardiac Resynchronization Therapy
CRT-D	CRT plus ICD
DASH	Dietary Approaches to Stop Hypertension
ESRD	End-Stage Renal Disease
GWAS	Genome-Wide Association Study
HDL	High-Density Lipoprotein Cholesterol
ICD	Implantable Cardioverter Defibrillator
KEEP	Kidney Early Evaluation Program
LDL	Low-Density Lipoprotein Cholesterol
LIFE	Losartan Intervention For Endpoint reduction
Lp-PLA2	Lipoprotein-Associated Phospholipase A2
LVH	Left Ventricular Hypertrophy
MESA	Multi-Ethnic Study of Atherosclerosis
MI	Myocardial Infarction
PAD	Peripheral Arterial Disease
REACH	Racial and Ethnic Approaches to Community Health
SNP	Single Nucleotide Polymorphism
SPECT	Single-Photon Emission Computed Tomography

STEMI   ST-Elevation Myocardial Infarction
TOHP   Trial of Hypertension Prevention

Introduction

CVD is the leading cause of morbidity and mortality in the United States with a prevalence that is disproportionately higher in African-Americans compared with whites. It is a major contributor to the reduced life expectancy observed in African-Americans. [1] Compared with any other race/ethnic group in the United States, African-Americans have the highest incidence of stroke, heart failure and CVD in general – with an earlier age of onset. [2] Risk of sudden cardiac death is particularly higher among African-Americans. [3].

Most African-Americans have at least one risk factor and overall, have higher total number of cardiovascular risk factors, and fewer ideal cardiovascular health parameters compared with European-Americans. [4-7] African-Americans have consistently been shown to have higher prevalence of hypertension, uncontrolled hypertension, diabetes, insulin resistance, obesity and albuminuria; and lower levels of triglycerides and LDL levels relative to Caucasians. [8, 9] The reason for the excess CVD risk in African-Americans is not completely understood, but economic, psychosocial, genetic and physiologic mechanisms have been proposed.

In this chapter, we discuss the cardiovascular risk in African-American patients - with a focus on recent advances in the understanding of pathophysiology, therapeutic considerations, and specific preventive strategies against CVD in African-Americans.

Specific Risk Factors and Pathophysiology

Hypertension

The prevalence of hypertension is significantly higher in African-Americans compared with any other racial/ethnic group within the United States. [2] Compared with Caucasians, African-Americans have higher prevalence of pre-hypertension, develop hypertension earlier in life, have higher and more severe blood pressures throughout life with significantly higher cardiovascular disease and mortality associated with hypertension. [2, 10-12] Compared with European Americans, African-Americans have 15-fold greater risk of ESRD related to hypertension. [13] Hypertension is a particularly strong predictor of CVD risk in African-American women, with 5-fold higher CV mortality versus African-American men with 2-fold greater CV mortality compared with whites. [13] African-American children with essential hypertension seemed to be at increased cardiovascular risk (with higher casual and 24-hour diastolic blood pressure; as well as higher daytime, nighttime and overall 24-hour blood pressure loads); and had significantly more co-morbidities including left ventricular hypertrophy, overweight/obesity and higher plasma renin activity compared with non-African-American children with essential hypertension. [14] Similarly, African-American adults exhibited blunted sleep-period systolic blood pressure dipping, and higher sleep-period systolic and diastolic blood pressure compared with white adults. [15] This appeared to be related to higher BMI and poorer sleep quality observed in African-Americans. [15] While systolic blood pressure was a better predictor of CHD mortality in older whites, systolic blood pressure was more indicative of CHD mortality in African-Americans across all age groups. [16].

Different mechanisms for higher prevalence and severity of hypertension in blacks have been described. There are likely differences in vasoreactivity between black and white individuals as observed in a study by Ergul *et al,* showing 4 to 8-fold higher endothelin-1 levels (a powerful vasoconstrictor) in black persons diagnosed with hypertension, compared with normotensive controls or white individuals with hypertension. [17] He also later showed both endothelin A and B receptors in saphenous vein grafts of black patients versus only endothelin A receptors in saphenous vein grafts of white persons, suggesting higher propensity for vasoconstriction in black individuals. [18] Black children from the Bogalusa heart study are shown to have lower renin levels, with lower 24-hour urinary potassium excretion relative to white children who had faster heart rates, higher glucose and lower insulin levels and a greater relation of blood pressure to body fat. [19] This possibly implicates the renin-angiotensin system and dietary sodium intake in the mechanism of hypertension in blacks, and more of metabolic and adrenergic influences on blood pressure levels in whites. [19] Indeed, the fact that the DASH diet demonstrated greater reductions in blood pressure in both hypertensive and non-hypertensive African-Americans more than Caucasians, possibly implicates diet and higher sodium levels in the mechanism of hypertension in African-Americans. [20] Similarly, potassium administration in black children resulted in lower blood pressures. [21] The stimulus response to orthostasis, handgrip and cold pressor blood pressure challenges was significantly greater in black compared with white children, [19] possibly suggesting a higher sympathetic, or less vagal tone in this population.

Hypertension seems to be more prevalent in black Africans compared with African-Americans, after adjusting for other risk factors,[22, 23] suggesting a possible role of the social environment in the pathophysiology of hypertension in blacks. In fact, neighborhood income, as well as individual income and education have been shown to be independent predictors of blood pressure in blacks. [24] With a more sedentary lifestyle and better access to fast foods than African blacks, the mechanism of hypertension in African-Americans could be mediated through increased BMI which has been shown to be an independent predictor of blood pressure in African-Americans. [25] More recent studies suggest vitamin D as a possible mediator of higher blood pressures in African-Americans relative to Caucasians. [26] In general, hypertension appears to contribute more to pathophysiology of CVD in African-American than Caucasians. Higher blood pressure levels are associated with microalbuminuria in black but not white children; and possibly relates to long-term burden of blood pressure causing rapidly advancing renal disease in blacks. [27] Nephrosclerosis occurring as a result of hypertension, happens more often in blacks than whites. [28].

Dyslipidemia

Relative to Caucasians, African-Americans have lower prevalence of elevated triglycerides and LDL, with a higher prevalence of low HDL. [29-32] This seemingly non-atherogenic lipid profile appears to be independent of diet in African-Americans, [33] and seems to exist relatively early in life in black children. [34] As such, elevated triglycerides contribute the least, while low HDL contributed the most to metabolic syndrome in African-Americans. [29-31, 35, 36] Consequently, other lipid measures such as ApoB/apoA-1 ratio have been suggested as a better prognosticator of CAD, and therefore a better assessor of the metabolic syndrome in African-Americans. [37].

Despite the lower prevalence of high LDL cholesterol, African-Americans with elevated levels of LDL cholesterol appear to have very high levels, and have more atherogenic LDL particle profile relative to Caucasians. African-Americans exhibited higher levels of oxidized LDL in a multi-ethnic sample of 879 non-statin users, [38] and in other studies, were shown to have small LDL particle size. [31, 32] In addition, elevated LDL cholesterol appears to have more negative CV effects in African-Americans compared with Caucasians. For example, the association between plasma lipids and PAD appear to be stronger in African-Americans. [39] Also, hypertensive African-American men and women have been shown to have lower LDL particle size relative to whites. [31] Although African-Americans have lower levels of triglycerides relative to Caucasians, those with elevated triglycerides exhibit worsening insulin resistance with increasing triglyceride levels. [40].

Obesity/Physical Activity

The prevalence of obesity continues to worsen in younger children of all races, and is fast becoming an epidemic in the United States. [2] For adults over 18 years of age, African-Americans exhibit a higher prevalence of obesity compared with European-Americans (~38% versus 27%). [2] This appears to be a major risk factor for CHD/CVD in this population. Although it does not explain all the differences in mechanism of disease in African-Americans, obesity constitutes a major risk factor for other CVD risk factors such as diabetes and hypertension, which then lead to overt CVD in African-Americans.

A major contributor to obesity in African-Americans is low physical fitness/activity levels. [41] Fitness is known to decrease cardiovascular mortality, and even alters the obesity paradox. [42] Obesity has been associated with clinical and subclinical atherosclerosis. [43] Although blacks generally have higher BMI relative to whites, black women appear to have less total body fat distribution and visceral adipose tissue compared with white women of similar BMI; [44, 45] and after adjusting for BMI, black children had lower waist circumference and subcutaneous adipose tissue relative to white children. [46] For a given waist circumference, blacks had less visceral adipose tissue than whites; [47] and within a BMI range, waist circumference cut-offs were shown to be higher for blacks than for whites. [48] Visceral adipose tissue correlated better with BMI in white more than black persons. [45].

Ethnic differences appear to exist in the association of obesity and CVD. Obesity (defined using BMI) appears to be related to elevated blood pressure in white, but not black children. [27] Furthermore, increased BMI was shown to be associated with increased risk for CVD mortality in white, but not black women; [49] and waist circumference was more strongly correlated with parameters of insulin resistance in white more than black participants. [47] In fact, a small study of 640 patients (~67% African-Americans) who underwent coronary angiography at a tertiary center showed an inverse relationship between angiographic CAD severity and BMI in African-American women. [50] Body fat distribution and BMI correlated less with lipid parameters and cardiovascular risk factors such as hypertension and diabetes in African-Americans compared with whites. [51, 52] As such, waist circumference is suggested to be a better indicator of CVD risk than BMI, particularly in African-Americans. [48].

There are also possible ethnic differences in effects of visceral obesity as suggested by an inverse association of the amount of visceral adipose tissue with adiponectin levels in African-Americans, but not in whites. [53] Adiponectin levels are independently negatively associated with CAD. [54].

Diabetes

In the ARIC study, African-Americans were shown to have a disproportionately higher incidence of type-2 diabetes compared with Caucasians. The incidence was 1.5 times higher in African-American men and 2.4 times higher in African-American women relative to their European-American counterparts. [55] The higher incidence of diabetes observed in the African-American population appears to be a significant contributor to CHD in this population. [13] Compared with European-Americans, African-Americans have significantly higher rates of MI, ESRD, stroke and CHF as complications of diabetes. [56] Risk factors such as hypertension and dyslipidemia are also higher in African-Americans compared with European-Americans with diabetes. [13] It is likely that the higher prevalence of obesity in African-Americans is a major contributor to elevated risk of type-2 diabetes in this population.

Other Risk Factors/Metabolic Syndrome

A lot of increased risk of CVD in the African-American population is related to higher total number of cardiovascular risk factors, and fewer ideal cardiovascular health parameters observed in this population. [4-7] African-Americans have consistently been shown to have higher prevalence of hypertension, uncontrolled hypertension, diabetes, insulin resistance, obesity and albuminuria; and lower levels of triglycerides and LDL cholesterol levels relative to Caucasians. [8, 9] This risk factor prevalence pattern holds through in childhood, and carries through adulthood, with black children exhibiting higher levels of hemoglobin A1c, insulin and CRP compared with white children. [57] The levels of HDL cholesterol in blacks are controversial with some studies suggesting higher and other suggesting lower levels relative to whites. In general, it appears African-American women have lower levels of HDL cholesterol, while African-American men have higher levels relative to Caucasian-American women and men, respectively. [58].

Because of low frequency of hypertriglyceridemia, African-Americans (even overweight/obese persons) have lower prevalence of the metabolic syndrome relative to whites, despite being at greater risk of CVD. [40, 59, 60] As such, calls have been made for a different definition of the metabolic syndrome in this population. [61] Of note, African-American women have 1.5 times higher prevalence of the metabolic syndrome relative to African-American men. [62] This has been attributed to higher prevalence of obesity, hypertension and diabetes, as well as lower physical activity levels in African-American women compared with African-American men. [63] Elevated blood pressure seems to be a major determinant of the definition of the metabolic syndrome in African-Americans. [60] It is noteworthy that the Framingham risk score made up of traditional cardiovascular risk factors predicts CVD risk equally in African-Americans and Caucasians, despite differing strengths of association between individual risk factors and CVD mortality. [64].

Major Disease Processes and Pathophysiology

Coronary Heart Disease (CHD) and Myocardial Infarction (MI]

African-Americans have the highest overall CHD mortality, sudden cardiac death and out-of-hospital coronary death rates. [65-70] Furthermore, African-Americans have an earlier age of onset; and the incidence of CHD is higher in African-Americans than whites. [69, 71, 72] The unadjusted risk for CHD is higher in blacks, particularly females. [69, 71, 72] Regardless, African-Americans have higher CHD death rates compared with white men within the younger age groups; [66, 67] and have the highest out-of-hospital coronary death rates (especially at younger ages), compared with any other racial/ethnic group in the United States. [13] This disturbing disparity trend has worsened in recent times. [66].

These trends in CHD mortality rates observed in (particularly young and middle-aged) African-Americans appear to be out of proportion to observed CHD risk burden including obesity, hypertension and diabetes. [73, 74] In fact, angiographic CAD occurs more frequently in whites and Hispanics compared with blacks. [75-80] The reason for this paradox may lie in the fact that different mechanisms have been suggested as regards ischemic heart disease in blacks compared with whites [81, 82].

The increase in incidence and prevalence of CHD events in African-Americans could be mediated through increased risk of thrombosis and inflammation as observed with thrombogenic factors and inflammatory markers in this population. Although African-Americans had lower Lp-PLA2 mass and activity levels,[83, 84] Lp-PLA2 index was independently associated with CHD in African-Americans, but not Caucasians. [85] Markers of inflammation such as CRP increased in blacks, but not whites with depression. [86] This suggests that increased risk of CVD observed in blacks could be mediated in part by psycho-social factors. Indeed, CRP levels are generally higher in African-Americans compared with any other racial/ethnic group within the United States [87, 88].

One study of 7849 patients undergoing pharmacologic stress testing found that African-Americans had higher SPECT myocardial perfusion abnormalities (21% vs. 13%), and higher annual CHD/CVD mortality rates for the same level of SPECT abnormalities compared with whites. [89] This could be mediated through microvascular disease and endothelial dysfunction and could be possible mechanisms for CHD in African-Americans. It is noteworthy that a study of 47 novel protein markers between blacks and whites, showed that African-Americans had significantly higher levels of 19 markers (including inflammatory markers, leptin, vasoconstrictor antidiuretic peptide, and markers of calcification and thrombosis), and lower levels of 6 markers (including adiponectin and vasodilator natriuretic peptide) relative to Caucasians. [90] Compared with Caucasians, African-Americans had higher levels of oxidative stress response compounds with acute exercise, [91] possibly suggesting that they may be more prone to vascular injury even with daily living activities.

A Nationwide Inpatient Sample database registry of over 1.3 million patients diagnosed with acute STEMI from 1988 to 2004 suggested the highest mortality rates from STEMI in African-Americans. [92] More recently however, despite slower revascularization times in African-Americans,[93] less use of angiography [94, 95] and percutaneous coronary intervention PCI, [96] and less use of beta-blockers and aspirin, [95] the 30-day survival after STEMI appears to be similar in blacks compared with whites, [93-95, 97]. However, long-term mortality rate was higher in African-Americans, [97] who also had higher likelihood of angina and worse quality of life at 1-year [98, 99] as well as higher incidence of MI, CHF and significantly lower survival compared with Caucasians at 5-year follow-up [100].

Heart Failure

Heart failure is a major cause of morbidity and mortality in the United States, with estimated direct and indirect costs of $37.2 billion in 2009. [69] The estimated annual mortality rate for heart failure is about 20%, with an average 5-year mortality rate of about 50%. [69, 101, 102] The incidence of heart failure in the U.S. is on the rise – singled out as an emerging epidemic. [102, 103] Heart failure is more common in blacks, affecting 3% of all black adults. [104, 105] This represents a 50% higher incidence in blacks, compared with the rest of the population. Data from the ARIC showed that the age-adjusted incidence rate (per 1000 person-years) for heart failure is significantly higher in African American men and women (9.1 and 8.1, respectively) compared with white men and women (6.0 and 3.4, respectively). [101] Other studies have reported similar findings with the incidence rate of heart failure in blacks being 20 times higher than that observed in whites in a CARDIA study. [106] In addition, blacks exhibit an earlier age of onset of heart failure compared with non-blacks, and demonstrate a rapidly progressive course once diagnosed. [104, 105] The reason for the greater risk and severity of heart failure in blacks is not fully understood. [106].

It appears heart failure in African-Americans is mostly mediated through hypertension which independently portends significantly increased risk of new heart failure in blacks. [107] After adjusting for cardiovascular risk factors, African-Americans with systolic heart failure had more hypertension, obesity and diabetes, [107-112] are younger and have lower ejection fraction [109, 111, 113] compared with Caucasians who tended to have more coronary heart disease and peripheral arterial disease. [108, 111, 113, 114] Hypertension also predicted heart failure admissions in African-Americans. [115] [107, 116] African-Americans have an impaired nitric oxide related vasodilation of smooth muscle and endothelial cells relative to Caucasians [117, 118], suggesting endothelial dysfunction as a possible mediator of heart failure and CVD in this population. This is because endothelial dysfunction leads to reduced production and bioavailability of nitric oxide, which in turn increases the production of reactive oxygen species and oxidative stress; thus altering myocyte function and increasing cardiac hypertrophy [119].

Mortality due to heart failure appears to be related to etiology. In the CHS of 1264 participants over 65 years old with incident heart failure, there was no racial difference cardiovascular mortality outcome over a 100-person year follow-up period. [108] However, when stratified by ischemic and non-ischemic etiologies, there was decreased survival in

African-Americans who had non-ischemic etiology of heart failure compared with blacks with ischemic etiology for their heart failure. [111] B-type natriuretic peptide appears to be equally predictive of dyspnea and heart failure severity in African-Americans and Caucasians. [120, 121] It should be noted that part of the etiology of heart failure deaths in African-Americans is the relatively lower prescription of recommended heart failure therapy in this population.

Although sudden cardiac death rates are much higher in the African-American population, and cardiac resynchronization and ICD therapies have been shown to be equally effective in whites and blacks, black patients are less likely to receive ICD or CRT-D relative to white patients. [122-126].

Renal Disease

Dialysis-dependent kidney failure is much more common in African-Americans compared with whites. [61, 127-132] Regardless, the survival advantage is higher in African-Americans once dialysis is initiated. [127] Heart failure and atherosclerotic CVD, including CAD (including fatal and non-fatal MI), PAD, CVD and CVD mortality are also more common in whites compared with African-Americans with ESRD on dialysis. [131, 133, 134] These findings appear to be independent of baseline traditional risk factors, duration of dialysis, pre-ESRD mortality, or other dialysis-related factors. [132, 133] Despite a higher incidence and risk of MI in the renal disease and dialysis population, African-Americans with chronic kidney disease and those with ESRD on dialysis have lower crude prevalence rates and lower incidence of fatal and non-fatal MI compared with their white counterparts. [135, 136] This pattern seems unchanged in the acute setting such that in-hospital mortality due to CABG, cardiac catheterization, acute MI, CHD, pneumonia, sepsis and gastrointestinal hemorrhage was also lower in African-Americans with acute renal failure relative to whites with the same. [137]. These observed racial differences in the renal disease population could be related to variations in mechanism of disease by race. For example, while white dialysis patients show paradoxical associations –increased risk of CVD mortality with *lower* LDL and total cholesterol levels, the opposite is true for blacks on dialysis who exhibit an almost two-fold increase in cardiovascular death risk with *higher* LDL cholesterol levels. [138] In the National Kidney Foundation's KEEP study of 37,107 obese participants with kidney disease (glomerular filtration rate <60mL/min/1.73m2), whites were more likely to have components of the metabolic syndrome – including hypertension, diabetes and dyslipidemia – compared with African-Americans; while African-Americans were more likely to have micro- and macro-albuminuria, anemia and hyperparathyroidism [130]. It has been suggested that the propensity for kidney disease and hypertension observed in African-Americans could be related to larger individual glomerular volumes and volume heterogeneity (leading to relative nephron deficiency) observed in this population. [139] Another mechanism related to lower urine volume and higher urine concentration in African-Americans relative to whites could be another explanation for the susceptibility of African-Americans to renal and cardiovascular disease. [140]. Albumin excretion rate is significantly higher and related to blood pressure only in blacks, particularly those African-Americans with impaired stress-induced pressure natriuresis. [141] Albumin excretion could therefore be a marker of vascular and renal injury even before clinically detectable hypertension.

Peripheral Vascular Disease and Subclinical Atherosclerosis

Stroke: Higher BMI is significantly associated increased risk of ischemic stroke. [142] The prevalence of obesity, and therefore ischemic stroke, is highest in the African-American relative to the Caucasian population. [142] Similarly, blacks have significantly greater incidence of first stroke (1.5 to 1) relative to whites. [143] This disparity in stroke risk between blacks and whites in the United States appears to be associated with excess risk of hypertension in blacks, in addition to social conditions and socio-economic status. [2, 143] Black patients with stroke are significantly younger, with higher prevalence of hypertension, diabetes and obesity; and lower prevalence of smoking, MI and atrial fibrillation. [144, 145] While white stroke patients are more likely to have large vessel and thromboembolic stroke, black patients are more predisposed to small vessel disease and lacunar infarcts. [144, 145].

Peripheral Arterial Disease: African-Americans have significantly higher prevalence of PAD [39, 146-149] and greater risk of CHD from PAD relative to whites. [146] Peripheral vascular resistance (and lower cardiac output) is shown to be greater in black patients who also have less brachial artery distensibility compared with white males. [27] This excess risk of PAD in African-Americans was only partially explained by traditional risk factors and novel markers [fibrinogen, lipoprotein(a), interleukin-6, D-dimer and homocysteine]; [147, 149, 150] however in one study, a third of this excess risk was explained by vitamin D status. [151] The prevalence of arterial stiffness and endothelial dysfunction is higher in blacks, [152-154] and African-Americans exhibited heart rate variability indices similar to those of older Caucasian Americans, [155-157] independent of clinical, psychological and behavioral factors. These could in part, explain the higher prevalence of hypertension and earlier vascular disease in this population. Subclinical atherosclerosis: Independent of worse cardiovascular risk profiles, African-Americans with CAD have higher prevalence of non-calcified plaque [158] and lower prevalence and extent of coronary calcium relative to whites. [158-166] Regardless, the prognostic value of CAC appears to be highest in African-Americans relative to any other ethnic group within the United States. [165] Depending on the study, the incidence of CAC progression, appears to be similar or less in African-Americans than whites. [159, 164] Gender differences do exist however such that while African-American men had less calcified coronary plaque, African-American women tended to have more or at least, similar amounts of CAC relative to white counterparts. [162, 163] African-Americans also appear to have less calcification in other facets of the cardiovascular system including the mitral annulus, mitral and aortic valves, aortic root, abdominal and thoracic aorta. [167-169] It is suggested that there is a possible genetic link between immune response and observed low CAC in African-Americans. [170] Stabilization of coronary plaque through fibrosis and calcification appears to be less common in blacks and could explain the higher rate of coronary-related deaths in African-Americans. Black patients have been reported to have greater prevalence of arterial fatty streaks and intimal thickness, while white patients have arterial fibrous plaques and higher calcium scores. [171] This might suggest that CHD in blacks is more related to small vessel disease and resulting cardiomyopathy versus CHD in whites mediated by epicardial atherosclerotic plaque. [171] In general, blacks have (up to 0.04cm) higher CIMT relative to whites. [162, 172, 173].

Other Disease Processes and Risk Factors

Atrial Fibrillation: Despite having higher prevalence of LVH and even after adjustments for conventional risk factors and other confounders, African-Americans have a lower prevalence of atrial fibrillation and less incidence of post-operative atrial fibrillation after CABG surgery compared with Caucasians. [174-177] It has been suggested that this could be related to smaller left atrial diameters observed in African-Americans [174].

Left Ventricular Hypertrophy: LVH is a major independent predictor of cardiovascular mortality and African-Americans are known to have higher left ventricular mass compared with whites. [27, 178, 179] In children, African-American race predicted LV mass independent of BMI. [180] In African-Americans, LVH is an independent predictor of CHD/CVD survival, [179, 181] and appears to be more important than single-vessel CAD, but similar to multi-vessel CAD in predicting survival in this population. [179] As such, LVH has been cited as a major player in black-white differential in CVD survival.

Depression: Another less cited risk factor associated with increased CVD risk in African-Americans is depression, [182, 183] which appears to be associated with CVD in blacks, but not in whites. [183] African American women appear to have more risk of depression compared with any other racial group. [184] This appears to affect cardiovascular risk as observed in the study by Lewis et al showing significant association between depressive symptoms and aortic calcification in African-American, but not white women. [185] Regardless, compared with whites with depression, African-Americans are less likely to be treated for depression compared with whites with depression. [186] A study showed that allostatic load was significantly higher in black women relative to white women, and that black women aged 40-49 years old had allostatic load that was higher than those for white women aged 50-59 years old; suggesting early health deterioration in black women. [187] A similar study showed that reported experiencing of racial discrimination was associated with higher risk of CVD in African-American men. [188]

The Role of Vitamin D in African-American CVD Risk: Vitamin D is associated with increased CVD mortality in blacks more than whites,[189] and may help explain the excess risk of CVD mortality observed in blacks. It has been suggested as a possible major mediator of hypertension and PAD in blacks. [26, 151] Compared with white teenagers, black teenagers living in year-round sunny climate had lower levels of vitamin D. In this population, vitamin D levels were inversely correlated with measures of adiposity. [190] It is possible that vitamin D could be a marker of physical activity, signifying individuals exposed to higher levels of sunshine by virtue of being outdoors and carrying out varying levels of physical activity during the day.

Relating Genetics and Genomics to Cardiovascular Disease Risk in African-Americans

It is clear that the processes which set the formation of plaque and progression of atherosclerosis in motion are already present in utero. [191] The GWAS for cardiovascular disease outcomes was first performed in 2007, and identified chromosome 9p21 as being the chromosome particularly linked to cardiovascular disease. [192] Some common genetic variants on this gene have been linked to different aspects of CVD in African-Americans. Particularly, CKDN2B has been linked to protection against CAD in African-Americans. [193] The angiotensinogen M235T mutation is shown to be associated with elevated circulating angiotensinogen concentrations and essential hypertension. The frequency of 235T allele is shown to be significantly higher in blacks compared with whites; and 235T homozygosity was independently associated with increased risk of coronary events in blacks, but not whites. [194] This finding in blacks was augmented by presence of hypertension. [194] The C825T genetic polymorphism of the G protein β-3 subunit which increases alpha adrenergic signaling and is associated with higher risk of hypertension, is more prevalent in African-Americans. [195] This is yet another genetic explanation for the increased risk of hypertension, particularly low renin hypertension, observed in blacks. [196].

The MYH9 gene locus is associated with 2 – 4 times higher risk of non-diabetic ESRD, and appears to explain most of the excess risk of ESRD (including focal segmental glomerulosclerosis and hypertensive ESRD) observed in African-Americans. [197] Another gene locus that has been associated with excess risk of ESRD in blacks is the APOL1 gene. Since apolipoprotein L1 is a serum factor that lyses trypanosomes, it is postulated that this gene evolved as a protective mechanism against trypanosomal infections in persons of African origin. [198].

Other genetic polymorphisms have been identified for other aspects of CVD in African-Americans. Loss of function mutations in the PCSK9 gene (gain of function associated with hypercholesterolemia) is much more common in African-Americans than whites, is associated with low LDL cholesterol and is implicated in higher prevalence of low LDL cholesterol observed in African-Americans. [199] In terms of arrhythmia, SCN5A genetic polymorphisms have been found to be more common in African-Americans and are implicated in cardiac arrhythmias independent of left ventricular size and function. This could explain the excess risk of arrhythmias and sudden cardiac deaths observed in African-Americans. [200-202].

Genetic admixture also has a major role to play in genetic findings related to CVD among African-Americans. Within the MESA cohort, each standard deviation increase in European ancestry was associated with an 8% higher CAC prevalence and 2% lower CIMT in African-Americans. So far, it appears that no major genetic loci particularly explain the high prevalence of CHD events observed in African-Americans. [203].

Therapeutic Considerations

Observed differences in genetic polymorphisms by race/ethnicity are likely to have far-reaching implications with respect to drug therapy for different aspects of cardiovascular disease. This in turn, has important implications for clinical decision-making for either a broad 'racial/ethnic' approach versus 'individualized/tailored' approach to drug therapy. The latter takes genetic admixture into account, realizing that most African-American individuals have varied racial makeup dating back to European, Spanish and Amerindian ancestries. Below, we discuss what we know so far about drug therapy for treating cardiovascular disease in African-Americans.

Heart Failure Therapy: Relative to whites, the use of spironolactone in African-Americans was associated with much less mean increase in potassium concentration,[204] suggesting African-Americans may be less responsive to potassium-sparing agents in the setting of heart failure. A meta-analysis of heart failure patients showed a 31% reduction in mortality versus only a 3% mortality reduction for whites and blacks on beta-blocker therapy, respectively. [205] On the other hand, carvedilol reduced hospitalizations, heart failure and death in African-American and Caucasian patients to the same extent in one community-based study. [206] The A-Heft study capitalized on the concept of decreased nitric oxide bioavailability as a major mechanism of CVD and heart failure in blacks. The study used a fixed-dose combination of hydralazine and nitrates in African-Americans with class III heart failure, resulting in significant mortality reduction, improvements in time to first hospitalization, measures of quality of life, and a composite of all 3 endpoints – on top of ACE inhibitor and beta blocker therapy. [207] This demonstrated the efficacy of increased nitric oxide bioavailability (using the combination of hydralazine and nitrates) in treating African-Americans with heart failure. [208] The prevalence of various genetic polymorphisms – including B1AR (Arg 389), NOS3 and aldosterone synthase – which influence heart failure therapeutics are different in whites and blacks, and have been put forward as possible explanations for observed racial variations in responses to ACE inhibitors, as well as hydralazine and nitrates. [209] Compared with whites, blacks appear to exhibit a reduced response to ACE inhibitors for heart failure hospitalization and mortality reduction. [210] In the LIFE study, despite greater LVH regression and similar blood pressure control, blacks on losartan therapy had increase in CV events relative to whites on the same therapy [211, 212].

Hypertension Therapy: In terms of hypertension control, blacks seem to do significantly better with CCBs and thiazide-type diuretics, compared with any other antihypertensive regimen. [213, 214] The ALLHAT trial enrolled more than 15,000 blacks and found that at similar doses, ACE inhibitors were less effective than thiazide diuretics or CCBs in lowering blood pressure; and was associated with significantly greater risk of stroke, heart failure and CVD in this population. However, at doses 4 times higher in blacks than whites, trandolapril appeared to control blood pressure to the same degree in both racial groups. [215] The lower response to ACE-inhibitors observed in blacks with hypertension is likely a result of lower renin and potassium and higher sodium levels in this population. [27] When salt is depleted, the vasodilatory response to ACE inhibitors is similar in blacks and whites. [13] Blacks with metabolic syndrome, had higher rates of heart failure with amlodipine, lisinopril and doxazosin compared with chlorthalidone; and higher rates of stroke, CVD and ESRD with lisinopril and doxazosin compared with chlorthalidone. [216] Currently, consensus guidelines recommend thiazides and CCBs as initial treatment for blacks, while using other approved blood pressure medications for compelling indications. [217, 218].

Coronary Heart Disease Therapy: Despite higher rates of CVD in black patients, cardioprotective drugs (such as ACE inhibitors, beta blockers, statin, glycoprotein IIb/IIIa inhibitors and clopidogrel) and cardiac procedures are used significantly less often in black relative to white patients with CVD. [219-224] This however, does not appear to fully explain the observed higher risk of CVD in black patients. [219, 225] ACE inhibitors demonstrate significantly reduced risk of CAD mortality in African-Americans;[226] and along with ARBs, appears to demonstrate equal efficacy in both whites and blacks with ischemic heart failure. [227].

Table 1. Black-White Therapeutic Differences for Specific Disease Processes

Heart Failure	Hydralazine plus nitrates	↑	
	Beta blockers	↓	Carvedilol appears to be equally effective in AAs and whites
	Potassium channel blockers	↓*	Less increase in potassium with spironolactone
	ACE inhibitors	↓	
	ARBs	↓	
Hypertension	Calcium channel blockers	↑	
	Thiazide diuretics	↑	
	ACE inhibitors	↓	Requires higher doses in AAs for effective BP control
CHD events	ACE inhibitors	↔	
	ARBs	↔	
	Beta blockers	↔	
	Aspirin	↔	
	Clopidogrel	↓	Higher risk of late stent thrombosis
	Statins	↑*	Possibly better CHD mortality reduction
	Thrombolytic therapy	↓*	Increased risk of bleeding
Lipid-lowering Therapy	Statins	↔	Pravastatin may possibly be more efficacious in AAs*
	Statins plus ezetimibe	↔	

AAs: African-Americans, ACE: Angiotensin Converting Enzyme, ARB: Angiotensin Receptor
    Blocker, BP: Blood pressure.
* Not a definite difference, may be controversial.
† Compared with whites.

Relative to whites, blacks have been shown to have higher risk of angioedema with ACE inhibitors [228] and higher risk of hemorrhage with thrombolytic and warfarin therapy. [228-230] Black race is significantly associated with late stent thrombosis compared with non-black race despite higher compliance with clopidogrel and after adjusting for socio-economic status. [231].

A possible explanation for this is described racial/ethnic variations in CYP2C19 and ABCB1 gene polymorphisms involved in metabolism and absorption of clopidogrel. [232] Similarly, variations in CYP2C9 and VKORC1 polymorphisms are likely involved in racial differences in response to warfarin therapy. [233] No racial differences in aspirin resistance have been noted. [234].

Lipid Lowering Therapy: Using atorvastatin alone, or in combination with ezetimibe appears to improve lipid profile to the same extent in whites and blacks. [235, 236] On the other hand, the ALLHAT-LLT showed that pravastatin had higher efficacy for lipid modification and CHD mortality reduction in blacks than whites. [237] This however, could have been related to study methodology rather than a racial variation in pravastatin effects on lipid modification.

The ARIES study showed rosuvastatin was superior to atorvastatin in increasing HDL cholesterol levels, and reducing LDL, triglycerides and non-HDL cholesterol levels in African-Americans [237, 238].

Specific Preventive Strategies for Cardiovascular Disease Reduction in African-Americans

Dietary Interventions: A diet made up of fruits, vegetables, whole grains, fat-free dairy, protein and seafood; and low in sodium, dietary cholesterol, saturated and/or trans fat and refined grains/sugars appears to be effective in reducing cardiovascular events. The DASH diet made up of fruits, vegetables, low fat dairy and reduced fats and cholesterol significantly reduced 10-year risk of CHD. [239] This effect of the DASH diet in reducing CHD risk was particularly noticeable in African-Americans. [239] The DASH diet emphasizing low sodium diet led to even greater reductions in blood pressure. [20] A multi-disciplinary approach emphasizing salt restriction, as well as weight loss and stress reduction led to significant decreases in blood pressure and long-term cardiovascular events in the TOHP studies. [240].

Weight Loss Strategies: Obesity is associated with higher risk of diabetes, hypertension and CVD in general. [241] As such intentional weight loss in obese persons should reverse this trend. Moderate physical activity levels, emotional support and less sugar-sweetened drinks consumption have been associated with higher odds of successful weight loss and weight loss maintenance in overweight men and women – particularly African-Americans. [242] A community and faith-based approach to weight loss has proved to be an effective approach particularly in African-American women, notably the most obese group in the nation. [243] Dietary approaches to weight loss have also proved to be effective. [244].

Physical Activity: A study of preadolescent African-American girls showed that average daily physical activity and time spent in moderate-to-vigorous physical activity were significantly correlated with body mass index and insulin. [245] Increased physical activity levels in children and teenagers may therefore represent an effective means to combat the current obesity epidemic – from childhood – in the United States. [2] Moderate-intensity exercise led to significant reductions in blood pressure in African-American men with severe hypertension. [246] Improvements in infrastructure geared towards making neighborhoods more suited for physical activity during regular activities of daily living (e.g. sidewalks for walking to school and the grocery store) appear to be effective in encouraging physical activity, and are actively advocated. [247] Community-based interventions seem to work very well to improve physical activity levels in African-Americans. [248].

Smoking Cessation: African-Americans have lower prevalence of cigarette smoking compared with European-Americans. [2] Nevertheless, cigarette smoking contributes significantly to increased risk of CVD observed in this population. Smoking cessation strategies which have been identified as being effective include behavioral counseling which includes identifying barriers to quitting and assessing patient's willingness to quit, then assisting the patient with the quitting process while ensuring adequate and close follow-up to avoid relapse. [249] Behavioral counseling can be combined with medical therapy. A meta-analysis of 83 smoking cessation studies showed varenicicline or the use of nicotine patch plus ad-lib gum or spray to be the most effective medical therapy strategies for sustained smoking cessation at 6 months. [249].

Medications Adherence: Medications such as aspirin, thienopyridines, statins, beta blockers, ACE inhibitors, hydralazine/nitrates have been shown to be effective in primary and secondary prevention of CVD events. Medications non-adherence appears to be a major deterrent to improvements in cardiovascular disease risk modification in African-Americans.

[250] Studies have proven nurse/community health worker-led interventions (with frequent phone calls by the nurses to discuss patient progress and plans for the future), as well as pharmacist-led interventions (to discuss medications side effects, interactions, drug coverage and patient beliefs) to be effective in improving adherence to medications. [251] Enlisting social support also helps improve medications adherence. [252].

Public Education: In one study made up mostly of African-Americans, knowledge of salt content of processed foods was associated with decreased frequency of adding salt at the table, and knowledge of effects of fat intake on heart disease led to consumption of low-fat dairy. [253] This underscores the importance of public education on heart disease and practical ways to avoid it. Educational programs geared towards heart disease reduction have been successfully initiated in the Mississippi delta. [254] The state of New York has partnered with the CDC to prevent heart disease and stroke by creating awareness through public education and community outreach, emphasizing such preventive strategies as heart healthy diet, exercise, weight loss, smoking cessation and cholesterol, blood pressure and/or fasting glucose screening.

Table 2. Specific Preventive Strategies Shown to be Effective for Cardiometabolic Risk Reduction in African-Americans

Diet	- Salt restriction - Diet rich in fruits, vegetables, whole grains, fat-free dairy, protein and seafood; and low in sodium, dietary cholesterol, saturated and/or trans fat and refined grains/sugars
Weight loss*	- Community-based interventions[†] - Moderate-intensity physical activity[‡] - Dietary approaches also emphasizing less use of sugar-sweetened drinks - Emotional support
Physical activity	- Infrastructure geared towards making neighborhoods more suited for physical activity - Community-based interventions*
Smoking cessation	- Behavioral counseling - Emotional support - Medications including varenicline, nicotine patch-plus[§]
Medication adherence	- Enlisting social support - Nurse/community health care worker interventions - Pharmacist-led interventions
Public education	- Through barber shops, church groups, social events: leads to better adherence to dietary interventions - On an individual basis, education on disease process and treatment leads to better adherence to medications, diet and follow-up
Health screening	- Through barber shops, faith-based groups, social events - Successful method of cardiometabolic disease screening and referral in African-Americans

* Compared with BMI, waist circumference is a better predictor of cardiovascular disease risk in African-Americans.
† E.g. counseling and health screening of community units such as barber shops and faith-based groups.
‡ Emphasis should be placed on initiating physical activity from childhood.
§ Nicotine patch combined with *ad lib* gum or spray.

Screening and Community-Based Outreach: In general, community-based interventions seem to work better in the African-American population. [243, 248] In one study, community-based interventions were associated with greater sustainability and less refractoriness for LDL cholesterol and blood pressure goals compared with enhanced usual care. [255] Community-based integrated risk counseling was associated with greater levels of self-efficacy for diet and physical activity, and significantly increased perceived risk of having a heart attack. [256]. Health screening (e.g. for cholesterol, blood pressure, ankle brachial index and/or fasting glucose) through barber shops have proved to be useful ways for cardiometabolic diseases referral and prevention in African-American men. [257] Faith-based interventions appear to be effective in African-American women. [243] The REACH project – a community-based intervention geared towards eliminating disparities in cholesterol screening in minority communities – has been particularly successful in black, Hispanic and Asian REACH communities. [258].

Imaging Modalities in CVD Prevention: Computed tomography and carotid ultrasonography have successfully been employed in the detection of subclinical atherosclerosis (CAC and CIMT/carotid plaque), and prediction of CVD events. [259, 260] CIMT is generally greater in blacks compared with other racial groups. [172, 173] While blacks generally have lower prevalence and severity of CAC relative to whites, [161, 164] CAC has been shown to be equally effective as a prognostic indicator of future cardiovascular events in African-Americans and European-Americans. [261] CAC is a better predictor of CHD events than CIMT, [262] but is associated with radiation exposure and related risks such as cancer. As such, the case can be made for employing either modality in CVD risk assessment, which would then help management decisions for further CVD prevention.

Cardiovascular Disease Prevention for the Future – Genetics, Genomics and Biomarkers

The problem with application of certain preventive strategies, particularly those involving medication administration based on race is that many African-Americans have diverse racial ancestry. As such, certain medical therapies thought to be effective for CVD prevention/treatment in African-Americans as a whole, may be partially successful or completely futile in some individuals depending on the ancestry line defining the pathophysiology of disease in that individual. Multiple SNPs within chromosome 9p21 have since been linked to different aspects of cardiovascular disease. [192] Since then, a freely accessible database of genetic material from thousands of participants with billions of SNPs has been created, making it easy for the scientific community to freely engage in genetics research and GWAS. Several SNPs from different gene loci have been linked to different phenotypes, and several genetic polymorphisms have been associated with pathophysiology of various disease processes. The result is that individuals can currently obtain a whole body genome scan which provides information on genetic ancestry, inherited traits and future risk of different diseases based on existing literature. This sets the pace for the future of preventive medicine which would likely involve individualized assessment of risk of different aspects of cardiovascular disease, with personally tailored specific preventive strategies to completely ameliorate this risk. This constitutes an especially useful disease management approach in African-Americans, who as a group are known to have diverse genetic makeup.

The use of biomarkers in risk prediction has been a recent topic of major interest. Similar to genomics, major advances in immunoassays have permitted the measurement of thousands of biomarkers. This has led to multiple biomarker research studies. Integration of emerging technologies from the 'omics' fields (proteomics, metabolomics, lipomics, ribomics, genomics and pharmacogenomics) will eventually enable the employment of these new technologies in the 'personalized' prediction – and therefore prevention – of disease. [263].

Conclusion

CVD is the major cause of morbidity and mortality in the United States, particularly in African-Americans where it is most prevalent. The very high prevalence of CVD in African-Americans is multifactorial, relating to economic, psychosocial, physiologic and genetic factors. In particular, African-Americans have higher prevalence of CVD risk factors, particularly hypertension which is much more severe in this population. The management of CVD risk in African-Americans should be a comprehensive, multi-faceted approach particularly geared towards educating and screening the community to achieve CVD prevention and overall improvement in community health. At the same time, one should bear in mind the various medical therapies which are proven to be more effective for CVD treatment/management in African-Americans – based on different pathophysiology of CVD in this population compared with European-Americans. Since African-Americans have varied genetic makeup due to diverse ancestry, and as the paradigm shifts to individually-tailored medicine based on an individual's risk for CVD, it is likely that in future, genomics and genetic admixture will play a major role in management of CVD in African-Americans.

References

[1]   Williams RA, Flack JM, Gavin JR, 3rd, Schneider WR, Hennekens CH. Guidelines for management of high-risk African Americans with multiple cardiovascular risk factors: recommendations of an expert consensus panel. *Ethnicity and disease.* 2007;17(2):214-20.

[2]   Roger VL, Go AS, Lloyd-Jones DM, Adams RJ, Berry JD, Brown TM, et al. Heart disease and stroke statistics--2011 update: a report from the American Heart Association. *Circulation.* 2011;123(4):e18-e209.

[3]   Foraker RE, Rose KM, Kucharska-Newton AM, Ni H, Suchindran CM, Whitsel EA. Variation in rates of fatal coronary heart disease by neighborhood socioeconomic status: the atherosclerosis risk in communities surveillance (1992-2002). *Annals of epidemiology.* 2011;21(8):580-8.

[4]   Bambs C, Kip KE, Dinga A, Mulukutla SR, Aiyer AN, Reis SE. Low prevalence of "ideal cardiovascular health" in a community-based population: the heart strategies concentrating on risk evaluation (Heart SCORE) study. *Circulation.* 2011;123(8):850-7.

[5]   Hayes DK, Denny CH, Keenan NL, Croft JB, Sundaram AA, Greenlund KJ. Racial/Ethnic and socioeconomic differences in multiple risk factors for heart disease and stroke in women: behavioral risk factor surveillance system, 2003. *Journal of women's health.* 2006;15(9):1000-8.

[6]   Henderson SO, Haiman CA, Wilkens LR, Kolonel LN, Wan P, Pike MC. Established risk factors account for most of the racial differences in cardiovascular disease mortality. *PloS one*. 2007;2(4):e377.

[7]   Mathur R, Hull SA, Badrick E, Robson J. Cardiovascular multimorbidity: the effect of ethnicity on prevalence and risk factor management. The British journal of general practice : *the journal of the Royal College of General Practitioners.* 2011;61(586):e262-70.

[8]   Sundaram AA, Ayala C, Greenlund KJ, Keenan NL. Differences in the prevalence of self-reported risk factors for coronary heart disease among American women by race/ethnicity and age: Behavioral Risk Factor Surveillance System, 2001. *American journal of preventive medicine*. 2005;29(5 Suppl 1):25-30.

[9]   Liu X, Liu M, Tsilimingras D, Schiffrin EL. Racial disparities in cardiovascular risk factors among diagnosed hypertensive subjects. *Journal of the American Society of Hypertension* : JASH. 2011;5(4):239-48.

[10]   Glasser SP, Judd S, Basile J, Lackland D, Halanych J, Cushman M, et al. Prehypertension, racial prevalence and its association with risk factors: Analysis of the REasons for Geographic And Racial Differences in Stroke (REGARDS) study. *American journal of hypertension*. 2011;24(2):194-9.

[11]   Harding S, Whitrow M, Lenguerrand E, Maynard M, Teyhan A, Cruickshank JK, et al. Emergence of ethnic differences in blood pressure in adolescence: the determinants of adolescent social well-being and health study. *Hypertension*. 2010;55(4):1063-9.

[12]   Park IU, Taylor AL. Race and ethnicity in trials of antihypertensive therapy to prevent cardiovascular outcomes: a systematic review. *Annals of family medicine.* 2007;5(5):444-52.

[13]   Watson KE. Cardiovascular risk reduction among African Americans: a call to action. *Journal of the National Medical Association*. 2008;100(1):18-26.

[14]   Brady TM, Fivush B, Parekh RS, Flynn JT. Racial differences among children with primary hypertension. *Pediatrics*. 2010;126(5):931-7.

[15]   Sherwood A, Routledge FS, Wohlgemuth WK, Hinderliter AL, Kuhn CM, Blumenthal JA. Blood Pressure Dipping: Ethnicity, Sleep Quality, and Sympathetic Nervous System Activity. *American journal of hypertension*. 2011.

[16]   Paultre F, Mosca L. The relation of blood pressure to coronary heart mortality in different age groups varies by ethnicity. *American journal of hypertension.* 2006;19(2):179-83.

[17]   Ergul S, Parish DC, Puett D, Ergul A. Racial differences in plasma endothelin-1 concentrations in individuals with essential hypertension. *Hypertension.* 1996;28(4):652-5.

[18]   Ergul A, Tackett RL, Puett D. Distribution of endothelin receptors in saphenous veins of African Americans: implications of racial differences. *Journal of cardiovascular pharmacology.* 1999;34(3):327-32.

[19]   Berenson GS, Chen W, Dasmahapatra P, Fernandez C, Giles T, Xu J, et al. Stimulus response of blood pressure in black and white young individuals helps explain racial divergence in adult cardiovascular disease: The Bogalusa Heart Study. *Journal of the American Society of Hypertension* : JASH. 2011;5(4):230-8.

[20]   Sacks FM, Svetkey LP, Vollmer WM, Appel LJ, Bray GA, Harsha D, et al. Effects on blood pressure of reduced dietary sodium and the Dietary Approaches to Stop

Hypertension (DASH) diet. DASH-Sodium Collaborative Research Group. *The New England journal of medicine.* 2001;344(1):3-10.

[21] Voors AW, Dalferes ER, Jr., Frank GC, Aristimuno GG, Berenson GS. Relation between ingested potassium and sodium balance in young Blacks and whites. *The American journal of clinical nutrition.* 1983;37(4):583-94.

[22] Cooper R, Rotimi C, Ataman S, McGee D, Osotimehin B, Kadiri S, et al. The prevalence of hypertension in seven populations of west African origin. *American journal of public health.* 1997;87(2):160-8.

[23] Fezeu L, Balkau B, Sobngwi E, Kengne AP, Vol S, Ducimetiere P, et al. Waist circumference and obesity-related abnormalities in French and Cameroonian adults: the role of urbanization and ethnicity. *International journal of obesity.* 2010;34(3):446-53.

[24] McGrath JJ, Matthews KA, Brady SS. Individual versus neighborhood socioeconomic status and race as predictors of adolescent ambulatory blood pressure and heart rate. *Social science and medicine.* 2006;63(6):1442-53.

[25] Javed F, Aziz EF, Sabharwal MS, Nadkarni GN, Khan SA, Cordova JP, et al. Association of BMI and cardiovascular risk stratification in the elderly African-American females. *Obesity.* 2011;19(6):1182-6.

[26] Fiscella K, Winters P, Tancredi D, Franks P. Racial Disparity in Blood Pressure: is Vitamin D a Factor? *Journal of general internal medicine.* 2011.

[27] Berenson G, Srinivasan S, Chen W, Li S, Patel D. Racial (black-white) contrasts of risk for hypertensive disease in youth have implications for preventive care: the Bogalusa Heart Study. *Ethnicity and disease.* 2006;16(3 Suppl 4):S4-2-9.

[28] Marcantoni C, Ma LJ, Federspiel C, Fogo AB. Hypertensive nephrosclerosis in African Americans versus Caucasians. *Kidney international.* 2002;62(1):172-80.

[29] Lin SX, Carnethon M, Szklo M, Bertoni A. Racial/ethnic differences in the association of triglycerides with other metabolic syndrome components: the Multi-Ethnic Study of Atherosclerosis. *Metabolic syndrome and related disorders.* 2011;9(1):35-40.

[30] Taylor H, Liu J, Wilson G, Golden SH, Crook E, Brunson CD, et al. Distinct component profiles and high risk among African Americans with metabolic syndrome: the Jackson Heart Study. *Diabetes care.* 2008;31(6):1248-53.

[31] Kullo IJ, Jan MF, Bailey KR, Mosley TH, Turner ST. Ethnic differences in low-density lipoprotein particle size in hypertensive adults. *Journal of clinical lipidology.* 2007;1(3):218-24.

[32] Aiyer AN, Kip KE, Marroquin OC, Mulukutla SR, Edmundowicz D, Reis SE. Racial differences in coronary artery calcification are not attributed to differences in lipoprotein particle sizes: the Heart Strategies Concentrating on Risk Evaluation (Heart SCORE) Study. *American heart journal.* 2007;153(2):328-34.

[33] Diaz VA, Mainous AG, 3rd, Koopman RJ, Carek PJ, Geesey ME. Race and diet in the overweight: association with cardiovascular risk in a nationally representative sample. *Nutrition.* 2005;21(6):718-25.

[34] Donin AS, Nightingale CM, Owen CG, Rudnicka AR, McNamara MC, Prynne CJ, et al. Ethnic differences in blood lipids and dietary intake between UK children of black African, black Caribbean, South Asian, and white European origin: the Child Heart and Health Study in England (CHASE). *The American journal of clinical nutrition.* 2010;92(4):776-83.

[35] Gaillard T, Schuster D, Osei K. Differential impact of serum glucose, triglycerides, and high-density lipoprotein cholesterol on cardiovascular risk factor burden in nondiabetic, obese African American women: implications for the prevalence of metabolic syndrome. Metabolism: *clinical and experimental*. 2010;59(8):1115-23.

[36] Anuurad E, Chiem A, Pearson TA, Berglund L. Metabolic syndrome components in african-americans and European-american patients and its relation to coronary artery disease. *The American journal of cardiology*. 2007;100(5):830-4.

[37] Enkhmaa B, Anuurad E, Zhang Z, Pearson TA, Berglund L. Usefulness of apolipoprotein B/apolipoprotein A-I ratio to predict coronary artery disease independent of the metabolic syndrome in African Americans. *The American journal of cardiology*. 2010;106(9):1264-9.

[38] Holvoet P, Jenny NS, Schreiner PJ, Tracy RP, Jacobs DR. The relationship between oxidized LDL and other cardiovascular risk factors and subclinical CVD in different ethnic groups: the Multi-Ethnic Study of Atherosclerosis (MESA). *Atherosclerosis*. 2007;194(1):245-52.

[39] Zheng ZJ, Rosamond WD, Chambless LE, Nieto FJ, Barnes RW, Hutchinson RG, et al. Lower extremity arterial disease assessed by ankle-brachial index in a middle-aged population of African Americans and whites: the Atherosclerosis Risk in Communities (ARIC) Study. *American journal of preventive medicine*. 2005;29(5 Suppl 1):42-9.

[40] Deboer MD. Underdiagnosis of Metabolic Syndrome in Non-Hispanic Black Adolescents: A Call for Ethnic-Specific Criteria. *Current cardiovascular risk reports*. 2010;4(4):302-10.

[41] Zeno SA, Kim-Dorner SJ, Deuster PA, Davis JL, Remaley AT, Poth M. Cardiovascular fitness and risk factors of healthy African Americans and Caucasians. *Journal of the National Medical Association*. 2010;102(1):28-35.

[42] McAuley PA, Kokkinos PF, Oliveira RB, Emerson BT, Myers JN. Obesity paradox and cardiorespiratory fitness in 12,417 male veterans aged 40 to 70 years. Mayo Clinic proccedings. *Mayo Clinic*. 2010;85(2):115-21.

[43] Lee CD, Jacobs DR, Jr., Schreiner PJ, Iribarren C, Hankinson A. Abdominal obesity and coronary artery calcification in young adults: the Coronary Artery Risk Development in Young Adults (CARDIA) Study. *The American journal of clinical nutrition*. 2007;86(1):48-54.

[44] Rahman M, Temple JR, Breitkopf CR, Berenson AB. Racial differences in body fat distribution among reproductive-aged women. *Metabolism: clinical and experimental*. 2009;58(9):1329-37.

[45] Araneta MR, Barrett-Connor E. Ethnic differences in visceral adipose tissue and type 2 diabetes: Filipino, African-American, and white women. *Obesity research*. 2005;13(8):1458-65.

[46] Sisson SB, Katzmarzyk PT, Srinivasan SR, Chen W, Freedman DS, Bouchard C, et al. Ethnic differences in subcutaneous adiposity and waist girth in children and adolescents. *Obesity*. 2009;17(11):2075-81.

[47] Desilets MC, Garrel D, Couillard C, Tremblay A, Despres JP, Bouchard C, et al. Ethnic differences in body composition and other markers of cardiovascular disease risk: study in matched Haitian and White subjects from Quebec. *Obesity*. 2006;14(6):1019-27.

[48] Zhu S, Heymsfield SB, Toyoshima H, Wang Z, Pietrobelli A, Heshka S. Race-ethnicity-specific waist circumference cutoffs for identifying cardiovascular disease risk factors. *The American journal of clinical nutrition.* 2005;81(2):409-15.

[49] Abell JE, Egan BM, Wilson PW, Lipsitz S, Woolson RF, Lackland DT. Age and race impact the association between BMI and CVD mortality in women. *Public health reports.* 2007;122(4):507-12.

[50] Afonso L, Niraj A, Veeranna V, Fakhry H, Pradhan J. Ethnic and sex differences in disease burden in patients undergoing coronary angiography: the confounding influence of obesity. *Ethn Dis.* 2008;18(1):53-8.

[51] Hosain GM, Rahman M, Williams KJ, Berenson AB. Racial differences in the association between body fat distribution and lipid profiles among reproductive-age women. *Diabetes and metabolism.* 2010;36(4):278-85.

[52] Taylor HA, Jr., Coady SA, Levy D, Walker ER, Vasan RS, Liu J, et al. Relationships of BMI to cardiovascular risk factors differ by ethnicity. *Obesity.* 2010;18(8):1638-45.

[53] Hanley AJ, Bowden D, Wagenknecht LE, Balasubramanyam A, Langfeld C, Saad MF, et al. Associations of adiponectin with body fat distribution and insulin sensitivity in nondiabetic Hispanics and African-Americans. *The Journal of clinical endocrinology and metabolism.* 2007;92(7):2665-71.

[54] Lu G, Chiem A, Anuurad E, Havel PJ, Pearson TA, Ormsby B, et al. Adiponectin levels are associated with coronary artery disease across Caucasian and African-American ethnicity. *Translational research : the journal of laboratory and clinical medicine.* 2007;149(6):317-23.

[55] Brancati FL, Kao WH, Folsom AR, Watson RL, Szklo M. Incident type 2 diabetes mellitus in African American and white adults: the Atherosclerosis Risk in Communities Study. *JAMA : the journal of the American Medical Association.* 2000;283(17):2253-9.

[56] Karter AJ, Ferrara A, Liu JY, Moffet HH, Ackerson LM, Selby JV. Ethnic disparities in diabetic complications in an insured population. *JAMA : the journal of the American Medical Association.* 2002;287(19):2519-27.

[57] Whincup PH, Nightingale CM, Owen CG, Rudnicka AR, Gibb I, McKay CM, et al. Early emergence of ethnic differences in type 2 diabetes precursors in the UK: the Child Heart and Health Study in England (CHASE Study). *PLoS medicine.* 2010;7(4):e1000263.

[58] Johnson CL, Rifkind BM, Sempos CT, Carroll MD, Bachorik PS, Briefel RR, et al. Declining serum total cholesterol levels among US adults. The National Health and Nutrition Examination Surveys. *JAMA.* 1993;269(23):3002-8.

[59] Walker SE, Gurka MJ, Oliver MN, Johns DW, Deboer MD. Racial/ethnic discrepancies in the metabolic syndrome begin in childhood and persist after adjustment for environmental factors. *Nutrition, metabolism, and cardiovascular diseases :* NMCD. 2010.

[60] Gaillard T, Schuster D, Osei K. Independent role of blood pressure on cardiovascular risk factors in nondiabetic, obese African-American women with family history of type 2 diabetes: Implications for metabolic syndrome components. *Journal of the American Society of Hypertension : JASH.* 2009;3(1):25-34.

[61] Lea JP, Greene EL, Nicholas SB, Agodoa L, Norris KC. Cardiorenal metabolic syndrome in the African diaspora: rationale for including chronic kidney disease in the metabolic syndrome definition. *Ethnicity and disease.* 2009;19(2 Suppl 2):S2-11-4.

[62] Ford ES, Giles WH, Dietz WH. Prevalence of the metabolic syndrome among US adults: findings from the third National Health and Nutrition Examination Survey. *JAMA : the journal of the American Medical Association.* 2002;287(3):356-9.

[63] Clark LT, El-Atat F. Metabolic syndrome in African Americans: implications for preventing coronary heart disease. *Clinical cardiology.* 2007;30(4):161-4.

[64] Hurley LP, Dickinson LM, Estacio RO, Steiner JF, Havranek EP. Prediction of cardiovascular death in racial/ethnic minorities using Framingham risk factors. *Circulation. Cardiovascular quality and outcomes.* 2010;3(2):181-7.

[65] Rosamond WD, Chambless LE, Folsom AR, Cooper LS, Conwill DE, Clegg L, et al. Trends in the incidence of myocardial infarction and in mortality due to coronary heart disease, 1987 to 1994. *N. Engl. J. Med.* 1998;339(13):861-7.

[66] Trends in ischemic heart disease death rates for blacks and whites--United States, 1981-1995. *MMWR Morb. Mortal Wkly Rep.* 1998;47(44):945-9.

[67] Traven ND, Kuller LH, Ives DG, Rutan GH, Perper JA. Coronary heart disease mortality and sudden death among the 35-44-year age group in Allegheny County, Pennsylvania. *Ann. Epidemiol.* 1996;6(2):130-6.

[68] Galea S, Blaney S, Nandi A, Silverman R, Vlahov D, Foltin G, et al. Explaining racial disparities in incidence of and survival from out-of-hospital cardiac arrest. *Am. J. Epidemiol.* 2007;166(5):534-43.

[69] Lloyd-Jones D, Adams R, Carnethon M, De Simone G, Ferguson TB, Flegal K, et al. Heart disease and stroke statistics--2009 update: a report from the American Heart Association Statistics Committee and Stroke Statistics Subcommittee. *Circulation.* 2009;119(3):480-6.

[70] Rea TD, Pearce RM, Raghunathan TE, Lemaitre RN, Sotoodehnia N, Jouven X, et al. Incidence of out-of-hospital cardiac arrest. *Am. J. Cardiol.* 2004;93(12):1455-60.

[71] Keil JE, Sutherland SE, Hames CG, Lackland DT, Gazes PC, Knapp RG, et al. Coronary disease mortality and risk factors in black and white men. Results from the combined Charleston, SC, and Evans County, Georgia, heart studies. *Arch. Intern. Med.* 1995;155(14):1521-7.

[72] Hozawa A, Folsom AR, Sharrett AR, Chambless LE. Absolute and attributable risks of cardiovascular disease incidence in relation to optimal and borderline risk factors: comparison of African American with white subjects--Atherosclerosis Risk in Communities Study. *Arch. Intern. Med.* 2007;167(6):573-9.

[73] Cooper RS, Liao Y, Rotimi C. Is hypertension more severe among U.S. blacks, or is severe hypertension more common? *Ann. Epidemiol.* 1996;6(3):173-80.

[74] Jones DW, Chambless LE, Folsom AR, Heiss G, Hutchinson RG, Sharrett AR, et al. Risk factors for coronary heart disease in African Americans: the atherosclerosis risk in communities study, 1987-1997. *Arch. Intern. Med.* 2002;162(22):2565-71.

[75] Onwuanyi AE, Abe O, Quarshie A, Al-Mahmoud A, Lapu-Bula R, Francis CK, et al. Comparative frequency of angiographic coronary artery disease in African Americans and Hispanics. *Ethnicity and disease.* 2006;16(1):58-63.

[76] Beohar N, Davidson CJ, Massaro EM, Srinivas VS, Sansing VV, Zonszein J, et al. The impact of race/ethnicity on baseline characteristics and the burden of coronary

atherosclerosis in the Bypass Angioplasty Revascularization Investigation 2 Diabetes trial. *American heart journal.* 2011;161(4):755-63.

[77] Chokshi NP, Iqbal SN, Berger RL, Hochman JS, Feit F, Slater JN, et al. Sex and race are associated with the absence of epicardial coronary artery obstructive disease at angiography in patients with acute coronary syndromes. *Clinical cardiology.* 2010;33(8):495-501.

[78] Shaw LJ, Shaw RE, Merz CN, Brindis RG, Klein LW, Nallamothu B, et al. Impact of ethnicity and gender differences on angiographic coronary artery disease prevalence and in-hospital mortality in the American College of Cardiology-National Cardiovascular Data Registry. *Circulation.* 2008;117(14):1787-801.

[79] Whittle J, Kressin NR, Peterson ED, Orner MB, Glickman M, Mazzella M, et al. Racial differences in prevalence of coronary obstructions among men with positive nuclear imaging studies. *Journal of the American College of Cardiology.* 2006;47(10):2034-41.

[80] Echols MR, Mahaffey KW, Banerjee A, Pieper KS, Stebbins A, Lansky A, et al. Racial differences among high-risk patients presenting with non-ST-segment elevation acute coronary syndromes (results from the SYNERGY trial). *The American journal of cardiology.* 2007;99(3):315-21.

[81] Whittle J, Conigliaro J, Good CB, Hanusa BH, Macpherson DS. Black-white differences in severity of coronary artery disease among individuals with acute coronary syndromes. *J. Gen. Intern. Med.* 2002;17(11):867-73.

[82] Clark LT. Anatomic substrate differences between black and white victims of sudden cardiac death: hypertension, coronary artery disease, or both? *Clin. Cardiol.* 1989;12(12 Suppl 4):IV13-7.

[83] Lee KK, Fortmann SP, Varady A, Fair JM, Go AS, Quertermous T, et al. Racial variation in lipoprotein-associated phospholipase A2 in older adults. *BMC cardiovascular disorders.* 2011;11:38.

[84] Brilakis ES, Khera A, McGuire DK, See R, Banerjee S, Murphy SA, et al. Influence of race and sex on lipoprotein-associated phospholipase A2 levels: observations from the Dallas Heart Study. *Atherosclerosis.* 2008;199(1):110-5.

[85] Anuurad E, Ozturk Z, Enkhmaa B, Pearson TA, Berglund L. Association of lipoprotein-associated phospholipase A2 with coronary artery disease in African-Americans and Caucasians. *The Journal of clinical endocrinology and metabolism.* 2010;95(5):2376-83.

[86] Deverts DJ, Cohen S, DiLillo VG, Lewis CE, Kiefe C, Whooley M, et al. Depressive symptoms, race, and circulating C-reactive protein: the Coronary Artery Risk Development in Young Adults (CARDIA) study. *Psychosomatic medicine.* 2010;72(8):734-41.

[87] Albert MA, Glynn RJ, Ridker PM. Effect of physical activity on serum C-reactive protein. *The American journal of cardiology.* 2004;93(2):221-5.

[88] LaMonte MJ, Durstine JL, Yanowitz FG, Lim T, DuBose KD, Davis P, et al. Cardiorespiratory fitness and C-reactive protein among a tri-ethnic sample of women. *Circulation.* 2002;106(4):403-6.

[89] Shaw LJ, Hendel RC, Cerquiera M, Mieres JH, Alazraki N, Krawczynska E, et al. Ethnic differences in the prognostic value of stress technetium-99m tetrofosmin gated single-photon emission computed tomography myocardial perfusion imaging. *Journal of the American College of Cardiology.* 2005;45(9):1494-504.

[90]   Kim CX, Bailey KR, Klee GG, Ellington AA, Liu G, Mosley TH, Jr., et al. Sex and ethnic differences in 47 candidate proteomic markers of cardiovascular disease: the Mayo Clinic proteomic markers of arteriosclerosis study. *PloS one.* 2010;5(2):e9065.

[91]   Feairheller DL, Diaz KM, Sturgeon KM, Williamson ST, Brown MD. Racial Differences in the Time-Course Oxidative Stress Responses to Acute Exercise. *Journal of exercise physiology online / American Society of Exercise Physiologists.* 2011;14(1):49-59.

[92]   Movahed MR, John J, Hashemzadeh M, Jamal MM. Trends in the age adjusted mortality from acute ST segment elevation myocardial infarction in the United States (1988-2004) based on race, gender, infarct location and comorbidities. *The American journal of cardiology.* 2009;104(8):1030-4.

[93]   Cooke CR, Nallamouthu B, Kahn JM, Birkmeyer JD, Iwashyna TJ. Race and timeliness of transfer for revascularization in patients with acute myocardial infarction. *Medical care.* 2011;49(7):662-7.

[94]   Pearte CA, Myerson M, Coresh J, McNamara RL, Rosamond W, Taylor H, et al. Variation and temporal trends in the use of diagnostic testing during hospitalization for acute myocardial infarction by age, gender, race, and geography (the Atherosclerosis Risk In Communities Study). *The American journal of cardiology.* 2008;101(9):1219-25.

[95]   Vaccarino V, Rathore SS, Wenger NK, Frederick PD, Abramson JL, Barron HV, et al. Sex and racial differences in the management of acute myocardial infarction, 1994 through 2002. *The New England journal of medicine.* 2005;353(7):671-82.

[96]   Casale SN, Auster CJ, Wolf F, Pei Y, Devereux RB. Ethnicity and socioeconomic status influence use of primary angioplasty in patients presenting with acute myocardial infarction. *American heart journal.* 2007;154(5):989-93.

[97]   Mehta RH, Marks D, Califf RM, Sohn S, Pieper KS, Van de Werf F, et al. Differences in the clinical features and outcomes in African Americans and whites with myocardial infarction. *The American journal of medicine.* 2006;119(1):70 e1-8.

[98]   Spertus JA, Jones PG, Masoudi FA, Rumsfeld JS, Krumholz HM. Factors associated with racial differences in myocardial infarction outcomes. *Annals of internal medicine.* 2009;150(5):314-24.

[99]   Spertus J, Safley D, Garg M, Jones P, Peterson ED. The influence of race on health status outcomes one year after an acute coronary syndrome. *Journal of the American College of Cardiology.* 2005;46(10):1838-44.

[100] Pradhan J, Schreiber TL, Niraj A, Veeranna V, Ramesh K, Saigh L, et al. Comparison of five-year outcome in African Americans versus Caucasians following percutaneous coronary intervention. Catheterization and cardiovascular interventions : *official journal of the Society for Cardiac Angiography and Interventions.* 2008;72(1):36-44.

[101] Loehr LR, Rosamond WD, Chang PP, Folsom AR, Chambless LE. Heart failure incidence and survival (from the Atherosclerosis Risk in Communities study). *Am. J. Cardiol.* 2008;101(7):1016-22.

[102] Roger VL, Weston SA, Redfield MM, Hellermann-Homan JP, Killian J, Yawn BP, et al. Trends in heart failure incidence and survival in a community-based population. *JAMA.* 2004;292(3):344-50.

[103] Schocken DD, Benjamin EJ, Fonarow GC, Krumholz HM, Levy D, Mensah GA, et al. Prevention of heart failure: a scientific statement from the American Heart Association

Councils on Epidemiology and Prevention, Clinical Cardiology, Cardiovascular Nursing, and High Blood Pressure Research; Quality of Care and Outcomes Research Interdisciplinary Working Group; and Functional Genomics and Translational Biology Interdisciplinary Working Group. *Circulation.* 2008;117(19):2544-65.

[104] Hunt SA, Abraham WT, Chin MH, Feldman AM, Francis GS, Ganiats TG, et al. ACC/AHA 2005 Guideline Update for the Diagnosis and Management of Chronic Heart Failure in the Adult: a report of the American College of Cardiology/American Heart Association Task Force on Practice Guidelines (Writing Committee to Update the 2001 Guidelines for the Evaluation and Management of Heart Failure): developed in collaboration with the American College of Chest Physicians and the International Society for Heart and Lung Transplantation: endorsed by the Heart Rhythm Society. *Circulation.* 2005;112(12):e154-235.

[105] Yancy CW. Heart failure in African Americans. *Am. J. Cardiol.* 2005;96(7B):3i-12i.

[106] Bibbins-Domingo K, Pletcher MJ, Lin F, Vittinghoff E, Gardin JM, Arynchyn A, et al. Racial differences in incident heart failure among young adults. *N. Engl. J. Med.* 2009;360(12):1179-90.

[107] Okin PM, Kjeldsen SE, Dahlof B, Devereux RB. Racial differences in incident heart failure during antihypertensive therapy. *Circulation. Cardiovascular quality and outcomes.* 2011;4(2):157-64.

[108] Parashar S, Katz R, Smith NL, Arnold AM, Vaccarino V, Wenger NK, et al. Race, gender, and mortality in adults > or =65 years of age with incident heart failure (from the Cardiovascular Health Study). *The American journal of cardiology.* 2009;103(8):1120-7.

[109] Thomas KL, Hernandez AF, Dai D, Heidenreich P, Fonarow GC, Peterson ED, et al. Association of race/ethnicity with clinical risk factors, quality of care, and acute outcomes in patients hospitalized with heart failure. *American heart journal.* 2011;161(4):746-54.

[110] Bahrami H, Kronmal R, Bluemke DA, Olson J, Shea S, Liu K, et al. Differences in the incidence of congestive heart failure by ethnicity: the multi-ethnic study of atherosclerosis. *Archives of internal medicine.* 2008;168(19):2138-45.

[111] Thomas KL, East MA, Velazquez EJ, Tuttle RH, Shaw LK, O'Connor CM, et al. Outcomes by race and etiology of patients with left ventricular systolic dysfunction. *The American journal of cardiology.* 2005;96(7):956-63.

[112] Bibbins-Domingo K, Pletcher MJ, Lin F, Vittinghoff E, Gardin JM, Arynchyn A, et al. Racial differences in incident heart failure among young adults. *The New England journal of medicine.* 2009;360(12):1179-90.

[113] Moe GW, Tu J. Heart failure in the ethnic minorities. *Current opinion in cardiology.* 2010;25(2):124-30.

[114] Hebert K, Lopez B, Michael C, Franco E, Dias A, Trahan P, et al. The prevalence of peripheral arterial disease in patients with heart failure by race and ethnicity. *Congestive heart failure.* 2010;16(3):118-21.

[115] Husaini BA, Mensah GA, Sawyer D, Cain VA, Samad Z, Hull PC, et al. Race, sex, and age differences in heart failure-related hospitalizations in a southern state: implications for prevention. *Circulation. Heart failure.* 2011;4(2):161-9.

[116] Singh H, Gordon HS, Deswal A. Variation by race in factors contributing to heart failure hospitalizations. *Journal of cardiac failure.* 2005;11(1):23-9.

[117] Cardillo C, Kilcoyne CM, Cannon RO, 3rd, Panza JA. Racial differences in nitric oxide-mediated vasodilator response to mental stress in the forearm circulation. *Hypertension.* 1998;31(6):1235-9.

[118] Kalinowski L, Dobrucki IT, Malinski T. Race-specific differences in endothelial function: predisposition of African Americans to vascular diseases. *Circulation.* 2004;109(21):2511-7.

[119] Yancy CW. Race-based therapeutics. *Current hypertension reports.* 2008;10(4):276-85.

[120] Krauser DG, Chen AA, Tung R, Anwaruddin S, Baggish AL, Januzzi JL, Jr. Neither race nor gender influences the usefulness of amino-terminal pro-brain natriuretic peptide testing in dyspneic subjects: a ProBNP Investigation of Dyspnea in the Emergency Department (PRIDE) substudy. *Journal of cardiac failure.* 2006;12(6):452-7.

[121] Daniels LB, Bhalla V, Clopton P, Hollander JE, Guss D, McCullough PA, et al. B-type natriuretic peptide (BNP) levels and ethnic disparities in perceived severity of heart failure: results from the Rapid Emergency Department Heart Failure Outpatient Trial (REDHOT) multicenter study of BNP levels and emergency department decision making in patients presenting with shortness of breath. *Journal of cardiac failure.* 2006;12(4):281-5.

[122] Farmer SA, Kirkpatrick JN, Heidenreich PA, Curtis JP, Wang Y, Groeneveld PW. Ethnic and racial disparities in cardiac resynchronization therapy. Heart rhythm : *the official journal of the Heart Rhythm Society.* 2009;6(3):325-31.

[123] Hernandez AF, Fonarow GC, Liang L, Al-Khatib SM, Curtis LH, LaBresh KA, et al. Sex and racial differences in the use of implantable cardioverter-defibrillators among patients hospitalized with heart failure. JAMA : *the journal of the American Medical Association.* 2007;298(13):1525-32.

[124] Thomas KL, Al-Khatib SM, Kelsey RC, 2nd, Bush H, Brosius L, Velazquez EJ, et al. Racial disparity in the utilization of implantable-cardioverter defibrillators among patients with prior myocardial infarction and an ejection fraction of <or=35%. *The American journal of cardiology.* 2007;100(6):924-9.

[125] Steiner HA, Miller JM. Disparity in utilization of implantable cardioverter-defibrillators in treatment of heart failure based on sex and race. Women's health. 2008;4:23-5.

[126] Echols MR, Felker GM, Thomas KL, Pieper KS, Garg J, Cuffe MS, et al. Racial differences in the characteristics of patients admitted for acute decompensated heart failure and their relation to outcomes: results from the OPTIME-CHF trial. *Journal of cardiac failure.* 2006;12(9):684-8.

[127] Buckalew VM, Jr., Freedman BI. Reappraisal of the impact of race on survival in patients on dialysis. American journal of kidney diseases : the *official journal of the National Kidney Foundation.* 2010;55(6):1102-10.

[128] Bash LD, Astor BC, Coresh J. Risk of incident ESRD: a comprehensive look at cardiovascular risk factors and 17 years of follow-up in the Atherosclerosis Risk in Communities (ARIC) Study. American journal of kidney diseases : the *official journal of the National Kidney Foundation.* 2010;55(1):31-41.

[129] Lea J, Cheek D, Thornley-Brown D, Appel L, Agodoa L, Contreras G, et al. Metabolic syndrome, proteinuria, and the risk of progressive CKD in hypertensive African Americans. American journal of kidney diseases: the *official journal of the National Kidney Foundation.* 2008;51(5):732-40.

[130] Bomback AS, Kshirsagar AV, Whaley-Connell AT, Chen SC, Li S, Klemmer PJ, et al. Racial differences in kidney function among individuals with obesity and metabolic syndrome: results from the Kidney Early Evaluation Program (KEEP). *American journal of kidney diseases : the official journal of the National Kidney Foundation*. 2010;55(3 Suppl 2):S4-S14.

[131] Kovesdy CP, Anderson JE, Derose SF, Kalantar-Zadeh K. Outcomes associated with race in males with nondialysis-dependent chronic kidney disease. *Clinical journal of the American Society of Nephrology*: CJASN. 2009;4(5):973-8.

[132] Newsome BB, McClellan WM, Allison JJ, Eggers PW, Chen SC, Collins AJ, et al. Racial differences in the competing risks of mortality and ESRD after acute myocardial infarction. American journal of kidney diseases : *the official journal of the National Kidney Foundation*. 2008;52(2):251-61.

[133] Parekh RS, Zhang L, Fivush BA, Klag MJ. Incidence of atherosclerosis by race in the dialysis morbidity and mortality study: a sample of the US ESRD population. *Journal of the American Society of Nephrology : JASN*. 2005;16(5):1420-6.

[134] Smith GL, Shlipak MG, Havranek EP, Masoudi FA, McClellan WM, Foody JM, et al. Race and renal impairment in heart failure: mortality in blacks versus whites. *Circulation*. 2005;111(10):1270-7.

[135] Young BA, Rudser K, Kestenbaum B, Seliger SL, Andress D, Boyko EJ. Racial and ethnic differences in incident myocardial infarction in end-stage renal disease patients: The USRDS. *Kidney international*. 2006;69(9):1691-8.

[136] Nguyen HT, Stack AG. Ethnic disparities in cardiovascular risk factors and coronary disease prevalence among individuals with chronic kidney disease: findings from the Third National Health and Nutrition Examination Survey. *Journal of the American Society of Nephrology : JASN*. 2006;17(6):1716-23.

[137] Waikar SS, Curhan GC, Ayanian JZ, Chertow GM. Race and mortality after acute renal failure. *Journal of the American Society of Nephrology*: JASN. 2007;18(10):2740-8.

[138] Kilpatrick RD, McAllister CJ, Kovesdy CP, Derose SF, Kopple JD, Kalantar-Zadeh K. Association between serum lipids and survival in hemodialysis patients and impact of race. *Journal of the American Society of Nephrology : JASN*. 2007;18(1):293-303.

[139] Hoy WE, Hughson MD, Diouf B, Zimanyi M, Samuel T, McNamara BJ, et al. Distribution of volumes of individual glomeruli in kidneys at autopsy: association with physical and clinical characteristics and with ethnic group. *American journal of nephrology*. 2011;33 Suppl 1:15-20.

[140] Perucca J, Bouby N, Valeix P, Jungers P, Bankir L. [Difference in urine concentration according to gender and ethnicity: possible involvement in the different susceptibility to various renal and cardiovascular diseases]. *Nephrologie and therapeutique*. 2008;4(3):160-72.

[141] Hanevold CD, Pollock JS, Harshfield GA. Racial differences in microalbumin excretion in healthy adolescents. *Hypertension*. 2008;51(2):334-8.

[142] Yatsuya H, Folsom AR, Yamagishi K, North KE, Brancati FL, Stevens J. Race- and sex-specific associations of obesity measures with ischemic stroke incidence in the Atherosclerosis Risk in Communities (ARIC) study. *Stroke; a journal of cerebral circulation*. 2010;41(3):417-25.

[143] Glymour MM, Avendano M, Haas S, Berkman LF. Lifecourse social conditions and racial disparities in incidence of first stroke. *Annals of epidemiology.* 2008;18(12):904-12.

[144] Markus HS, Khan U, Birns J, Evans A, Kalra L, Rudd AG, et al. Differences in stroke subtypes between black and white patients with stroke: the South London Ethnicity and Stroke Study. *Circulation.* 2007;116(19):2157-64.

[145] Singh R, Cohen SN, Krupp R, Abedi AG. Racial differences in ischemic cerebrovascular disease. Journal of stroke and cerebrovascular diseases : *the official journal of National Stroke Association.* 1998;7(5):352-7.

[146] Weatherley BD, Nelson JJ, Heiss G, Chambless LE, Sharrett AR, Nieto FJ, et al. The association of the ankle-brachial index with incident coronary heart disease: the Atherosclerosis Risk In Communities (ARIC) study, 1987-2001. *BMC cardiovascular disorders.* 2007;7:3.

[147] Ix JH, Allison MA, Denenberg JO, Cushman M, Criqui MH. Novel cardiovascular risk factors do not completely explain the higher prevalence of peripheral arterial disease among African Americans. The San Diego Population Study. *Journal of the American College of Cardiology.* 2008;51(24):2347-54.

[148] Aboyans V, Criqui MH, McClelland RL, Allison MA, McDermott MM, Goff DC, Jr., et al. Intrinsic contribution of gender and ethnicity to normal ankle-brachial index values: the Multi-Ethnic Study of Atherosclerosis (MESA). *Journal of vascular surgery : official publication, the Society for Vascular Surgery [and] International Society for Cardiovascular Surgery, North American Chapter.* 2007;45(2):319-27.

[149] Criqui MH, Vargas V, Denenberg JO, Ho E, Allison M, Langer RD, et al. Ethnicity and peripheral arterial disease: the San Diego Population Study. *Circulation.* 2005;112(17):2703-7.

[150] Allison MA, Criqui MH, McClelland RL, Scott JM, McDermott MM, Liu K, et al. The effect of novel cardiovascular risk factors on the ethnic-specific odds for peripheral arterial disease in the Multi-Ethnic Study of Atherosclerosis (MESA). *Journal of the American College of Cardiology.* 2006;48(6):1190-7.

[151] Reis JP, Michos ED, von Muhlen D, Miller ER, 3rd. Differences in vitamin D status as a possible contributor to the racial disparity in peripheral arterial disease. *The American journal of clinical nutrition.* 2008;88(6):1469-77.

[152] Mulukutla SR, Venkitachalam L, Bambs C, Kip KE, Aiyer A, Marroquin OC, et al. Black race is associated with digital artery endothelial dysfunction: results from the Heart SCORE study. *European heart journal.* 2010;31(22):2808-15.

[153] Duprez DA, Jacobs DR, Jr., Lutsey PL, Herrington D, Prime D, Ouyang P, et al. Race/ethnic and sex differences in large and small artery elasticity--results of the multi-ethnic study of atherosclerosis (MESA). *Ethnicity and disease.* 2009;19(3):243-50.

[154] Shah AS, Dolan LM, Gao Z, Kimball TR, Urbina EM. Racial differences in arterial stiffness among adolescents and young adults with type 2 diabetes. *Pediatric diabetes.* 2011.

[155] Choi JB, Hong S, Nelesen R, Bardwell WA, Natarajan L, Schubert C, et al. Age and ethnicity differences in short-term heart-rate variability. *Psychosomatic medicine.* 2006;68(3):421-6.

[156] Wang X, Thayer JF, Treiber F, Snieder H. Ethnic differences and heritability of heart rate variability in African- and European American youth. *The American journal of cardiology*. 2005;96(8):1166-72.

[157] Lampert R, Ickovics J, Horwitz R, Lee F. Depressed autonomic nervous system function in African Americans and individuals of lower social class: a potential mechanism of race- and class-related disparities in health outcomes. *American heart journal*. 2005;150(1):153-60.

[158] Nance JW, Jr., Bamberg F, Schoepf UJ, Kang DK, Barraza JM, Jr., Abro JA, et al. Coronary Atherosclerosis in African American and White Patients with Acute Chest Pain: Characterization with Coronary CT Angiography. *Radiology*. 2011;260(2):373-80.

[159] Taylor AJ, Wu H, Bindeman J, Bauer K, Byrd C, O'Malley PG, et al. Comparison of coronary artery calcium progression in African American and white men. *Journal of cardiovascular computed tomography*. 2009;3(2):71-7.

[160] Fair JM, Kiazand A, Varady A, Mahbouba M, Norton L, Rubin GD, et al. Ethnic differences in coronary artery calcium in a healthy cohort aged 60 to 69 years. *The American journal of cardiology*. 2007;100(6):981-5.

[161] Loria CM, Liu K, Lewis CE, Hulley SB, Sidney S, Schreiner PJ, et al. Early adult risk factor levels and subsequent coronary artery calcification: the CARDIA Study. *Journal of the American College of Cardiology*. 2007;49(20):2013-20.

[162] Freedman BI, Hsu FC, Langefeld CD, Rich SS, Herrington DM, Carr JJ, et al. The impact of ethnicity and sex on subclinical cardiovascular disease: the Diabetes Heart Study. *Diabetologia*. 2005;48(12):2511-8.

[163] Budoff MJ, Nasir K, Mao S, Tseng PH, Chau A, Liu ST, et al. Ethnic differences of the presence and severity of coronary atherosclerosis. *Atherosclerosis*. 2006;187(2):343-50.

[164] Kawakubo M, LaBree L, Xiang M, Doherty TM, Wong ND, Azen S, et al. Race-ethnic differences in the extent, prevalence, and progression of coronary calcium. *Ethnicity and disease*. 2005;15(2):198-204.

[165] Nasir K, Shaw LJ, Liu ST, Weinstein SR, Mosler TR, Flores PR, et al. Ethnic differences in the prognostic value of coronary artery calcification for all-cause mortality. *Journal of the American College of Cardiology*. 2007;50(10):953-60.

[166] Bild DE, Detrano R, Peterson D, Guerci A, Liu K, Shahar E, et al. Ethnic differences in coronary calcification: the Multi-Ethnic Study of Atherosclerosis (MESA). *Circulation*. 2005;111(10):1313-20.

[167] Allison MA, Budoff MJ, Nasir K, Wong ND, Detrano R, Kronmal R, et al. Ethnic-specific risks for atherosclerotic calcification of the thoracic and abdominal aorta (from the Multi-Ethnic Study of Atherosclerosis). *The American journal of cardiology*. 2009;104(6):812-7.

[168] Kanjanauthai S, Nasir K, Katz R, Rivera JJ, Takasu J, Blumenthal RS, et al. Relationships of mitral annular calcification to cardiovascular risk factors: the Multi-Ethnic Study of Atherosclerosis (MESA). *Atherosclerosis*. 2010;213(2):558-62.

[169] Nasir K, Katz R, Takasu J, Shavelle DM, Detrano R, Lima JA, et al. Ethnic differences between extra-coronary measures on cardiac computed tomography: multi-ethnic study of atherosclerosis (MESA). *Atherosclerosis*. 2008;198(1):104-14.

[170] Huang CC, Lloyd-Jones DM, Guo X, Rajamannan NM, Lin S, Du P, et al. Gene expression variation between African Americans and whites is associated with coronary

artery calcification: the multiethnic study of atherosclerosis. *Physiol Genomics.* 2011;43(13):836-43.

[171] Hravnak M, Ibrahim S, Kaufer A, Sonel A, Conigliaro J. Racial disparities in outcomes following coronary artery bypass grafting. *The Journal of cardiovascular nursing.* 2006;21(5):367-78.

[172] Breton CV, Wang X, Mack WJ, Berhane K, Lopez M, Islam TS, et al. Carotid artery intima-media thickness in college students: Race/ethnicity matters. *Atherosclerosis.* 2011;217(2):441-6.

[173] Bennett PC, Gill PS, Silverman S, Blann AD, Lip GY. Ethnic differences in common carotid intima-media thickness, and the relationship to cardiovascular risk factors and peripheral arterial disease: the Ethnic-Echocardiographic Heart of England Screening Study. QJM : *monthly journal of the Association of Physicians.* 2011;104(3):245-54.

[174] Marcus GM, Olgin JE, Whooley M, Vittinghoff E, Stone KL, Mehra R, et al. Racial differences in atrial fibrillation prevalence and left atrial size. *The American journal of medicine.* 2010;123(4):375 e1-7.

[175] Sun X, Hill PC, Lowery R, Lindsay J, Boyce SW, Bafi AS, et al. Comparison of Frequency of Atrial Fibrillation After Coronary Artery Bypass Grafting in African Americans Versus European Americans. *The American journal of cardiology.* 2011.

[176] Lahiri MK, Fang K, Lamerato L, Khan AM, Schuger CD. Effect of race on the frequency of postoperative atrial fibrillation following coronary artery bypass grafting. *The American journal of cardiology.* 2011;107(3):383-6.

[177] Michael Smith J, Soneson EA, Woods SE, Engel AM, Hiratzka LF. Coronary artery bypass graft surgery outcomes among African-Americans and Caucasian patients. *International journal of surgery.* 2006;4(4):212-6.

[178] Hebert K, Lopez B, Dias A, Steen DL, Colombo RA, Franco E, et al. Prevalence of electrocardiographic abnormalities in a systolic heart failure disease management population by race, ethnicity, and sex. *Congestive heart failure.* 2010;16(1):21-6.

[179] Liao Y, Cooper RS, McGee DL, Mensah GA, Ghali JK. The relative effects of left ventricular hypertrophy, coronary artery disease, and ventricular dysfunction on survival among black adults. JAMA : *the journal of the American Medical Association.* 1995;273(20):1592-7.

[180] Crowley DI, Khoury PR, Urbina EM, Ippisch HM, Kimball TR. Cardiovascular impact of the pediatric obesity epidemic: higher left ventricular mass is related to higher body mass index. *The Journal of pediatrics.* 2011;158(5):709-14 e1.

[181] Havranek EP, Froshaug DB, Emserman CD, Hanratty R, Krantz MJ, Masoudi FA, et al. Left ventricular hypertrophy and cardiovascular mortality by race and ethnicity. *The American journal of medicine.* 2008;121(10):870-5.

[182] Collins-McNeil J, Holston EC, Edwards CL, Carbage-Martin J, Benbow DL, Dixon TD. Depressive symptoms, cardiovascular risk, and diabetes self-care strategies in African American women with type 2 diabetes. *Archives of psychiatric nursing.* 2007;21(4):201-9.

[183] Lewis TT, Guo H, Lunos S, Mendes de Leon CF, Skarupski KA, Evans DA, et al. Depressive symptoms and cardiovascular mortality in older black and white adults: evidence for a differential association by race. Circulation. *Cardiovascular quality and outcomes.* 2011;4(3):293-9.

[184] Knox S, Barnes A, Kiefe C, Lewis CE, Iribarren C, Matthews KA, et al. History of depression, race, and cardiovascular risk in CARDIA. *International journal of behavioral medicine.* 2006;13(1):44-50.

[185] Lewis TT, Everson-Rose SA, Colvin A, Matthews K, Bromberger JT, Sutton-Tyrrell K. Interactive effects of race and depressive symptoms on calcification in African American and white women. *Psychosomatic medicine.* 2009;71(2):163-70.

[186] Waldman SV, Blumenthal JA, Babyak MA, Sherwood A, Sketch M, Davidson J, et al. Ethnic differences in the treatment of depression in patients with ischemic heart disease. *American heart journal.* 2009;157(1):77-83.

[187] Chyu L, Upchurch DM. Racial and ethnic patterns of allostatic load among adult women in the United States: findings from the National Health and Nutrition Examination Survey 1999-2004. *Journal of women's health.* 2011;20(4):575-83.

[188] Chae DH, Lincoln KD, Adler NE, Syme SL. Do experiences of racial discrimination predict cardiovascular disease among African American men? The moderating role of internalized negative racial group attitudes. *Social science and medicine.* 2010;71(6):1182-8.

[189] Fiscella K, Franks P. Vitamin D, race, and cardiovascular mortality: findings from a national US sample. *Annals of family medicine.* 2010;8(1):11-8.

[190] Dong Y, Pollock N, Stallmann-Jorgensen IS, Gutin B, Lan L, Chen TC, et al. Low 25-hydroxyvitamin D levels in adolescents: race, season, adiposity, physical activity, and fitness. *Pediatrics.* 2010;125(6):1104-11.

[191] Napoli C. Developmental mechanisms involved in the primary prevention of atherosclerosis and cardiovascular disease. *Curr. Atheroscler Rep.* 2011;13(2):170-5.

[192] Samani NJ, Erdmann J, Hall AS, Hengstenberg C, Mangino M, Mayer B, et al. Genomewide association analysis of coronary artery disease. *N. Engl. J. Med.* 2007;357(5):443-53.

[193] Kral BG, Mathias RA, Suktitipat B, Ruczinski I, Vaidya D, Yanek LR, et al. A common variant in the CDKN2B gene on chromosome 9p21 protects against coronary artery disease in Americans of African ancestry. *J. Hum. Genet.* 2011;56(3):224-9.

[194] Goldenberg I, Moss AJ, Ryan D, McNitt S, Eberly SW, Zareba W. Polymorphism in the angiotensinogen gene, hypertension, and ethnic differences in the risk of recurrent coronary events. *Hypertension.* 2006;48(4):693-9.

[195] Siffert W, Rosskopf D, Siffert G, Busch S, Moritz A, Erbel R, et al. Association of a human G-protein beta3 subunit variant with hypertension. *Nat. Genet.* 1998;18(1):45-8.

[196] Sagnella GA. Why is plasma renin activity lower in populations of African origin? *J. Hum. Hypertens.* 2001;15(1):17-25.

[197] Kao WH, Klag MJ, Meoni LA, Reich D, Berthier-Schaad Y, Li M, et al. MYH9 is associated with nondiabetic end-stage renal disease in African Americans. *Nat. Genet.* 2008;40(10):1185-92.

[198] Genovese G, Friedman DJ, Ross MD, Lecordier L, Uzureau P, Freedman BI, et al. Association of trypanolytic ApoL1 variants with kidney disease in African Americans. *Science.* 2010;329(5993):841-5.

[199] Cohen J, Pertsemlidis A, Kotowski IK, Graham R, Garcia CK, Hobbs HH. Low LDL cholesterol in individuals of African descent resulting from frequent nonsense mutations in PCSK9. *Nat. Genet.* 2005;37(2):161-5.

[200] Sun AY, Koontz JI, Shah SH, Piccini JP, Nilsson KR, Jr., Craig D, et al. The S1103Y cardiac sodium channel variant is associated with implantable cardioverter-defibrillator events in blacks with heart failure and reduced ejection fraction. *Circ Cardiovasc Genet.* 2011;4(2):163-8.

[201] Splawski I, Timothy KW, Tateyama M, Clancy CE, Malhotra A, Beggs AH, et al. Variant of SCN5A sodium channel implicated in risk of cardiac arrhythmia. *Science.* 2002;297(5585):1333-6.

[202] Burke A, Creighton W, Mont E, Li L, Hogan S, Kutys R, et al. Role of SCN5A Y1102 polymorphism in sudden cardiac death in blacks. *Circulation.* 2005;112(6):798-802.

[203] Lettre G, Palmer CD, Young T, Ejebe KG, Allayee H, Benjamin EJ, et al. Genome-wide association study of coronary heart disease and its risk factors in 8,090 African Americans: the NHLBI CARe Project. *PLoS genetics.* 2011;7(2):e1001300.

[204] Cavallari LH, Groo VL, Momary KM, Fontana D, Viana MA, Vaitkus P. Racial differences in potassium response to spironolactone in heart failure. *Congestive heart failure.* 2006;12(4):200-5.

[205] Shekelle PG, Rich MW, Morton SC, Atkinson CS, Tu W, Maglione M, et al. Efficacy of angiotensin-converting enzyme inhibitors and beta-blockers in the management of left ventricular systolic dysfunction according to race, gender, and diabetic status: a meta-analysis of major clinical trials. *Journal of the American College of Cardiology.* 2003;41(9):1529-38.

[206] Abraham WT, Massie BM, Lukas MA, Lottes SR, Nelson JJ, Fowler MB, et al. Tolerability, safety, and efficacy of beta-blockade in black patients with heart failure in the community setting: insights from a large prospective beta-blocker registry. *Congestive heart failure.* 2007;13(1):16-21.

[207] Taylor AL, Ziesche S, Yancy C, Carson P, D'Agostino R, Jr., Ferdinand K, et al. Combination of isosorbide dinitrate and hydralazine in blacks with heart failure. *The New England journal of medicine.* 2004;351(20):2049-57.

[208] Ferdinand KC. African American heart failure trial: role of endothelial dysfunction and heart failure in African Americans. *The American journal of cardiology.* 2007;99(6B):3D-6D.

[209] McNamara DM. Emerging role of pharmacogenomics in heart failure. *Curr. Opin. Cardiol.* 2008;23(3):261-8.

[210] Exner DV, Dries DL, Domanski MJ, Cohn JN. Lesser response to angiotensin-converting-enzyme inhibitor therapy in black as compared with white patients with left ventricular dysfunction. *N. Engl. J. Med.* 2001;344(18):1351-7.

[211] Lindholm LH, Ibsen H, Dahlof B, Devereux RB, Beevers G, de Faire U, et al. Cardiovascular morbidity and mortality in patients with diabetes in the Losartan Intervention For Endpoint reduction in hypertension study (LIFE): a randomised trial against atenolol. *Lancet.* 2002;359(9311):1004-10.

[212] Dahlof B, Devereux RB, Kjeldsen SE, Julius S, Beevers G, de Faire U, et al. Cardiovascular morbidity and mortality in the Losartan Intervention For Endpoint reduction in hypertension study (LIFE): a randomised trial against atenolol. *Lancet.* 2002;359(9311):995-1003.

[213] Major outcomes in high-risk hypertensive patients randomized to angiotensin-converting enzyme inhibitor or calcium channel blocker vs diuretic: The Antihypertensive and Lipid-Lowering Treatment to Prevent Heart Attack Trial

(ALLHAT). *JAMA : the journal of the American Medical Association.* 2002;288(23):2981-97.

[214] Cushman WC, Reda DJ, Perry HM, Williams D, Abdellatif M, Materson BJ. Regional and racial differences in response to antihypertensive medication use in a randomized controlled trial of men with hypertension in the United States. Department of Veterans Affairs Cooperative Study Group on Antihypertensive Agents. *Archives of internal medicine.* 2000;160(6):825-31.

[215] Weir MR, Gray JM, Paster R, Saunders E. Differing mechanisms of action of angiotensin-converting enzyme inhibition in black and white hypertensive patients. *The Trandolapril Multicenter Study Group. Hypertension.* 1995;26(1):124-30.

[216] Wright JT, Jr., Harris-Haywood S, Pressel S, Barzilay J, Baimbridge C, Bareis CJ, et al. Clinical outcomes by race in hypertensive patients with and without the metabolic syndrome: Antihypertensive and Lipid-Lowering Treatment to Prevent Heart Attack Trial (ALLHAT). *Archives of internal medicine.* 2008;168(2):207-17.

[217] Flack JM, Sica DA, Bakris G, Brown AL, Ferdinand KC, Grimm RH, Jr., et al. Management of high blood pressure in Blacks: an update of the International Society on Hypertension in Blacks consensus statement. Hypertension. 2010;56(5):780-800.

[218] Jones DW, Hall JE. Seventh report of the Joint National Committee on Prevention, Detection, Evaluation, and Treatment of High Blood Pressure and evidence from new hypertension trials. *Hypertension.* 2004;43(1):1-3.

[219] Mehta JL, Bursac Z, Mehta P, Bansal D, Fink L, Marsh J, et al. Racial disparities in prescriptions for cardioprotective drugs and cardiac outcomes in Veterans Affairs Hospitals. *The American journal of cardiology.* 2010;105(7):1019-23.

[220] Mathur R, Badrick E, Boomla K, Bremner S, Hull S, Robson J. Prescribing in general practice for people with coronary heart disease; equity by age, sex, ethnic group and deprivation. *Ethnicity and health.* 2011;16(2):107-23.

[221] Ma J, Sehgal NL, Ayanian JZ, Stafford RS. National trends in statin use by coronary heart disease risk category. *PLoS medicine.* 2005;2(5):e123.

[222] Palmeri ST, Lowe AM, Sleeper LA, Saucedo JF, Desvigne-Nickens P, Hochman JS. Racial and ethnic differences in the treatment and outcome of cardiogenic shock following acute myocardial infarction. *The American journal of cardiology.* 2005;96(8):1042-9.

[223] Sonel AF, Good CB, Mulgund J, Roe MT, Gibler WB, Smith SC, Jr., et al. Racial variations in treatment and outcomes of black and white patients with high-risk non-ST-elevation acute coronary syndromes: insights from CRUSADE (Can Rapid Risk Stratification of Unstable Angina Patients Suppress Adverse Outcomes With Early Implementation of the ACC/AHA Guidelines?). *Circulation.* 2005;111(10):1225-32.

[224] Cram P, Bayman L, Popescu I, Vaughan-Sarrazin MS. Racial disparities in revascularization rates among patients with similar insurance coverage. *Journal of the National Medical Association.* 2009;101(11):1132-9.

[225] Clark LT, Maki KC, Galant R, Maron DJ, Pearson TA, Davidson MH. Ethnic differences in achievement of cholesterol treatment goals. Results from the National Cholesterol Education Program Evaluation Project Utilizing Novel E-Technology II. *Journal of general internal medicine.* 2006;21(4):320-6.

[226] Papademetriou V, Kaoutzanis C, Dumas M, Pittaras A, Faselis C, Kokkinos P, et al. Protective effects of angiotensin-converting enzyme inhibitors in high-risk African

American men with coronary heart disease. *Journal of clinical hypertension.* 2009;11(11):621-6.

[227] Prisant LM, Thomas KL, Lewis EF, Huang Z, Francis GS, Weaver WD, et al. Racial analysis of patients with myocardial infarction complicated by heart failure and/or left ventricular dysfunction treated with valsartan, captopril, or both. *Journal of the American College of Cardiology.* 2008;51(19):1865-71.

[228] McDowell SE, Coleman JJ, Ferner RE. Systematic review and meta-analysis of ethnic differences in risks of adverse reactions to drugs used in cardiovascular medicine. *BMJ.* 2006;332(7551):1177-81.

[229] Mehta RH, Stebbins A, Lopes RD, Rao SV, Bates ER, Pieper KS, et al. Race, Bleeding, and Outcomes in STEMI Patients Treated with Fibrinolytic Therapy. *The American journal of medicine.* 2011;124(1):48-57.

[230] Hannan EL, Racz M, Walford G, Clark LT, Holmes DR, King SB, 3rd, et al. Differences in utilization of drug-eluting stents by race and payer. *The American journal of cardiology.* 2007;100(8):1192-8.

[231] Collins SD, Torguson R, Gaglia MA, Jr., Lemesle G, Syed AI, Ben-Dor I, et al. Does black ethnicity influence the development of stent thrombosis in the drug-eluting stent era? *Circulation.* 2010;122(11):1085-90.

[232] Santos PC, Soares RA, Santos DB, Nascimento RM, Coelho GL, Nicolau JC, et al. CYP2C19 and ABCB1 gene polymorphisms are differently distributed according to ethnicity in the Brazilian general population. *BMC Med. Genet.* 2011;12:13.

[233] Scott SA, Jaremko M, Lubitz SA, Kornreich R, Halperin JL, Desnick RJ. CYP2C9*8 is prevalent among African-Americans: implications for pharmacogenetic dosing. *Pharmacogenomics.* 2009;10(8):1243-55.

[234] Gum PA, Kottke-Marchant K, Poggio ED, Gurm H, Welsh PA, Brooks L, et al. Profile and prevalence of aspirin resistance in patients with cardiovascular disease. *Am. J. Cardiol.* 2001;88(3):230-5.

[235] Chapman N, Chang CL, Caulfield M, Dahlof B, Feder G, Sever PS, et al. Ethnic variations in lipid-lowering in response to a statin (EVIREST): a substudy of the Anglo-Scandinavian Cardiac Outcomes Trial (ASCOT). *Ethnicity and disease.* 2011;21(2):150-7.

[236] Bays HE, Conard SE, Leiter LA, Bird SR, Lowe RS, Tershakovec AM. Influence of age, gender, and race on the efficacy of adding ezetimibe to atorvastatin vs. atorvastatin up-titration in patients at moderately high or high risk for coronary heart disease. *International journal of cardiology.* 2010.

[237] Major outcomes in moderately hypercholesterolemic, hypertensive patients randomized to pravastatin vs usual care: The Antihypertensive and Lipid-Lowering Treatment to Prevent Heart Attack Trial (ALLHAT-LLT). JAMA : *the journal of the American Medical Association.* 2002;288(23):2998-3007.

[238] Ferdinand KC, Clark LT, Watson KE, Neal RC, Brown CD, Kong BW, et al. Comparison of efficacy and safety of rosuvastatin versus atorvastatin in African-American patients in a six-week trial. *The American journal of cardiology.* 2006;97(2):229-35.

[239] Chen ST, Maruthur NM, Appel LJ. The effect of dietary patterns on estimated coronary heart disease risk: results from the Dietary Approaches to Stop Hypertension (DASH) trial. *Circ. Cardiovasc. Qual.* Outcomes. 2010;3(5):484-9.

[240] Cook NR, Cutler JA, Obarzanek E, Buring JE, Rexrode KM, Kumanyika SK, et al. Long term effects of dietary sodium reduction on cardiovascular disease outcomes: observational follow-up of the trials of hypertension prevention (TOHP). *BMJ.* 2007;334(7599):885-8.

[241] Lew EA. Mortality and weight: insured lives and the American Cancer Society studies. *Ann. Intern. Med.* 1985;103(6 (Pt 2)):1024-9.

[242] Phelan S, Wing RR, Loria CM, Kim Y, Lewis CE. Prevalence and predictors of weight-loss maintenance in a biracial cohort: results from the coronary artery risk development in young adults study. *Am. J. Prev. Med.* 2010;39(6):546-54.

[243] Thompson E, Berry D, Nasir L. Weight management in African-Americans using church-based community interventions to prevent type 2 diabetes and cardiovascular disease. *J Natl Black Nurses Assoc.* 2009;20(1):59-65.

[244] Flechtner-Mors M, Ditschuneit HH, Johnson TD, Suchard MA, Adler G. Metabolic and weight loss effects of long-term dietary intervention in obese patients: four-year results. *Obes Res.* 2000;8(5):399-402.

[245] Alhassan S, Robinson TN. Objectively measured physical activity and cardiovascular disease risk factors in African American girls. *Ethn Dis.* 2008;18(4):421-6.

[246] Kokkinos PF, Narayan P, Colleran JA, Pittaras A, Notargiacomo A, Reda D, et al. Effects of regular exercise on blood pressure and left ventricular hypertrophy in African-American men with severe hypertension. *N. Engl. J. Med.* 1995;333(22):1462-7.

[247] Cornell CE, Littleton MA, Greene PG, Pulley L, Brownstein JN, Sanderson BK, et al. A Community Health Advisor Program to reduce cardiovascular risk among rural African-American women. *Health Educ. Res.* 2009;24(4):622-33.

[248] Plescia M, Herrick H, Chavis L. Improving health behaviors in an African American community: the Charlotte Racial and Ethnic Approaches to Community Health project. *Am. J. Public Health.* 2008;98(9):1678-84.

[249] A clinical practice guideline for treating tobacco use and dependence: 2008 update. A U.S. Public Health Service report. *Am. J. Prev Med.* 2008;35(2):158-76.

[250] Wu JR, Lennie TA, De Jong MJ, Frazier SK, Heo S, Chung ML, et al. Medication adherence is a mediator of the relationship between ethnicity and event-free survival in patients with heart failure. *Journal of cardiac failure.* 2010;16(2):142-9.

[251] Davis AM, Vinci LM, Okwuosa TM, Chase AR, Huang ES. Cardiovascular health disparities: a systematic review of health care interventions. *Med. Care Res. Rev.* 2007;64(5 Suppl):29S-100S.

[252] Haynes RB, McDonald HP, Garg AX. Helping patients follow prescribed treatment: clinical applications. *JAMA : the journal of the American Medical Association.* 2002;288(22):2880-3.

[253] Pace R, Dawkins N, Wang B, Person S, Shikany JM. Rural African Americans' dietary knowledge, perceptions, and behavior in relation to cardiovascular disease. *Ethn Dis.* 2008;18(1):6-12.

[254] Low AK, Grothe KB, Wofford TS, Bouldin MJ. Addressing disparities in cardiovascular risk through community-based interventions. *Ethn Dis.* 2007;17(2 Suppl 2):S2-55-9.

[255] Cene CW, Yanek LR, Moy TF, Levine DM, Becker LC, Becker DM. Sustainability of a multiple risk factor intervention on cardiovascular disease in high-risk African American families. *Ethn Dis.* 2008;18(2):169-75.

[256] Halbert CH, Bellamy S, Bowman M, Briggs V, Delmoor E, Purnell J, et al. Effects of integrated risk counseling for cancer and cardiovascular disease in African Americans. *J. Natl. Med. Assoc.* 2010;102(5):396-402.

[257] Releford BJ, Frencher SK, Jr., Yancey AK, Norris K. Cardiovascular disease control through barbershops: design of a nationwide outreach program. *J. Natl. Med. Assoc.* 2010;102(4):336-45.

[258] Liao Y, Tucker P, Siegel P, Liburd L, Giles WH. Decreasing disparity in cholesterol screening in minority communities--findings from the racial and ethnic approaches to community health 2010. *J. Epidemiol. Community Health.* 2010;64(4):292-9.

[259] Greenland P, Bonow RO, Brundage BH, Budoff MJ, Eisenberg MJ, Grundy SM, et al. ACCF/AHA 2007 clinical expert consensus document on coronary artery calcium scoring by computed tomography in global cardiovascular risk assessment and in evaluation of patients with chest pain: a report of the American College of Cardiology Foundation Clinical Expert Consensus Task Force (ACCF/AHA Writing Committee to Update the 2000 Expert Consensus Document on Electron Beam Computed Tomography) developed in collaboration with the Society of Atherosclerosis Imaging and Prevention and the Society of Cardiovascular Computed Tomography. *J. Am. Coll Cardiol.* 2007;49(3):378-402.

[260] Stein JH, Korcarz CE, Hurst RT, Lonn E, Kendall CB, Mohler ER, et al. Use of carotid ultrasound to identify subclinical vascular disease and evaluate cardiovascular disease risk: a consensus statement from the American Society of Echocardiography Carotid Intima-Media Thickness Task Force. Endorsed by the Society for Vascular Medicine. *J. Am. Soc. Echocardiogr.* 2008;21(2):93-111; quiz 89-90.

[261] Detrano R, Guerci AD, Carr JJ, Bild DE, Burke G, Folsom AR, et al. Coronary calcium as a predictor of coronary events in four racial or ethnic groups. *N. Engl. J. Med.* 2008;358(13):1336-45.

[262] Folsom AR, Kronmal RA, Detrano RC, O'Leary DH, Bild DE, Bluemke DA, et al. Coronary artery calcification compared with carotid intima-media thickness in the prediction of cardiovascular disease incidence: the Multi-Ethnic Study of Atherosclerosis (MESA). *Arch. Intern. Med.* 2008;168(12):1333-9.

[263] Parikh NI, Vasan RS. Assessing the clinical utility of biomarkers in medicine. *Biomark Med.* 2007;1(3):419-36.

In: Current Advances in Cardiovascular Risk. Volume 2   ISBN: 978-1-62081-746-9
Editor: Sandeep Ajoy Saha   © 2012 Nova Science Publishers, Inc.

Chapter XXIV

Unique Challenges in the Management of Cardiovascular Disease in Asian Americans

*Ariel T. Holland and Latha P. Palaniappan**

Palo Alto Medical Foundation Research Institute, Palo Alto, CA, US

Abstract

Asian Americans (Asian Indian, Chinese, Filipino, Japanese, Korean, Vietnamese) are the fastest growing of the racial/ethnic groups in the United States, with a population of over 13 million in 2008, and projected to reach nearly 34 million by 2050. Although the Asian American population continues to grow, data on risk, incidence and treatment of cardiovascular disease (CVD) for Asian Americans are limited. Data collection and interpretation for CVD in Asian Americans has suffered from three major flaws — omission, aggregation, and extrapolation. Some studies, such as the National Health and Nutrition Examination Survey, which provides health information for a nationally representative population sample of the U.S., have omitted Asian Americans entirely. Some data sources, such as the National Registry of Myocardial Infarction, have collected data on Asians, but have aggregated disparate subgroups, making interpretation and clinical application difficult. In some cases, results of a study in just one Asian race/ethnic group, such as the Ni-Hon-San study in Japanese, are extrapolated to all Asians generally, resulting in inaccurate assumptions regarding disease risk for the other Asian subgroups. Due to these challenges of existing data, conventional knowledge has assumed that all Asian American subgroups are at low risk for CVD. In recent years more studies have examined Asian American subgroups separately, indicating that there is substantial variability in cardiovascular risk and incidence of coronary artery disease (CAD), stroke, and peripheral vascular disease across subgroups. Prevalence of traditional risk factors, such as diabetes and obesity, varies greatly across the Asian subgroups, which affects risk prediction models commonly used in the U.S. Recent research has identified certain subgroups as demonstrating higher rates of CAD, with

* Corresponding author: Latha Palaniappan, 795 El Camino Real, Palo Alto, CA 94301, Ames Building, Fax: 650-853-4835, Tel: 650-853-4752, Email: lathap@pamfri.org.

higher prevalence rates found for Asian Indians and Filipinos. In addition to heterogeneity in CVD risk and incidence, Asian Americans differ in responsiveness to treatment and adverse effects. The field of pharmacogenetics has offered some important findings regarding drug responsiveness in Asian Americans. This chapter examines the current understanding of CVD risk factors, incidence, and treatment in Asian Americans, emphasizing the impact of these unique differences on CVD management in this population.

List of Abbreviations

AHA	American Heart Association
BMI	Body Mass Index
CABG	Coronary Artery Bypass Grafting
CAC	Coronary Artery Calcification
CAD	Coronary Artery Disease
CCHRC	Chinese Community Health Resource Center
CVD	Cardiovascular Diseases
CYP	cytochrome P450
ICH	Intracerebral hemorrhage
IDF	International Diabetes Federation
INR	international normalized ratio
INTERHEART	A Global Case-Control Study of Risk Factors for Acute Myocardial Infarction
HDL	High-Density Lipoprotein Cholesterol
hsCRP	High sensitivity C-reactive Protein
JUPITER	Justification for the Use of Statins in Prevention: An Intervention Trial Evaluating Rosuvastatin
Lp(a)	Lipoprotein (a)
LDL	Low-Density Lipoprotein Cholesterol
MESA	Multi-Ethnic Study of Atherosclerosis
MI	Myocardial Infarction
NHANES	National Health and Nutrition Examination Survey
NHIS	National Health Interview Survey
NHLBI	National Heart Lung and Blood Institute
NHWs	Non-Hispanic Whites
Ni-Hon-San Study	Nippon-Honolulu-San Francisco Study of Japanese men and cardiovascular risk factors
NRMI	National Registry of Myocardial Infarction
PCI	Percutaneous Coronary Intervention
PRANA	Prevention and AwareNess for South Asians
PVD	Peripheral Vascular Disease
SAH	Subarachnoid hemorrhage
VKORC1	vitamin K epoxide reductase complex subunit 1 enzyme
WC	Waist Circumference
WHO	World Health Organization.

Introduction

Conventional wisdom has held that Asian Americans are healthier on average than other racial/ethnic groups. With higher average education and income levels compared to other racial/ethnic groups, Asian Americans have been labeled the "model minority" [1]. The myth of the model minority has often led to the interpretation that Asian Americans have fewer barriers to healthcare than other racial/ethnic groups. In addition, our current knowledge of CVD among Asian Americans has either been based on one relatively healthy Asian group, with results extrapolated to all Asian subgroups, or on studies of Asians as a group, potentially masking differences among subgroups.

In recent years more studies have been devoted to investigating CVD among Asian American subgroups. These data indicate that there is substantial variability in cardiovascular risk and incidence of coronary artery disease (CAD), stroke, and peripheral vascular disease across subgroups. Certain Asian subgroups, Asian Indians and Filipinos, have been identified as demonstrating higher risk of CAD [2, 3] compared to non-Hispanic whites (NHWs). Prevalence of traditional risk factors for CVD, such as diabetes and obesity, varies greatly across the Asian subgroups, which affects risk prediction models commonly used in the U.S [4].

In addition to heterogeneity in CVD risk, Asian Americans differ in responsiveness to treatment for commonly used CVD drugs such as clopidogrel, warfarin and rosuvastatin. There is also some evidence that CVD drug dosing differs among Asian American subgroups, and that some subgroups may be at greater risk for treatment complications.

Knowledge and management of cardiovascular disease (CVD) in Asian Americans has the potential for impact on a global scale, with the populations of these Asian countries making up almost half of the 6 billion people living in the world [5]. Asian Americans are the fastest growing racial/ethnic group in the United States, with a population of over 13 million in 2008, and projected to reach nearly 34 million by 2050 [6]. The six largest Asian subgroups (Asian Indian, Chinese, Filipino, Japanese, Korean, Vietnamese) comprise over 90% of all Asians living in the U.S. [7]. This article will examine the current understanding of cardiovascular disease risk factors, outcomes, and treatment in Asian Americans, emphasizing the impact of these unique differences on cardiovascular disease management in this population.

CVD Incidence and Prevalence in Asians

Examining Asian Americans as a group would indicate that their prevalence of CVD is lower compared to that of NHWs. According to telephone survey data from the 2008 National Health Interview Survey (NHIS), national prevalence estimates of CAD and stroke, among adults 18 years of age and older, are 2.9% and 1.8%, respectively, for Asian Americans, compared to 6.5% and 2.7% for NHWs [8].

While CVD data for Asian Americans are not as complete compared to that of other racial/ethnic groups, there is growing evidence that incidence and prevalence of CVD is quite varied across Asian subgroups (see Table 1).

Table 1. Asian Populations at High and Low Risk of Cardiovascular Disease

Cardiovascular Disease	High Risk Populations	Low Risk Populations
CAD	Asian Indians, [2, 3] Filipinos [2, 3]	Chinese [2, 10]
Stroke	--	--
Ischemic Stroke	--	--
Hemorrhagic Stroke	Chinese [16]	--
Subarachnoid Hemorrhage	Japanese [14]	--
Intracerebral Hemorrhage	Filipinos [14]	--
PVD	--	All subgroups [2, 21-23]

National stroke prevalence estimates also vary widely, and due to small sample sizes many of the estimates for stroke are either unreported or indicated as unreliable. Nationally representative prevalence rates for PVD are unavailable for Asian Americans as a group or Asian American subgroups.

Coronary Artery Disease (CAD)

Because annual prevalence rates of CAD from NHIS data are not available by Asian American subgroup, due to small sample sizes, Barnes and colleagues grouped data from years 2004-2006 to produce stable estimates of self-reported heart disease (which includes CAD, angina pectoris, heart attack, or any other heart condition or disease) [9]. According to this data, prevalence rates of heart disease vary considerably by Asian American subgroup, ranging from 4.4% for Koreans to 9.2% for Asian Indians, compared to 12.2% for NHWs [9]. Hospitalization and outpatient data from Northern California have identified higher rates of CAD for Asian Indians and Filipinos [2, 3] and lower rates of CAD for Chinese [2, 10], compared to NHWs.

Some of the differences in CAD prevalence among Asian American subgroups may be related to differences in presentation and detection of vascular disease. One study of chest pain demonstrated that Korean Americans present with the atypical symptoms of dyspnea, perspiration and fatigue more often than NHWs [11]. In addition, left ventricular mass and volume [12] and coronary artery calcification prevalence [13] may differ in Asian Americans compared with other racial/ethnic groups. It is unclear if these differences play any role in the varying prevalence of CAD in Asians.

Stroke

The prevalence of stroke among Asian American subgroups is largely unstudied. Self-report data from NHIS for the years 2004-2006 indicate that the prevalence of stroke for Chinese (2.4%) is similar to that of NHWs (2.4%) [9]. Stroke prevalence estimates for other subgroups were not reported due to small sample sizes. Clinical data from Northern California, revealed no difference in stroke prevalence rates for Asian subgroups, compared to NHWs [2]. However, racial/ethnic differences emerge when stroke prevalence is examined by subtype. In populations of European ancestry, approximately 15–20% of all strokes are hemorrhagic strokes, whereas that percentage is even higher (25-40%) in those of Asian ancestry [14, 15]. While no studies have examined differences in ischemic stroke among Asian Americans, clinical data demonstrate higher risk of hemorrhagic stroke for Chinese [16]. For hemorrhagic stroke subtypes, Japanese are more likely to have a subarachnoid hemorrhage (RR=3.7), compared to Whites, while Filipinos are more likely to have an intracerebral hemorrhage (RR=2.8) [14].

While differences in prevalence of stroke subtype among Asian American subgroups are not entirely understood, the etiology of ischemic stroke has been found to more closely mirror that of coronary artery disease. Cholesterol and diabetes are more strongly associated with increased risk of ischemic stroke, whereas hypertension appears to play a greater role in hemorrhagic stroke [17]. In an autopsy study of Japanese men, ischemic stroke accompanied myocardial infarction in 58% of cases and were associated with CAD risk factors (high serum cholesterol, hypertension, severe atherosclerosis of the coronary arteries and aorta) [18]. In contrast, hypertension, cigarette use, and alcohol consumption were found to be strongly associated with hemorrhagic stroke [18]. Intracerebral hemorrhage (ICH) comprises a majority of hemorrhagic stroke cases, with higher risk associated with increasing age, systemic hypertension, and cigarette smoking [14]. While hypertension, cigarette smoking, and alcohol consumption are important risk factors for SAH, genetic factors may be especially important for SAH [14, 19].

Peripheral Vascular Disease (PVD)

The MESA study, one of the few studies of PVD in an Asian American subgroup (Chinese), found that Chinese Americans had a lower prevalence (2.0%) of peripheral arterial disease (defined by ankle-brachial index ≤ 0.90) compared to NHWs (3.6%) [20]. Lower risk of peripheral arterial disease has been reported in Asians as a group as well, although these findings were not significantly different from NHWs [21]. Similarly, low prevalence rates have been found for venous thromboembolism [22, 23], and lower risk of secondary venous thromboembolism in Asians as a group [22]. Most recently, using electronic health record data from a Northern California outpatient clinic, researchers found lower risk of PVD (including peripheral arterial disease, venous thromboembolism, and deep venous thrombosis) for all six major Asian subgroups, compared to NHWs [2].

The low risk of PVD in Asian Americans is not well understood. The MESA study demonstrated lower risk of peripheral arterial disease for Chinese, even after adjusting for traditional and novel risk factors, suggesting factors inherent to race may contribute to low risk [20]. Genetic factors relating to coagulability have been posited as a possible explanation [24-26]. The Factor V Leiden mutation and prothrombin G20210A mutation have been identified as the major genetic risk factors for PVD. The Factor V Leiden [2-15%] mutation and prothrombin G20210A (1-3%) mutation are very prevalent in NHWs [27, 28], but virtually absent in Asians [29], which may explain the lower risk of PVD in Asians.

Although CVD research for Asian American subgroups is limited, the studies that have examined specific subgroups demonstrate marked differences in the prevalence of CAD, stroke, and PVD (see Table 1). Higher rates of CAD have been found in Asian Indians and Filipinos, higher rates of hemorrhagic stroke among Chinese Americans, more intracerebral hemorrhage in Filipino Americans, more subarachnoid hemorrhage in Japanese Americans, and lower rates of CAD among Chinese Americans, and lower rates of PVD for most Asian

American subgroups. Studies using a nationally representative sample of Asian Americans with precise case ascertainment are needed to confirm these initial findings.

Using Body Mass Index (BMI) and Waist Circumference to Predict CVD Risk

There is currently some debate about the appropriate body mass index (BMI) cut points for Asians. International studies have found strong, positive associations for BMI and cardio-metabolic disorders, at low mean BMI (22.0-24.0 kg/m^2) in Chinese and Indian populations [30]. In addition, BMI does not predict percentage of body fat equally for all racial ethnic groups, with Chinese [31] and Asian Indians [32] demonstrating lower BMI values when compared to NHWs with similar body fat percentages [30]. These and other comparisons of Chinese, Japanese, and Asian Indians with Europeans underlie World Health Organization recommendations to lower the BMI thresholds defining overweight (>23.0 vs. >25.0 kg/m^2) and obesity (>27.5 vs. 30.0 kg/m^2) in Asians worldwide, compared to other racial/ethnic groups [33]. While lower BMI cut-points for Asian Americans would be an improvement over a single cut-point, these guidelines may still underestimate cardio-metabolic risk. BMI fails to account for differential distribution of body fat distribution among racial/ethnic groups, with a greater proportion of body fat stored in central visceral deposits in Chinese, Filipinos, and Asian Indians, versus NHWs and other racial/ethnic groups [34, 35]. Other measures, such as waist circumference, may provide a better measure of the distribution of fatness in Chinese and Asian Indians [36]. Race/ethnicity- and sex- specific cut points for waist circumference thresholds for abdominal obesity have been recommended by several organizations (see Table 2), with some organizations recommending lower cut-points (<80-90 cm) for Asian subgroups compared to U.S. NHWs (<88-102 cm) [37].

Table 2. Population- and sex- specific waist circumference (WC)
cut-points for obesity [37]

Organization	Population	Cut-Points for Obesity BMI	Waist Circumference Men	Women
WHO	European	≥ 30.0 kg/m^2	≥ 94 cm	≥ 80 cm
	Asian	≥ 27.5 kg/m^2	≥ 90 cm	≥ 80 cm
AHA/NHLBI (ATP III)	U.S.	≥ 30.0 kg/m^2	≥ 102 cm	≥ 88 cm
Japanese Obesity Society	Japanese	-	≥ 85 cm	≥ 90 cm
Cooperative Task Force	China	-	≥ 85 cm	≥ 80 cm
IDF	European		≥ 94 cm	≥ 80 cm
	South Asian		≥ 90 cm	≥ 80 cm
	Chinese		≥ 90 cm	≥ 80 cm
	Japanese		≥ 90 cm	≥ 80 cm

While the ATP III guidelines do not recommend specific obesity cut-points for waist circumference in Asians, they do note that some individuals with only 2 other metabolic syndrome criteria appear to be insulin resistant even when the waist circumference is only slightly elevated, (94 to 101 cm for men or 80 to 87 cm for women) [38]. Using the lower

BMI and waist circumference cut-points may be beneficial in addressing CVD risk for Asian patients.

Traditional Risk Factors for CVD

Whereas the majority of knowledge regarding CVD risk factors is largely based on European populations, the INTERHEART study was designed to determine the strength of association between traditional risk factors (smoking, hypertension, diabetes, waist/hip ratio, dietary patterns, physical activity, consumption of alcohol, blood apolipoproteins (Apo), and psychosocial factors such as depression, locus of control, perceived stress, and life events)) and acute MI in a geographically and ethnically diverse population [39]. The INTEHREART study included over 12,000 cases of acute MI and over 14,000 age- and sex- matched controls from 52 countries in Asia, Europe, the Middle East, Africa, Australia, North America, and South America. Traditional risk factors accounted for 90% of the population attributable risk for MI in men and 94% in women [39]. Current smoking and raised ApoB/ApoA1 ratio (top vs. lowest quintile) were the two strongest risk factors, followed by history of diabetes, hypertension, and psychosocial factors [39]. Daily consumption of fruits or vegetables, moderate or strenuous physical exercise, and consumption of alcohol three or more times per week, was protective [39]. These results suggest that CVD prevention efforts that target the same set of risk factors can be implemented worldwide.

While the same set of risk factors explained over 90% of the risk of MI for all ethnic populations in the INTERHEART study, risk factor prevalence and their relative impact on CVD risk may vary among ethnic groups. The INTERHEART study published a follow-up analysis that examined lipid abnormalities among Asian subgroups. Mean LDL-C, HDL-C, and TG levels were lower for Asians compared to non-Asians [40]. Lipid levels differed substantially by Asian subgroup. Southeast Asians had the highest mean LDL-C and TG levels and Chinese the lowest LDL-C and TG levels compared to both aggregated Asians and non-Asians [40]. The relative risk of MI associated with elevations in LDL-C levels was similar to that observed in the rest of the INTERHEART population [40]. However, for a given LDL-C level, the risk of acute MI may be higher among Asians compared with non-Asian populations. Despite lower mean levels, the risk of acute MI was proportionately higher with higher LDL-C in all of the Asian subgroups [40]. However, TG levels were not found to be associated with risk of acute MI for the INTERHEART population [40].

In contrast to the lower LDL-C levels among Asian subgroups, HDL-C levels were generally higher or similar compared to the non-Asian population [40]. However, substantially lower HDL-C levels were found for South Asians compared to all other Asian subgroups and the non-Asian population [40]. In contrast, Japanese appeared to have substantially higher HDL-C levels, although these findings were based on a relatively small sample size (n=247) [40]. Elevations in HDL-C were associated with a decreased risk of AMI, but this effect was weaker in South Asian population [40]. Previous research has shown that at any given HDL-C level, Asian Indians have a higher prevalence of small HDL-C particles compared with Caucasians, which may be a marker of impaired reverse cholesterol transport, which has been associated with CAD [40].

Similar to the rest of the INTERHEART population, the ApoB to ApoA1 ratio was found to have the strongest association with risk of acute MI for Asians [40]. Lower ApoB and similar ApoA1 levels were found for Asians, with lowest ApoB levels found for Chinese, compared to non-Asians [40]. For South Asians, however, ApoB levels were much higher and ApoA1 levels much lower compared to other Asians and the non-Asian population. ApoB levels may indicate a larger atherogenic particle load and possibly smaller LDL-C particle size [40]. Among South Asians changes in ApoA1 levels may be better determinants of risk than changes in HDL-C levels [40]. And given the lower levels of HDL-C among South Asians, efforts to increase HDL-C may also be beneficial in this population [40].

The INTERHEART study has contributed to better understanding CVD and its risk factors in Asian populations. While the same set of risk factors explained over 90% of the risk of MI for all ethnic populations, risk factor prevalence and their relative impact on CVD risk may vary among ethnic groups. Lipid patterns, in particular, have been shown to differ for Asians compared to non-Asians, with marked heterogeneity among the Asian subgroups. Despite lower LDL-C levels, for a given level of LDL-C the risk of acute MI may be higher for Asians compared to non-Asians.

Using CVD Risk Prediction Models in Asians

Differences in risk factor prevalence and CVD incidence are important to note, because they affect risk prediction models used in the U.S. Risk prediction models tend to overestimate risk in subgroups in which risk factor prevalence and CVD incidence is lower, and underestimate risk in subgroups in which risk factor prevalence and CVD incidence is higher than the reference (usually NHW) population. For instance, the Framingham risk score has been shown to systematically overestimate CAD events among Japanese American men. However, when the lower prevalence of specific risk factors and CAD incidence in Japanese men is taken into account, this overestimation is corrected [41, 42]. Similar results have been found in studies of Asian populations in China, Singapore, and Japan [43]. One study of South Asians in the UK found that the Framingham stroke model underestimated stroke rates, when compared to national data [44]. Modifications to the Framingham risk score, such as multiplying the TC:HDL cholesterol ratio by a factor of 1.5 or multiplying the overall score by a factor of 1.79 (the increased risk of CAD compared to NHWs), have been suggested for South Asians in the UK [45]. While similar modifications to the Framingham risk score have been recommended in other countries [45, 46], risk prediction models should be developed and validated for all Asian American subgroups, especially those in which CVD risk factor prevalence and incidence is higher (i.e., Asian Indian, Filipinos).

The prevalence of CVD risk factors and their relative importance varies greatly across the Asian subgroups. This variation is highlighted in the association of diabetes with CAD as an example. Higher prevalence rates have been reported for type 2 diabetes among Filipinos [47-48] and Asian Indians [50-52], compared to NHWs. These two Asian subgroups are also noted to have higher rates of CAD [2, 3, 10]. However, the role of diabetes in CAD may differ by Asian subgroup. Despite high prevalence rates of diabetes in Japanese [49], Japanese appear to have similar rates of CAD [2, 10], compared to NHWs. There may be some protective factors in some Asian American subgroups that mitigate the CAD risks associated with diabetes. High levels of protective HDL has been observed in Japanese Americans (unlike Asian Indians and Filipinos) compared to NHWs [53, 54]. While HDL levels appear to be higher in Japanese Americans compared to NHWs, these levels are not as high compared to native Japanese [55]. This may explain why rates of CAD for Japanese Americans are more similar to NHWs, than to native Japanese. Thus, HDL may be a protective factor, mitigating the negative effects of Type 2 diabetes in the Japanese American population. However, studies in which a comprehensive set of risk factors are tested in a cohort of Asian Americans followed prospectively are needed to support or refute this hypothesis.

Emerging Risk Factors

While the INTERHEART study demonstrated that over 90% of risk of MI can be explained by traditional risk factors [39], recent research has been devoted to finding novel risk factors for CVD. Emerging risk factors, such as lipoprotein (a) [Lp(a)], high sensitivity C-reactive protein (hsCRP), and coronary artery calcification (CAC), may provide further tools for risk stratification in Asian American populations in which the prognostic value of traditional risk scores are somewhat limited.

Inflammation/Thrombosis

Lipoprotein (a) [Lp(a)] is an independent risk factor for CVD [56], and more than 90% of the variation is accounted for by the Apo(a) gene [57]. Lp(a) levels differ significantly by racial/ethnic group; for example, African-Americans have higher Lp(a) levels than Whites, but nevertheless have a lower risk of CVD [58]. While the distribution of Lp(a) levels in Asians in the U.S. is poorly characterized, because most studies failed to distinguish Asian subgroups, higher Lp(a) levels have been reported in Asian Indians compared to other Asian populations (Chinese and Koreans) and NHWs [58]. Some reports have found no association between Lp(a) and CVD in Chinese [59]. A proposed possible reason for these conflicting results is that Lp(a) interacts with age with respect to further cardiovascular events [59]. Additionally differences in gender and the presence of high LDL-cholesterol and triglyceride concentrations may modify the association between Lp(a) and CVD outcomes [59]. Therefore, study samples that differ with respect to those characteristics may report different results [59].

High Sensitivity C-Reactive Protein

In the Women's Health Study, Asian women overall were found to have the lowest median high sensitivity C-reactive protein (hsCRP) levels when compared to NHW, Black, and Hispanic women [60]. International studies of Asian subgroups demonstrated that Japanese men and women had much lower hsCRP levels [61], while Asian Indians in the United Kingdom were found to have higher levels of hsCRP as compared to their European counterparts [62]. There are no prospective studies of Asian American subgroups that have examined the effects of aspirin or statin use on hsCRP levels. The recent international JUPITER trial for treatment of elevated hsCRP expressly limited recruitment of Asians, due to concerns of rosuvastatin dosage safety and higher risk of adverse side effects, such as rhabdomylosis and myopathy [63].

Coronary Artery Calcification (CAC)

Racial/ethnic differences for coronary artery calcification (CAC) are not well-defined. In one study, Asian Americans (excluding Asian Indians) were less likely to have any CAC than NHWs, despite higher prevalence of diabetes [13]. Asian Indians were reported to have higher median CAC scores as compared with NHWs, despite having younger age and lower hypertension prevalence [13]. In a Northern California study, East Asian (Japanese and Chinese) women were more likely to have any CAC, and East Asian men were less likely to have any CAC compared with NHW women and men respectively, after adjustment for multiple CVD risk factors [64]. Other studies have reported lower CAC scores for Chinese, compared to NHWs [13]. Despite higher prevalence of diabetes and hypertension, comparable CAC prevalence was found for Filipino women compared to than NHWs [65]. Prospective studies have confirmed the prognostic value of CAC in Chinese [66], and Asian Americans (excluding Asian Indians) [13].

These studies highlight the need to study emerging risk factors in Asian American subgroups, as levels of association may differ. More studies are needed to develop risk stratification tools using Lp(a), hsCRP, and CAC in Asians.

Pharmacogenetics

A patient's drug response has been found to vary considerably according to their race/ethnicity. While variability in drug response differences can be attributed to a number of factors, including diet, body weight, age, and co-morbid conditions, in the past couple of decades the fields of pharmacogenetics and pharmacogenomics have attributed this difference to different genetic polymorphisms that affect drug metabolism, transport, and target, and these polymorphism distributions in populations [67]. The FDA has made safety labeling changes highlighting pharmacogenomic differences in Asians for three common cardiovascular drugs: warfarin, clopidogrel, and statins.

Warfarin

Warfarin, one of the most commonly prescribed drugs [68], is used to prevent thromboembolic events in patients with chronic or paroxysmal atrial fibrillation, prosthetic valves, pulmonary emboli or deep venous thrombosis. However, its utility is limited by the narrow therapeutic range, risk of bleeding, and need for international normalized ratio (INR) monitoring [68]. In 2007, the FDA revised the warning label on warfarin, stating that "lower initiation doses should be considered for patients with certain genetic variations in CYP2C9 and VKORC1 enzymes" [69]. Two mutations in CYP2C9 have been identified in NHWs as contributing to poor metabolism of warfarin, CYP2C9*2 and CYP2C9*3, leading to lower dose requirements. However, these mutations that result in poor warfarin metabolism and lower dose requirements are extremely rare or absent (1-5%) in Asians (Chinese, Japanese, Korean), and may not explain all of the observed therapeutic variation [70].

Recent research has demonstrated that polymorphisms in the vitamin K epoxide reductase complex subunit 1 gene (VKORC1) plays a greater role in responsiveness to warfarin, compared to CYP2C9 polymorphisms, particularly in Asians [70]. Warfarin acts by inhibiting the synthesis of vitamin K-dependent coagulation factors [71]. VKORC1 genotype frequencies requiring lower warfarin dose are higher (~80% v. ~30%) for Asian (Chinese, Japanese) patients than Caucasian and African-American [70-72]. VKORC1 variants requiring higher maintenance dose of warfarin are more commonly found in Asian Indians, but less so in Chinese [70, 73]. Clinicians should start with lower doses of warfarin (generally 3mg or approximately 40 to 50% of the dose required by NHWs) for some Asian subgroups, including Chinese, Japanese, and Korean, to achieve the same level of anticoagulation [70]. Higher warfarin doses may be required for Asian Indians.

Clopidogrel (Plavix)

Clopidogrel (Plavix) is a platelet inhibitor commonly prescribed to patients with acute coronary syndrome undergoing percutaneous coronary intervention in order to reduce and prevent further cardiovascular events. In March of 2010, the FDA added a black box warning to clopidogrel in describing the dangers of treatment in patients carrying polymorphisms in the cytochrome P450 2C19 gene (CYP2C19) [74]. The CYP2C19 *2 and CYP2C19 *3 alleles are associated with less inhibition of platelets due to an inability to convert clopidogrel to its active form [74, 75]. African and Asian (Chinese and Japanese) American patients are at especially high risk with 30-50% having one variant gene [76], and a larger proportion (14% v. 2%) of Chinese patients having two variant genes compared to NHWs [74]. Patients with one CYP2C19 variants have a 1.57 times, and those with two CYP2C19 variants a 1.76 times, greater risk for major adverse cardiovascular events such as death, heart attack, and stroke [74]. A study from the TRITON-TIMI 38 trial found that the CYP2C19 *2 polymorphism that affects metabolism of clopidogrel does not affect prasugrel [77]. Further research is needed to identify alternative therapeutic treatments to clopidogrel [77], and more clinically applicable measures of treatment response.

Statins

The recent international JUPITER trial for treatment of elevated hsCRP expressly limited recruitment of Asians, due to concerns of rosuvastatin safety in the context of dosages administered [63]. The FDA has included a statement on the label insert for rosuvastatin (Crestor) stating that "initiation of Crestor therapy with 5 mg once daily (instead of 10 mg) should be considered for Asian patients." Pharmacokinetic studies have demonstrated an approximate 2-fold increase in median exposure to rosuvastatin in Japanese subjects when compared with Caucasian controls [78]. The dosage recommendation was based on studies of Japanese, but this data on one Asian subgroup was subsequently inaccurately extrapolated to all Asians [78, 79]. However, more recent studies have confirmed the safety of rosuvastatin in Japanese, Chinese, and Koreans [79].

Polymorphisms in the ATP-binding cassette G2 (ABCG2) have been found to play a significant role in the pharmacokinetics of rosuvastatin in Chinese and Japanese [79]. The ABCG2 variant, c.421A, is associated with reduced ability to export substrates, leading to an increase in drug accumulation in the hepatocytes and blood serum. Chinese and Japanese have higher frequencies (~35%) of this variant compared with NHWs (14%). This variant may contribute to the pharmacokinetic and treatment outcomes differences of rosuvastatin [79].

Two genetic haplotypes, SLCO1B1*5 and SLCO1B1*15, have been implicated in the lower recommended statin dosage due to decreased activity of an organic anion-transporting polypeptide, OATP1B1 [80-83]. These low activity haplotypes have a frequency of ~15–20% in Caucasians, ~10–15% in Asians [83]. Carriers of these SCLO1B1 variants are at high risk of myopathy during high-dose simvastatin therapy [83]. High-dose statin therapy of atorvastatin and pitavastatin, particularly, and probably for rosuvastatin and pravastatin should be avoided in carriers of the SCLO1B1 variants previously mentioned [83].

Certain Asian subgroups appear to have different responses to warfarin, clopidogrel, and/or statins. Although pharmacogenomics has the potential to alter drug dosing, pretreatment genetic testing for all patients has not been explicitly recommended by the FDA. Currently there are no clinically recommended dosing algorithms that account for genetic variations. Recent studies using pharmacogenetic guided algorithms have reported shorter times to stable anticoagulation and therapeutic warfarin doses [84-86]. However, these dosing algorithms for warfarin treatment have not been shown to improve the percent of patients within therapeutic INR range [70, 84, 87]. Clinicians should be aware that some Asian subgroups require lower warfarin doses (Chinese, Japanese, Korean) and others higher (Asian Indian) warfarin doses for therapeutic effect. Chinese and Japanese patients are at higher risk of carrying a polymorphism known to decrease the efficacy of clopidogrel, and increase blood serum concentrations of statins, leading to increased risk of cardiovascular events (myocardial infarction, stroke) and adverse events (myopathy and rhabdomylosis). Genetic tests are readily available for these variants, and testing may be appropriate for these high-risk populations.

Treatment Differences in Asians

Treatment patterns and outcomes for CAD in Asian Americans have only been studied in Asian Americans as a group as Asian subgroup information was not collected in these studies.

Asian Americans hospitalized for non–ST-segment elevation acute coronary syndromes may have significantly higher bleeding risk even after adjusting for risk factors such as aspirin use [88]. Higher risk of bleeding complications may be related to lower body mass index and slightly higher rates of renal impairment in Asians, which have previously been shown to increase vulnerability to excess antithrombotic overdosing [88].

Similarly, Asian Americans and Pacific Islanders may have longer "door-to-drug" times for acute reperfusion therapy after correction for clinical characteristics, socio-demographic factors, insurance status, or structural hospital characteristics [89]. While these differences are not entirely understood, there may be other unmeasured patient and hospital characteristics (e.g., communication, institutional biases) that influence quality of care [89]. Male Asian Americans are less likely to undergo percutaneous coronary intervention (PCI) and more likely to undergo coronary artery bypass grafting (CABG) than Caucasians [90]. Our understanding of CVD treatment outcomes in Asian subgroups is limited as research continues to examine Asians as a single group.

Culturally Competent Cardiovascular Care

The concept of heterogeneity among Asian American subgroups is not only important in the context of cardiovascular outcomes and treatment, but with respect to cultural behaviors and attitudes. Culture is a multi-dimensional construct, encompassing language, social structure, environment, economy, technology, religion/world view, and belief and values, which is passed on from one generation to the next [91].

There is great cultural diversity among Asian Americans, and culture is important to cardiovascular care as it defines patient perceptions of health, self-care behaviors, and lifestyle risk factors [91]. These cultural differences between clinician and patient are important to recognize in that they may result in barriers to health care.

In the context of health care, language is often the most easily identifiable cultural difference between patient and clinician. In the U.S., 62% of Vietnamese, 50% of Chinese, 24% of Filipinos, and 23% of Asian Indians are not fluent in English [92]. Language is cited as a common barriers to health care by Chinese, [93, 94] Vietnamese [93-95] and Korean [93, 94] patients. Studies have shown that limited English proficient (LEP) patients receive fewer preventive health screenings and demonstrate lower rates of medication adherence [96]. Bilingual physicians and professional interpreters, as opposed to family or friends, have been shown to improve care delivery to LEP patients [97].

While translation and interpretation services can improve communication between patient and physician, they may not resolve cultural differences. Asian Americans report frustration with translated education materials that often only provide Western examples for lifestyle changes such as diet or physical activity [93].

Few studies have examined cultural and language barriers to cardiovascular care in Asian Americans specifically. However, recent studies indicate that cultural and language barriers may impede knowledge of CVD symptoms among Asian Americans.

New immigrant Asian populations were been found to have incomplete knowledge about CVD, compared with more those who had lived in the U.S. longer [93, 95]. Limited knowledge of CVD symptoms and risk factors may prevent patients from seeking proper medical care and ultimately lead to poor health outcomes.

Culturally competent care has been implemented in many healthcare settings to improve health care for racial/ethnic minorities, including Asian Americans. "Culturally competent providers consistently and systematically: understand and respect their patients' values, beliefs, and expectations; understand the disease-specific epidemiology and treatment efficacy of different population groups; adapt the way they deliver care to each patient's needs and expectations" [98]. Resources for providing culturally competent care for Asian American subgroups are available in the appendix.

Conclusion

As the Asian American population continues to grow, it is imperative to accurately assess and address CVD health disparities in Asian American subgroups.

The limited data currently available suggest substantial variability in CVD risk and incidence across Asian American subgroups. Asian Indians and Filipinos appear to be at higher risk of CAD, Chinese at higher risk of hemorrhagic stroke, Japanese at higher risk of subarachnoid hemorrhage and Filipinos at higher risk of intracerebral hemorrhage compared to NHWs. There is also considerable heterogeneity with regards to risk factor prevalence among Asian subgroups, which alters the accuracy of common risk assessment tools, such as the Framingham risk score.

Additionally, Asians respond differently to drug treatment due to pharmacogenomic differences. While the majority of studies continue to examine Asian Americans as a single group, it is vital that researchers study Asian American subgroups separately in order to target high risk populations for prevention and treatment efforts.

Acknowledgments

The authors would like to thank Kathy Orrico and Mick O'Keefe for their assistance in reviewing the literature on pharmacogenomics.

Appendix 1.
Culturally Competent Resources for Clinicians

Clinicians treating Asian patients should strive for culturally competent care. Certain risk factors are more prevalent in some Asian subgroups. In addition, lifestyle behaviors (e.g., diet, physical activity, smoking, drinking) that are associated with increased CVD risk and poor CVD outcomes are often tied closely to cultural beliefs and values. To improve patient-clinician communication and patient care, it is important to understand prevention and treatment of CVD among Asian Americans from a cultural competence perspective. Resources are available to aid clinicians serving Asian populations.

The Palo Alto Medical Foundation's PRANA (PRevention and AwareNess for South Asians)

The PRANA (PRevention and AwareNess for South Asians) wellness program was developed by physicians at the Palo Alto Medical Foundation to educate South Asian patients about risk factors and ways to lead healthier lives. Audiovisual resources regarding risk factor modification are available in Hindi, as well as English.

www.pamf.org/prana/

The Chinese Community Health Resource Center (CCHRC)

The Chinese Community Health Resource Center (CCHRC) was established in 1989 as a private, non-profit community center by the Chinese Community Health Care Association (a physicians' independent practice association), Chinese Community Health Plan, and Chinese Hospital. The CCHRC provides culturally and linguistically competent preventive health and disease management education resources for patients.

http://www.cchrchealth.org/

Kaiser Permanente

Kaiser Permanente has developed modules of culturally targeted health care delivery at their San Francisco facility. The multilingual Chinese module provides care and services to all patients but have specific cultural and linguistic capacity to care for Chinese. The Chinese module contributed to an increase in annualized membership growth and patient satisfaction. For more information on implementing institutional cultural and linguistic competence programs, please visit:

http://xnet.kp.org/permanentejournal/sum09/language_challenge.html

Curriculum in Ethnogeriatrics

The curriculum in ethnogeriatrics was developed by the Collaborative of Ethnogeriatric Education in 1999, 2000 and 2001, with support from the Bureau of Health Professions, Health Resources and Services Administration. The modules are designed to increase cultural competence in geriatric health care of Asian elders. Eight different modules are available for the following Asian subgroups: Asian Indian, Chinese, Filipino, Japanese, Korean, Native Hawaiian/Pacific Islander, Pakistani, and Southeast Asian.

http://www.stanford.edu/group/ethnoger/

The National Library of Medicine, Asian American Health

The National Library of Medicine offers multiple educational resources for Asian Americans, including risk assessment tools, language-specific reading materials for cardiovascular disease, as well as many other health issues.

http://asianamericanhealth.nlm.nih.gov/

References

[1]   Sohn L. The health and health status of older Korean Americans at the 100-year anniversary of Korean immigration. *J. Cross Cult Gerontol*. 2004, 19, 203-19.

[2]   Holland AT, Wong EC, Lauderdale DS, Palaniappan LP. Spectrum of Cardiovascular Diseases in Asian-American Racial/Ethnic Subgroups. *Ann. Epidemiol.* 2011, 21, 608-14.

[3]   Klatsky AL, Tekawa I. Health problems and hospitalizations among Asian-American ethnic groups. *Ethn Dis.* 2005, 15, 753-60.

[4]   Palaniappan LP, Araneta MR, Assimes TL, Barrett-Connor EL, Carnethon MR, Criqui MH, Fung GL, Narayan KM, Patel H, Taylor-Piliae RE, Wilson PW, Wong ND. Call to action: cardiovascular disease in Asian Americans: a science advisory from the American Heart Association. *Circulation.* 2010, 122, 1242-52.

[5]   Population Division of the Department of Economic and Social Affairs of the United Nations Secretariat. World Population Prospects: The 2008 Revision. 2008 [January 3, 2010]; Available from: http://esa.un.org/unpp.

[6]   Population Division U.S. Census Bureau. Table 17. Projections of the Asian Alone Population by Age and Sex for the United States: 2010 to 2050 (NO-2008-T17). August 14, 2008.

[7]   U.S. Census Bureau, American Community Survey. Table C02006. Asian Alone by Selected Groups. 2006-2008.

[8]   Pleis JR, Lucas JW, Ward BW. Summary health statistics for U.S. adults: National Health Interview Survey, 2008. *Vital Health Stat* 10. 2009, 242, 1-157.

[9]   Barnes PM, Adams PF, Powell-Griner E. Health characteristics of the Asian adult population: United States, 2004-2006. *Adv. Data.* 2008, 394, 1-22.

[10] Klatsky AL, Tekawa I, Armstrong MA, Sidney S. The risk of hospitalization for ischemic heart disease among Asian Americans in northern California. *Am. J. Public Health.* 1994, 84, 1672-5.

[11] Lee H, Bahler R, Park OJ, Kim CJ, Lee HY, Kim YJ. Typical and atypical symptoms of myocardial infarction among African-Americans, whites, and Koreans. *Crit. Care Nurs. Clin. North Am.* 2001,13, 531-9.

[12] Natori S, Lai S, Finn JP, Gomes AS, Hundley WG, Jerosch-Herold M, et al. Cardiovascular function in multi-ethnic study of atherosclerosis: normal values by age, sex, and ethnicity. *AJR Am. J. Roentgenol.* 2006, 186, S357-65.

[13] Orakzai SH, Orakzai RH, Nasir K, Santos RD, Edmundowicz D, Budoff MJ, Blumenthal RS. Subclinical coronary atherosclerosis: racial profiling is necessary! *Am. Heart J.* 2006, 152, 819-27.

[14] Klatsky AL, Friedman GD, Sidney S, Kipp H, Kubo A, Armstrong MA. Risk of hemorrhagic stroke in Asian American ethnic groups. *Neuroepidemiology.* 2005, 25, 26-31.

[15] Burke TA, Venketasubramanian RN. The epidemiology of stroke in the East Asian region: a literature-based review. *Int. J. Stroke.* 2006, 1, 208-15.

[16] Fang J, Foo SH, Jeng JS, Yip PK, Alderman MH. Clinical characteristics of stroke among Chinese in New York City. *Ethn Dis.* 2004, 14, 378-83.

[17] McCarron MO, Davey Smith G, McCarron P. Secular stroke trends: early life factors and future prospects. *QJM.* 2006, 99, 117-22.

[18] Stemmermann GN, Hayashi T, Resch JA, Chung CS, Reed DM, Rhoads GG. Risk factors related to ischemic and hemorrhagic cerebrovascular disease at autopsy: the Honolulu Heart Study. *Stroke.* 1984, 15, 23-8.

[19] Olsson S, Csajbok LZ, Jood K, Nylen K, Nellgard B, Jern C. Association between genetic variation on chromosome 9p21 and aneurysmal subarachnoid haemorrhage. *J. Neurol. Neurosurg. Psychiatry.* 2011, 82, 384-8.

[20] Allison MA, Criqui MH, McClelland RL, Scott JM, McDermott MM, Liu K, et al. The effect of novel cardiovascular risk factors on the ethnic-specific odds for peripheral arterial disease in the Multi-Ethnic Study of Atherosclerosis (MESA). *J. Am. Coll Cardiol.* 2006, 48, 1190-7.

[21] Criqui MH, Vargas V, Denenberg JO, Ho E, Allison M, Langer RD, Bergan J, Golomb BA. Ethnicity and peripheral arterial disease: the San Diego Population Study. *Circulation.* 2005, 112, 2703-7.

[22] White RH, Zhou H, Romano PS. Incidence of idiopathic deep venous thrombosis and secondary thromboembolism among ethnic groups in California. *Ann. Intern. Med.* 1998, 128, 737-40.

[23] Klatsky AL, Armstrong MA, Poggi J. Risk of pulmonary embolism and/or deep venous thrombosis in Asian-Americans. *Am. J. Cardiol.* 2000, 85, 1334-7.

[24] Ridker PM, Miletich JP, Hennekens CH, Buring JE. Ethnic distribution of factor V Leiden in 4047 men and women. Implications for venous thromboembolism screening. *JAMA.* 1997, 277, 1305-7.

[25] White RH. The epidemiology of venous thromboembolism. *Circulation.* 2003, 107, I4-8.

[26] Gregg JP, Yamane AJ, Grody WW. Prevalence of the factor V-Leiden mutation in four distinct American ethnic populations. *Am. J. Med. Genet.* 1997, 73, 334-6.

[27] Rees DC, Cox M, Clegg JB. World distribution of factor V Leiden. *Lancet.* 1995, 346, 1133-4.

[28] Rosendaal FR, Doggen CJ, Zivelin A, Arruda VR, Aiach M, Siscovick DS, Hillarp A, Watzke HH, Bernardi F, Cumming AM, Preston FE, Reitsma PH. Geographic distribution of the 20210 G to A prothrombin variant. *Thromb. Haemost.* 1998, 79, 706-8.

[29] Jun ZJ, Ping T, Lei Y, Li L, Ming SY, Jing W. Prevalence of factor V Leiden and prothrombin G20210A mutations in Chinese patients with deep venous thrombosis and pulmonary embolism. *Clin. Lab. Haematol.* 2006, 28, 111-6.

[30] Deurenberg-Yap M, Chew SK, Deurenberg P. Elevated body fat percentage and cardiovascular risks at low body mass index levels among Singaporean Chinese, Malays and Indians. *Obes. Rev.* 2002, 3, 209-15.

[31] Deurenberg P, Yap M, van Staveren WA. Body mass index and percent body fat: a meta analysis among different ethnic groups. *Int. J. Obes. Relat. Metab. Disord.* 1998, 22, 1164-71.

[32] Enas EA, Mohan V, Deepa M, Farooq S, Pazhoor S, Chennikkara H. The metabolic syndrome and dyslipidemia among Asian Indians: a population with high rates of diabetes and premature coronary artery disease. *J. Cardiometab. Syndr.* 2007, 2, 267-75.

[33] WHO expert consultation. Appropriate body-mass index for Asian populations and its implications for policy and intervention strategies. *Lancet.* 2004, 363, 157-63.

[34] Araneta MR, Barrett-Connor E. Ethnic differences in visceral adipose tissue and type 2 diabetes: Filipino, African-American, and white women. *Obes. Res.* 2005, 13, 1458-65.

[35] Lear SA, Humphries KH, Kohli S, Chockalingam A, Frohlich JJ, Birmingham CL. Visceral adipose tissue accumulation differs according to ethnic background: results of the Multicultural Community Health Assessment Trial (M-CHAT). *Am. J. Clin. Nutr.* 2007, 86, 353-9.

[36] Lear SA, Humphries KH, Kohli S, Birmingham CL. The use of BMI and waist circumference as surrogates of body fat differs by ethnicity. *Obesity* (Silver Spring). 2007, 15, 2817-24.

[37] Alberti KG, Eckel RH, Grundy SM, Zimmet PZ, Cleeman JI, Donato KA, Fruchart JC, James WP, Loria CM, Smith SC Jr; International Diabetes Federation Task Force on Epidemiology and Prevention; Hational Heart, Lung, and Blood Institute; American Heart Association; World Heart Federation; International Atherosclerosis Society; International Association for the Study of Obesity. Harmonizing the metabolic syndrome: a joint interim statement of the International Diabetes Federation Task Force on Epidemiology and Prevention; National Heart, Lung, and Blood Institute; American Heart Association; World Heart Federation; International Atherosclerosis Society; and International Association for the Study of Obesity. *Circulation.* 2009, 120, 1640-5.

[38] Grundy SM, Cleeman JI, Merz CN, Brewer HB, Jr., Clark LT, Hunninghake DB, Pasternak RC, Smith SC Jr, Stone NJ; National Heart, Lung, and Blood Institute; American College of Cardiology Foundation; American Heart Association. Implications of recent clinical trials for the National Cholesterol Education Program Adult Treatment Panel III guidelines. *Circulation.* 2004, 110, 227-39.

[39] Yusuf S, Hawken S, Ounpuu S, Dans T, Avezum A, Lanas F, McQueen M, Budaj A, Pais P, Varigos J, Lisheng L. Effect of potentially modifiable risk factors associated with myocardial infarction in 52 countries (the INTERHEART study): case-control study. *Lancet.* 2004, 364, 937-52.

[40] Karthikeyan G, Teo KK, Islam S, McQueen MJ, Pais P, Wang X, Sato H, Lang CC, Sitthi-Amorn C, Pandey MR, Kazmi K, Sanderson JE, Yusuf S. Lipid profile, plasma apolipoproteins, and risk of a first myocardial infarction among Asians: an analysis from the INTERHEART study. *JACC.* 2009, 53, 244-253.

[41] D'Agostino RB, Sr., Grundy S, Sullivan LM, Wilson P. Validation of the Framingham coronary heart disease prediction scores: results of a multiple ethnic groups investigation. *JAMA.* 2001, 286, 180-7.

[42] Dodani S. Excess coronary artery disease risk in South Asian immigrants: can dysfunctional high-density lipoprotein explain increased risk? *Vasc. Health Risk Manag.* 2008, 4, 953-61.

[43] Barzi F, Patel A, Gu D, Sritara P, Lam TH, Rodgers A, Woodward M. Cardiovascular risk prediction tools for populations in Asia. *J. Epidemiol. Community Health.* 2007, 61, 115-21.

[44] Bhopal R, Fischbacher C, Vartiainen E, Unwin N, White M, Alberti G. Predicted and observed cardiovascular disease in South Asians: application of FINRISK, Framingham and SCORE models to Newcastle Heart Project data. *J. Public Health* (Oxf). 2005, 27, 93-100.

[45] Aarabi M, Jackson PR. Predicting coronary risk in UK South Asians: an adjustment method for Framingham-based tools. *Eur. J. Cardiovasc. Prev. Rehabil.* 2005, 12, 46-51.

[46] Lip GY, Barnett AH, Bradbury A, Cappuccio FP, Gill PS, Hughes E, Imray C, Jolly K, Patel K. Ethnicity and cardiovascular disease prevention in the United Kingdom: a practical approach to management. *J. Hum. Hypertens.* 2007, 21, 183-211.

[47] Tanchoco CC, Cruz AJ, Duante CA, Litonjua AD. Prevalence of metabolic syndrome among Filipino adults aged 20 years and over. *Asia Pac. J. Clin. Nutr.* 2003, 12, 271-6.

[48] Araneta MR, Wingard DL, Barrett-Connor E. Type 2 diabetes and metabolic syndrome in Filipina-American women : a high-risk nonobese population. *Diabetes Care.* 2002, 25, 494-9.

[49] Choi SE, Chow VH, Chung SJ, Wong ND. Do Risk Factors Explain the Increased Prevalence of Type 2 Diabetes Among California Asian Adults? *J. Immigr. Minor Health.* 2011, 13, 803-8.

[50] Oza-Frank R, Ali MK, Vaccarino V, Narayan KM. Asian Americans: diabetes prevalence across U.S. and World Health Organization weight classifications. *Diabetes Care.* 2009, 32, 1644-6.

[51] Kanaya AM, Wassel CL, Mathur D, Stewart A, Herrington D, Budoff MJ, Ranpura V, Liu K. Prevalence and correlates of diabetes in South asian indians in the United States: findings from the metabolic syndrome and atherosclerosis in South asians living in america study and the multi-ethnic study of atherosclerosis. *Metab Syndr Relat. Disord.* 2010, 8, 157-64.

[52] Ye J, Rust G, Baltrus P, Daniels E. Cardiovascular risk factors among Asian Americans: results from a National Health Survey. *Ann. Epidemiol.* 2009, 19, 718-23.

[53] Carr MC, Brunzell JD, Deeb SS. Ethnic differences in hepatic lipase and HDL in Japanese, black, and white Americans: role of central obesity and LIPC polymorphisms. *J. Lipid. Res.* 2004, 45, 466-73.

[54] Palaniappan LP, Wong EC, Shin JJ, Fortmann SP, Lauderdale DS. Asian Americans have greater prevalence of metabolic syndrome despite lower body mass index. *Int. J. Obes.* (Lond). 2011, 35, 393-400.

[55] Ucshima H, Okayama A, Saitoh S, Nakagawa H, Rodriguez B, Sakata K, et al. Differences in cardiovascular disease risk factors between Japanese in Japan and Japanese-Americans in Hawaii: the INTERLIPID study. *J. Hum. Hypertens.* 2003, 17, 631-9.

[56] Danesh J, Collins R, Peto R. Lipoprotein(a) and coronary heart disease. Meta-analysis of prospective studies. *Circulation.* 2000, 102, 1082-5.

[57] Snieder H, van Doornen LJ, Boomsma DI. Dissecting the genetic architecture of lipids, lipoproteins, and apolipoproteins: lessons from twin studies. *Arterioscler Thromb. Vasc. Biol.* 1999, 19, 2826-34.

[58] Enas EA, Chacko V, Senthilkumar A, Puthumana N, Mohan V. Elevated lipoprotein(a)- -a genetic risk factor for premature vascular disease in people with and without standard risk factors: a review. *Dis. Mon.* 2006, 52, 5-50.

[59] Chien KL, Hsu HC, Su TC, Sung FC, Chen MF, Lee YT. Lipoprotein(a) and cardiovascular disease in ethnic Chinese: the Chin-Shan Community Cardiovascular Cohort Study. *Clin. Chem.* 2008, 54, 285-91.

[60] Albert MA, Glynn RJ, Buring J, Ridker PM. C-Reactive Protein Levels Among Women of Various Ethnic Groups Living in the United States (from the Women's Health Study). *Am. J. Cardiol.* 2004, 93, 1238-42.

[61] Yamada S, Gotoh T, Nakashima Y, Kayaba K, Ishikawa S, Nago N, et al. Distribution of serum C-reactive protein and its association with atherosclerotic risk factors in a Japanese population: Jichi Medical School Cohort Study. *Am. J. Epidemiol.* 2001, 153, 1183-90.

[62] Forouhi NG, Sattar N, McKeigue PM. Relation of C-reactive protein to body fat distribution and features of the metabolic syndrome in Europeans and South Asians. *Int. J. Obes. Relat. Metab. Disord.* 2001, 25, 1327-31.

[63] Gibbons RJ. Rosuvastatin in patients with elevated C-reactive protein. *N. Engl. J. Med.* 2009, 360, 1038; author reply 41-2.

[64] Fair JM, Kiazand A, Varady A, Mahbouba M, Norton L, Rubin GD, Iribarren C, Go AS, Hlatky MA, Fortmann SP. Ethnic differences in coronary artery calcium in a healthy cohort aged 60 to 69 years. *Am. J. Cardiol.* 2007, 100, 981-5.

[65] Araneta MR, Barrett-Connor E. Subclinical coronary atherosclerosis in asymptomatic Filipino and white women. *Circulation.* 2004, 110, 2817-23.

[66] Ueshima H, Sekikawa A, Miura K, Turin TC, Takashima N, Kita Y, Watanabe M, Kadota A, Okuda N, Kadowaki T, Nakamura Y, Okamura T. Cardiovascular disease and risk factors in Asia: a selected review. *Circulation.* 2008, 118, 2702-9.

[67] Morrison A, Levy R. Toward individualized pharmaceutical care of East Asians: the value of genetic testing for polymorphisms in drug-metabolizing genes. *Pharmacogenomics.* 2004, 5, 673-89.

[68] Hirsh J, Dalen J, Guyatt G. The sixth (2000) ACCP guidelines for antithrombotic therapy for prevention and treatment of thrombosis. American College of Chest Physicians. *Chest.* 2001, 119, 1S-2S.

[69] Food and Drug Administration. Label and Approval History: Coumadin. 2007 [January 17, 2011]; Available from: http://www.accessdata.fda.gov/scripts/cder/drugsatfda/index.cfm?fuseaction=Search.Label_ApprovalHistory.

[70] Tan GM, Wu E, Lam YY, Yan BP. Role of warfarin pharmacogenetic testing in clinical practice. *Pharmacogenomics.* 2010, 11, 439-48.

[71] Yang L, Ge W, Yu F, Zhu H. Impact of VKORC1 gene polymorphism on interindividual and interethnic warfarin dosage requirement--a systematic review and meta analysis. *Thromb. Res.* 2010, 125, e159-66.

[72] Rieder MJ, Reiner AP, Gage BF, Nickerson DA, Eby CS, McLeod HL, Blough DK, Thummel KE, Veenstra DL, Rettie AE. Effect of VKORC1 haplotypes on transcriptional regulation and warfarin dose. *N. Engl. J. Med.* 2005, 352, 2285-93.

[73] Lee SC, Ng SS, Oldenburg J, Chong PY, Rost S, Guo JY, Yap HL, Rankin SC, Khor HB, Yeo TC, Ng KS, Soong R, Goh BC. Interethnic variability of warfarin maintenance requirement is explained by VKORC1 genotype in an Asian population. *Clin. Pharmacol. Ther.* 2006, 79, 197-205.

[74] Mega JL, Simon T, Collet JP, Anderson JL, Antman EM, Bliden K, Cannon CP, Danchin N, Giusti B, Gurbel P, Horne BD, Hulot JS, Kastrati A, Montalescot G, Neumann FJ, Shen L, Sibbing D, Steg PG, Trenk D, Wiviott SD, Sabatine MS. Reduced-function CYP2C19 genotype and risk of adverse clinical outcomes among patients treated with clopidogrel predominantly for PCI: a meta-analysis. *JAMA.* 2010, 304, 1821-30.

[75] George J, Doney A, Palmer CN, Lang CC. Pharmacogenetics testing: implications for cardiovascular therapeutics with clopidogrel and warfarin. *Cardiovasc. Ther.* 2010, 28, 135-8.

[76] Shuldiner AR, O'Connell JR, Bliden KP, Gandhi A, Ryan K, Horenstein RB, Damcott CM, Pakyz R, Tantry US, Gibson Q, Pollin TI, Post W, Parsa A, Mitchell BD, Faraday N, Herzog W, Gurbel PA. Association of cytochrome P450 2C19 genotype with the antiplatelet effect and clinical efficacy of clopidogrel therapy. *JAMA.* 2009, 302, 849-57.

[77] Brandt JT, Close SL, Iturria SJ, Payne CD, Farid NA, Ernest CS, 2nd, Lachno DR, Salazar D, Winters KJ. Common polymorphisms of CYP2C19 and CYP2C9 affect the pharmacokinetic and pharmacodynamic response to clopidogrel but not prasugrel. *J .Thromb. Haemost.* 2007, 5, 2429-36.

[78] Food and Drug Administration. FDA Public Health Advisory for Crestor (rosuvastatin). 2005 [November 22, 2010]; Available from: <http://www.fda.gov/Drugs/DrugSafety/ PostmarketDrugSafetyInformationforPatientsandProviders/DrugSafetyInformationforH eathcareProfessionals/PublicHealthAdvisories/ucm051756.htm>.

[79] Tomlinson B, Hu M, Lee VW, Lui SS, Chu TT, Poon EW, Ko GT, Baum L, Tam LS, Li EK. ABCG2 polymorphism is associated with the low-density lipoprotein cholesterol response to rosuvastatin. *Clin. Pharmacol. Ther.* 2010, 87, 558-62.

[80] Lee E, Ryan S, Birmingham B, Zalikowski J, March R, Ambrose H, Moore R, Lee C, Chen Y, Schneck D. Rosuvastatin pharmacokinetics and pharmacogenetics in white and Asian subjects residing in the same environment. *Clin. Pharmacol. Ther.* 2005, 78, 330-41.

[81] Tirona RG. Ethnic differences in statin disposition. *Clin. Pharmacol. Ther.* 2005 , 78, 311-6.

[82] Choi JH, Lee MG, Cho JY, Lee JE, Kim KH, Park K. Influence of OATP1B1 genotype on the pharmacokinetics of rosuvastatin in Koreans. *Clin. Pharmacol. Ther.* 2008, 83, 251-7.

[83] Niemi M. Transporter pharmacogenetics and statin toxicity. *Clin. Pharmacol. Ther.* 2010 , 87, 130-3.

[84] Anderson JL, Horne BD, Stevens SM, Grove AS, Barton S, Nicholas ZP, Kahn SF, May HT, Samuelson KM, Muhlestein JB, Carlquist JF. Randomized trial of genotype-guided versus standard warfarin dosing in patients initiating oral anticoagulation. *Circulation.* 2007, 116, 2563-70.

[85] Schwarz UI, Ritchie MD, Bradford Y, Li C, Dudek SM, Frye-Anderson A, Kim RB, Roden DM, Stein CM. Genetic determinants of response to warfarin during initial anticoagulation. *N. Engl. J. Med.* 2008, 358, 999-1008.

[86] Wadelius M, Chen LY, Lindh JD, Eriksson N, Ghori MJ, Bumpstead S, Holm L, McGinnis R, Rane A, Deloukas P. The largest prospective warfarin-treated cohort supports genetic forecasting. *Blood.* 2009, 113, 784-92.

[87] Takahashi H, Wilkinson GR, Caraco Y, Muszkat M, Kim RB, Kashima T, Kimura S, Echizen H. Population differences in S-warfarin metabolism between CYP2C9 genotype-matched Caucasian and Japanese patients. *Clin. Pharmacol. Ther.* 2003, 73, 253-63.

[88] Wang TY, Chen AY, Roe MT, Alexander KP, Newby LK, Smith SC Jr, Bangalore S, Gibler WB, Ohman EM, Peterson ED. Comparison of baseline characteristics,

treatment patterns, and in-hospital outcomes of Asian versus non-Asian white Americans with non-ST-segment elevation acute coronary syndromes from the CRUSADE quality improvement initiative. *Am. J. Cardiol.* 2007, 100, 391-6.

[89] Bradley EH, Herrin J, Wang Y, McNamara RL, Webster TR, Magid DJ, Blaney M, Peterson ED, Canto JG, Pollack CV Jr, Krumholz HM. Racial and ethnic differences in time to acute reperfusion therapy for patients hospitalized with myocardial infarction. *JAMA.* 2004, 292, 1563-72.

[90] Taira DA, Seto TB, Marciel C. Ethnic disparities in care following acute coronary syndromes among Asian Americans and Pacific Islanders during the initial hospitalization. *Cell Mol. Biol.* (Noisy-le-grand). 2001, 47, 1209-15.

[91] Kagawa-Singer M, Kassim-Lakha S. A strategy to reduce cross-cultural miscommunication and increase the likelihood of improving health outcomes. *Acad. Med.* 2003, 78, 577-87.

[92] Office of Minority Health, U.S. Department of Health and Human Services. Asian American/Pacific Islander Profile. 2010. Retrieved February 8, 2011, (http://minorityhealth.hhs.gov/templates/browse.aspx? lvl=3andlvlid=29).

[93] Bryant LL, Chin NP, Cottrell LA, Duckles JM, Fernandez ID, Garces DM, Keyserling TC, McMilin CR, Peters KE, Samuel-Hodge CD, Tu SP, Vu MB, Fitzpatrick AL. Perceptions of cardiovascular health in underserved communities. *Prev. Chronic Dis.* 2010, 7, A30.

[94] Ton TG, Steinman L, Yip MP, Ly KA, Sin MK, Fitzpatrick AL, Tu SP. Knowledge of cardiovascular health among Chinese, Korean and Vietnamese immigrants to the US. *J. Immigr Min. Health.* 2011, 13, 127-39.

[95] Nguyen TT, Liao Y, Gildengorin G, Tsoh J, Bui-Tong N, McPhee SJ. Cardiovascular risk factors and knowledge of symptoms among Vietnamese Americans. *J. Gen. Int. Med.* 2009, 24, 238-43.

[96] Flores, Glenn. Language barriers to health care in the United States. *N. Engl. J. Med.* 2006, 355, 229-31.

[97] Diamond LC, Wilson-Stronks A, Jacobs EA. Do hospitals measure up to the national culturally and linguistically appropriate services standards? *Med. Care.* 2010, 48, 1080-7.

[98] Office of Minority Health and Bureau of Primary Health Care, Health Resources and Services Administration. Reducing Health Disparities in Asian American and Pacific Islander Populations: What is Cultural Competence. 2005. Retrieved February 8, 2011, (http://erc.msh.org/ aapi/cc4.html).

In: Current Advances in Cardiovascular Risk. Volume 2
Editor: Sandeep Ajoy Saha

ISBN: 978-1-62081-746-9
© 2012 Nova Science Publishers, Inc.

Chapter XXV

Heart Failure in Ethnic Minority Patients – Focus on Risk Factors, Clinical Presentation and Therapeutic Considerations

*Gordon W. Moe**

Li Ka Shing Knowledge Institute, St Michael's Hospital,
University of Toronto, Toronto, Canada

Abstract

Introduction: Ethnic minority groups constitute increasing proportions of the population in Western countries. Heart failure is increasingly prevalent world wide and is associated with significant morbidity and mortality. The aim of this chapter is to discuss the epidemiology, etiologies as well as the still limited research/evidence on management of heart failure among the ethnic minority groups.

Key findings: South Asians have more coronary risk factors that may increase the risk for premature coronary heart disease leading to development of heart failure at a younger age. In the Chinese, hypertension remains an important aetiology of heart failure and available data suggest that heart failure with preserved systolic function is common. African Americans have a higher prevalence of heart failure than Caucasians, present with heart failure at younger ages, and are less likely to be due to coronary heart disease. Findings from a randomized controlled trial conducted specifically in African Americans support the addition of the combination of isosorbide dinitrate and hydralazine to standard medical regimen for black patients with heart failure. Hispanics comprise the largest and fastest-growing ethnic group in the United States. Hispanics with heart failure are more likely to be younger and underinsured than non-Hispanic whites. They have higher rates of readmissions but appear to have lower short-term mortality. Hispanics have excessive rates of diabetes, obesity, dyslipidemia, and metabolic syndrome and encounter multiple barriers to health care influenced by socioeconomic factors that in

* Correspondence to Gordon W. Moe, MD, St. Michael's Hospital, 30 Bond Street, Toronto, Ontario, Canada, M5B 1W8 Tel: +1 416 8645615; fax: +1 416 8645941; e-mail: moeg@smh.ca.

turn have an adverse impact on disease prognosis. Finally, aboriginal people are more likely than non-aboriginal people to have less access to health care and to have a higher disease burden for atherosclerosis. Heart failure is more prevalent in aboriginal than in the non-aboriginal counterparts.

Conclusion: There are important differences across ethnic groups in the etiologies of heart failure and the response to selected treatments. Given the likely increasing frequency of heart failure in these populations and an increasingly multiethnic world, additional studies on heart failure across different ethnic groups are warranted.

Keywords: Heart failure, ethnic minority, ethnic diversity

Abbreviations

ACE   angiotensin-converting –enzyme
CVD   cardiovascular disease
LVEF   left ventricular ejection fraction.

Introduction

By the middle of the 21st century, ethnic minorities are projected to approach the majority in many Western industrialized countries. Among the industrialized countries, few places possess the ethnic diversity that is present in Canada. Based on a Statistics Canada 2006 census, [1] the visible minority population surpassed the 5 million, reaching 16.2% of the population. In the Canadian province of Ontario, over 1.5 million people are of Chinese, South Asian, Black, or Aboriginal descent. In the United States (U.S.), the Census Bureau projects that by 2042, non-Hispanic whites will no longer constitute the majority of the population. [2] Hispanic and Latino populations will increase to an estimated 30% of the population, and Black populations will rise to an estimated 15%. Populations of Asian and Hispanic origin are among the fastest growing populations in every region of the U.S.

Ethnicity is a rather catch-all term that refers to the culture, customs and traditions acquired from the environment one belongs to. There is often confusion in distinguishing race from ethnicity. While race refers to the biological aspects of a person including skin color, hair color and eye color, ethnicity is defined more on the lines of social grouping. While races may be altered over generations due to crossovers, the ethnicity of a person can easily change if he/she chooses to adopt the customs and traditions of another ethnic group, as may happen in the ethnic minority groups in the industrialized nations. It is therefore important to recognize ethnocultural differences when managing patients with heart failure. In order to understand and manage a person's illness it is necessary to appreciate the effects of the person's culture and social environment. This is perhaps most relevant in the healthcare management of minority groups. Hope and morale are invariably crucial to the patients' adaptation and their maintenance of involvement in their management [3] and gaps in communications as a result of ethnocultural differences may have detrimental effect on their adaptation to their illness. Additionally, healthcare providers may contribute to the ethnic care disparities through clinical uncertainty and stereotyping of health behaviours related to minority patients. [4] On the other hand, the use of race or ethnicity as a way to differentiate patients is potentially tricky and differential medical treatment based on the color of one's skin has been associated with detrimental outcomes for ethnic minorities [5].

Although there are many underlying causes of healthcare disparities, [6,7] a significant contributor is the paucity of research to clearly identify the sources of differences in outcomes in ethnic groups and to distinguish among biological, environmental, or social causes of disease differences. [6] Evaluation of disease differences in subsegments of the population is needed to understand the variety of mechanisms of pathophysiology, as well as to optimally target therapeutic responses. Thus, effective research that would contribute to a reduction in healthcare disparities requires collection of data on health status in ethnic populations and assessment of differences in disease patterns. It also requires clinical trials with the inclusion of adequate numbers of diverse populations to probe for differences in pathophysiology including environmental or social factors contributing to disease and responses to treatment. Where differences are observed among population segments, clinical trials focused in these population groups are warranted [6,7].

Heart failure in Ethnic Minority Groups: General Considerations

To date, there have been very few published population-based epidemiological studies or large-scale randomized controlled studies of heart failure in countries outside North America, Europe and Australasia, in regions where most of the minority groups that reside in the Western countries emigrated from. For example, it is generally believed that rheumatic heart disease and congenital heart disease remain important causes of heart failure in sub-Saharan Africa and certain parts of Asia and South America. Hypertension is thought to be an important cause of heart failure in Asia, and in the African and African American population, whereas Chagas' disease is an important aetiology in subjects from South America. [8] Hispanics comprise the largest and fastest growing ethnic group in the U.S. and a recent review has suggested Hispanics with heart failure are more likely to be younger and underinsured than non-Hispanic whites and have higher rates of readmissions but lower in-hospital mortality rates. Hispanics have excessive rates of diabetes, obesity, dyslipidemia, and metabolic syndrome that may predispose to heart failure. [9] Although it is useful to remember region-specific aetiologies of heart failure particularly when managing recent immigrants from the regions where the minority groups were resident, it should be recognized that as these regions also constantly undergo epidemiological and economic transitions and the epidemiology of heart failure is likely to be increasing similar to that of the Western world. The large international case-controlled INTERHEART study has demonstrated that the impact of conventional and potentially preventable risk factors of myocardial infarctions is consistent across different geographical regions and different ethnic groups. [10] This implies that simple measures that can prevent myocardial infarction and the subsequent development of heart failure are equally applicable to different ethnic populations in different geographic locations. There is little evidence to indicate that criteria used to diagnose heart failure differ substantially between ethnic populations. For example, a recent study from the US has demonstrated that the diagnostic performance of the biomarker N-terminal *pro*B-type natriuretic peptide is similar in African Americans and non-African Americans. [11] Evidence that different ethnic groups have the same mortality benefit from current standard therapy is slim as very few large randomized controlled intervention trials have included regions outside Europe and the US. There have been much smaller trials that confirmed the effectiveness of ACE inhibitors and β-blockers in patients from Africa and Asia. [12,13] Given the fundamental nature of the derangements in heart failure, it is likely that the current treatment approach such as blockade of neurohormonal activation and the judicious use of devices will be similarly effective, although one cannot rule out the possibility that the degree of response to treatment may vary among ethnic groups.

Heart Failure in Specific Ethnic Minority Populations

The South Asian Population

The South Asians are currently the largest and fastest growing minority group, representing 25% of all minority and 4% of the total population in Canada. [1] South Asians have increased susceptibility to premature mortality from coronary heart disease. [14-17] A higher disease burden of coronary heart disease in South Asian subjects might be expected to result in a higher prevalence of heart failure. In a study conducted in Leicestershire in United Kingdom involving 5789 consecutive patients, [18] admission rates for heart failure were higher among South Asian patients than white patients.

South Asian patients were younger and more frequently had concomitant diabetes than white patients. Despite differences in personal characteristics and risk factors, clinical outcome was similar. In a matched historical cohort study of patients hospitalized for heart failure conducted also in Leicestershire, [19] when compared to Caucasian patients the South Asian patients had similar rates of prior coronary artery disease but more often had hypertension and diabetes.

South Asian patients had a lower mortality than Caucasian patients. A retrospective sequential chart review of South Asians and non-South Asian whites hospitalized with heart failure at two Toronto-area community hospitals in Canada demonstrated that South Asians were younger, of lower body mass index and were more often diabetic. [20] In-hospital mortality was also not different although South Asians were more likely to experience atrial and ventricular arrhythmias.

These data therefore suggest that South Asians have more risk factors thereby increasing the risk for premature coronary heart disease which may lead to development of heart failure at a younger age. As in other ethnic groups, in order to understand and manage a person's illness it is necessary to appreciate the effects of their culture, experiences and environment on the illness.

Thus, to prevent heart failure in the South Asians, healthcare professionals and the South Asian community should be made aware of their unique risk profile so that appropriate ethnocultural-specific screening procedures and support programs can be implemented.

The Chinese Population

The Chinese represent the second largest visible minority comprising of 24% of the minority population in Canada. [1] When managing Chinese patients, their ability to comprehend and speak English and their family values should be considered. Chinese is the third most commonly spoken language in Canada and many Chinese do not speak or understand English well, particularly in technical terms. The modern Chinese continue to emphasize the values of family and there is a strong bond between parents, children and family members. A recent survey conducted in Toronto and Vancouver where the majority of Chinese reside revealed that there is a general lack of awareness of the symptoms of stroke and myocardial infarction and risk factors for cardiovascular disease among the Chinese Canadians. [21] These social and ethnocultural factors may therefore confound the management of the Chinese patients.

There are very few long-term prospective studies defining specifically etiologic factors for heart failure in the Chinese. Available data, which are by no means definitive, point to hypertension being the most important identifiable risk factor in Chinese with heart failure. [8,22] In a prospective study of 730 consecutive Hong Kong Chinese patients admitted to hospital with heart failure, the main identifiable risk factors were hypertension (37%), coronary heart disease (31%), valvular heart disease (15%), cor pulmonale (27%), idiopathic dilated cardiomyopathy (4%), and miscellaneous (10%). In women, hypertension was the commonest cause of heart failure at all ages but in men aged <70 years, coronary heart disease was equal in frequency to hypertension (36% and 35% respectively). Twenty-one percent had diabetes compared to a community rate of 10% for this age group. [23] A subsequent study reported by the same group evaluated 200 consecutive patients with heart failure using Doppler echocardiography. [24] A left ventricular ejection fraction (LVEF) >45% was considered normal. The results showed that 12.5% had significant valvular heart disease. Of the remaining 175 patients, 132 had a LVEF >45%. Therefore, 66% of patients with a clinical diagnosis of heart failure had a normal LVEF. Heart failure with normal left ventricular systolic function was more common than systolic heart failure in those >70 years old. Most (57%) had an abnormal relaxation pattern in diastole and 14% had a restrictive filling pattern. In the systolic heart failure group, a restrictive filling pattern was more common (46%). There were no significant differences in the sex distribution, aetiology, or prevalence of left ventricular hypertrophy between these two heart failure groups. These investigators conclude that heart failure with a normal LVEF is more common than systolic heart failure in Chinese patients and that this may be related to an older age at presentation and the high prevalence of hypertension. In a case-mix study from a tertiary care center in Toronto, LVEF of Chinese (n=47) and Caucasian patients (n=243) with a diagnosis of heart failure were compared. [25] Among these patients with a primary diagnosis of heart failure, there were more Chinese patients with LVEF > 40% than Caucasian patients. The median LVEF was also greater in Chinese (34 vs. 28%, p = 0.031) and the Chinese patients were older. With the most rapid economic growth in the world and the associated socioeconomic changes, a large proportion of Chinese adults now have the metabolic syndrome and obesity has become an important public health problem in China. [26] A recent review [27] from China indicated that in contrast to the Western countries, the prevalence of heart failure is greater in women than in men which might in turn be related to higher prevalence of rheumatic heart disease which affected women more than men. It is therefore more than likely that antecedent factors for incident heart failure in the Chinese will rapidly approach those of the Western world.

Our group recently examined the clinical profile of ethnic minority groups among patients with heart failure managed in two specialized heart failure clinics that follow a large number of Chinese and South Asian patients respectively. [28] Detailed medical records of 1266 non-Chinese, non-South Asians, 215 South Asians and 151 Chinese patients managed in two specialized heart failure clinics in Ontario that follow large numbers of South Asian and Chinese patients were reviewed. Compared to non-Chinese, non-South Asians, there were more women in the Chinese heart failure patients. South Asian patients had highest frequency of a history of previous myocardial infarctions and hypertension and the least frequency of concurrent atrial fibrillation. A smaller proportion of Chinese patients had left ventricular dysfunction that was categorized as Grade 2 or worse. Chinese patients had the least frequent use of angiotensin-converting enzyme (ACE) inhibitors but on the other hand had the most frequent use in angiotensin receptor blockers (Figure 1). Our data therefore indicate that among patients managed in heart failure clinics in Ontario, Canada, Chinese and South Asian patients have different patterns of demographics, comorbid conditions, proportion of patients with preserved left ventricular systolic function and medication use when compared to non-Chinese, non-South Asian patients with heart failure. Awareness of these differences may help to design future studies and develop differential strategies to prevent and manage heart failure among the largest and increasing ethnic minority groups in the Western countries.

There are currently no large scale randomized controlled trials of pharmacologic and device therapy conducted specifically in Chinese patients with heart failure. Indeed, the recommendations from the Chinese guidelines on the diagnosis and treatment of chronic heart failure closely resemble those contained in guidelines in the Western world. [29].

The recently published Hong Kong Diastolic Heart Failure Study studied 150 Chinese patients with heart failure and preserved systolic function and reported no significant additional benefit by adding irbesartan or ramipril to diuretic treatment. [30] It has been stated that Chinese subjects experience a high incidence of cough when treated with ACE inhibitors [31-33].

However, most of these studies that reported high incidence of ACE inhibitor-induced cough in Chinese patients had involved very small number of patients and did not compare simultaneously Chinese and Caucasian patients. In the Perindopril Protection Against Recurrent Stroke Study (PROGRESS), there were no differences in cough among the Asian and non-Asian participants [34,35]. Given the compelling data in support of the benefit of ACE inhibition in heart failure with systolic dysfunction, a Chinese patient with heart failure should not be denied the initiation of an ACE inhibitor based on anticipated intolerance. The doses of antihypertensive agents prescribed in Asian patients are frequently lower than in Caucasian patients, due in part to a perception of greater sensitivity [36] and therefore higher risk of hypotension in the Asian patients. Although this is by no means a uniform finding, in a frail Chinese patient with more advanced symptoms of heart failure, it may be appropriate to start vasodilator medications at lower doses and uptitrate the dose slower than in a Caucasian patient, but with a goal of eventually reaching the evidence-based dose. Unless strong evidence that can change the management of Chinese patients with heart failure is available, it is prudent to follow the recommendations from guidelines in the Western countries when managing Chinese heart failure patients.

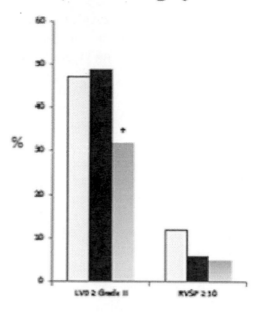

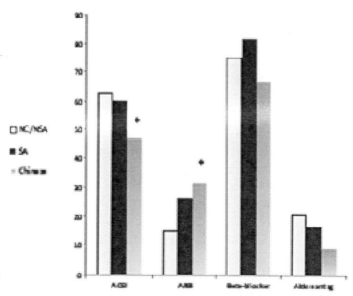

NC/NSA, Non-Chinese/Non-South Asian; SA, South Asians; LVD, left ventricular dysfunction, RVSP, right ventricular systolic pressure; ACEi, ACE inhibitors; ARB, angiotensin receptor blockers; Aldos antag, aldosterone receptor angatonists; *p<0.05 vs. NC/NSA.

Figure 1. Left ventricular function and medication use in heart failure patients from different ethic groups.

The Black Population

In the US, the black population has a higher prevalence of heart failure than persons of other races, and they present with symptoms of heart failure at younger ages, and are less likely to be due to coronary heart disease than in Caucasians. [37-39] Two recently published studies have reported on the contemporary epidemiology of heart failure among African Americans. Observations from the Coronary Artery Risk Development in Young Adult (CARDIA) study have indicated that 1 in 100 African-American men and women develop heart failure at an average age of 39, 20 times the rate in Caucasians. Incident heart failure in the African Americans before 50 years of age was associated with hypertension, obesity, chronic kidney disease and systolic dysfunction that were already present before age of 35. [40] The incidence, risk factors, and outcomes of heart failure among African Americans were also examined in the 2934 older individuals without heart failure in the Health, Aging, and Body Composition (Health ABC) Study. [41] African Americans were more likely than Whites to develop heart failure. Population-attributable-risks for independent risk factors for incident heart failure revealed that coronary heart disease and uncontrolled blood pressure carried the highest risks in both races. Smoking, left ventricular hypertrophy, fasting glucose levels, systolic blood pressure, decreased albumin, and increased heart rate were more prevalent in African Americans. Indeed, hypertension, the key aetiology of heart failure in the black population, disproportionately affects African Americans, with a prevalence that is among the highest globally and it is steadily increasing [42].

These data imply that young black subjects with risk factors should be a target of more aggressive intervention for heart failure prevention. Analysis of outcome data from the Studies of Left Ventricular Dysfunction (SOLVD) trials has shown higher mortality and morbidity rates in blacks compared to Caucasians with heart failure. [43] Whether this reflects differences in baseline characteristics, access of care or socioeconomic factors is not entirely clear. There have been reports which point to access to care and unfavourable clinical characteristics that are independent of heart failure as factors for poor outcomes. [44,45] A recently published study from the US reported that non-Hispanic blacks were more likely to be anxious and depressed than Hispanics and non-Hispanic whites with advanced chronic heart failure [46].

Long-standing clinical observations have suggested that blacks with hypertension respond less well than Caucasians to ACE inhibitors. [47] Concerns remain that differences in the effectiveness of blockade of the renin-angiotensin system might also be present. Several retrospective subgroup analyses of data from randomized trials have added some support to the concept that the response of blacks and Caucasians with heart failure and left ventricular systolic dysfunction to ACE inhibition may differ. [48] However, these *post hoc* analyses do not provide sufficient evidence to support a strategy other than routine use of ACE inhibitors in black subjects with heart failure and systolic dysfunction. Although the Beta-Blocker Evaluation of Survival *Trial* (BEST) with bucindolol did not find a beneficial effect of β-blockade in blacks, [49] subgroup analysis of data from the US Carvedilol Trials suggests that the beneficial effect of β-blockers on outcomes in blacks is similar to the effects in the larger population [50] and these findings are supported by other analyses. [51,52] The totality of data to date therefore still support the use of β-blockers in black patients with heart failure with systolic dysfunction.

Data from the earlier Vasodilator-Heart Failure Trial (VHeFT) I and II first suggested a racial difference in treatment response between white and black patients with symptomatic systolic left ventricular dysfunction treated with hydralazine-isosorbide dinitrate. [53] It is noteworthy that the observations reported in these retrospective analyses occurred 10 to 15 years after the trials were completed, and they were only possible because these studies fortuitously included a sufficient number of black patients to be able to identify differences. Representation of blacks, women, and other minorities in other heart failure trials has been so poor that even meaningful retrospective subgroup analyses have been precluded; thus, the opportunities to define the mechanisms for important population differences may have been missed. On the basis of the ethnic differences observed in these retrospective analyses, the African-American Heart Failure Trial (A-HeFT) was designed as the first heart failure trial in an all-black cohort. A-HeFT enrolled 1050 black patients with New York Heart Association class III or IV symptoms and with dilated ventricles and systolic dysfunction. [54] Subjects were assigned to receive a fixed combination of isosorbide dinitrate plus hydralazine or placebo in addition to standard therapy. The primary end point was a composite score made up of weighted values for death from any cause, a first hospitalization for heart failure and change in the quality of life. The study was terminated early due to a higher mortality rate in the placebo group. The mean primary composite score was significantly better in the group given nitrate and hydralazine than in the placebo group, as well as its components: 43% relative reduction in the rate of death from any cause, 33% reduction in first heart failure hospitalization, and an improvement in the quality of life. These data therefore form the basis for the support of recent recommendations for the addition of the combination of isosorbide dinitrate and hydralazine to the standard medical regimen for black patients with heart failure, [55,56] and is an example that heart failure can treated differently based on ethnicity. On the other hand, while A-HeFT showed a clear benefit, the trial design leaves unanswered the question of whether the response actually differs between whites and blacks.

The Hispanic Population

"Hispanic" broadly refers to a relatively heterogeneous group of populations who are ancestrally linked to Spain and the Spanish-speaking nations of the Caribbean and Central and South America. [57,58] Observational and retrospective studies have reported that compared with non-Hispanic whites, Hispanics with heart failure tended to be younger, [59,60], underinsured, [59] and to have higher rates of dyslipidemia, diabetes, and kidney disease, [59-61] as well as impaired left ventricular systolic function. [60-62] Hispanics overall are affected more frequently by known etiologic conditions for the development of heart failure. This includes obesity, diabetes, hypertension and dyslipidemia, diabetes, hypertension and dyslipidemia. [60-64] On the other hand, previous studies have suggested a lower coronary artery disease burden and cardiovascular mortality in the Hispanic. [65,66] However, more recent studies that prospectively ascertained vital status information have reported similar or higher all-cause and cardiovascular death rates in Hispanic in non-Hispanic white subjects. [67] The incidence of rheumatic heart disease continues to decline but appears to remain relatively high in a few populations including Hispanics, particularly Mexican Americans. [64,68] Age-adjusted mortality rates for rheumatic heart disease in New Mexico over a 25-year period were higher in Hispanics than in non-Hispanic whites. [68]

These observations may, however, be attributable to their poorer economic status and access to public health care. [68,69] Chagas' disease is an important cause of heart failure in endemic regions including Mexico and Central and South America, where approximately 16 to 18 million people are infected. [70] In the U.S., an estimated 50,000 to 350,000 Hispanic immigrants may have chronic, asymptomatic *T. cruzi* infection [70,71] with a 20% likelihood of progression to chronic cardiomyopathy in this population. [72] Chagas' disease in the U.S. is principally driven by immigration, although disease transmission can also occur via blood transfusion or organ transplant, or congenitally in pregnant women. [70] Misdiagnosis of idiopathic dilated cardiomyopathy or coronary artery disease is common due to poor disease recognition in both patients and medical professionals especially in nonendemic areas. [71].

A study of Medicare beneficiaries examining ethnic disparities in quality of heart failure care reported that compared with Hispanics were least likely to have an assessment of LVEF and to be discharged on ACE inhibitor treatment. [73].

The OPTIMIZE-HF (Organized Program to Initiate Lifesaving Treatment in Hospitalized Patients with Heart Failure) study showed that Hispanic ethnicity was an independent predictor for non-delivery of complete discharge instructions, even among hospitals serving the highest proportion of this population [74].

Barriers to health care may be an important issue that hampers the management of Hispanic subjects with heart failure in the US. [75] Across populations in the U.S., Hispanics have the poorest health insurance access: over one-third of them have no medical insurance. [76] In addition, they are most likely to have no usual place of care and to have the most difficulty paying for medical care, irrespective of insurance status. [77] In the U.S., Hispanics have the lowest level of education, [77] a well-known correlate of health risk. Another significant variable of acculturation and health care impediment for many Hispanics is the language barrier. About 8 million Hispanics in the U.S. do not speak English fluently. Monolingual Spanish speakers have a higher prevalence of cardiovascular risk factors and poorer recognition of coronary symptoms. [78].

On the other hand, exclusively English-speaking physicians engage Hispanic patients less effectively in their medical care than do bilingual physicians [75].

The Aboriginal Population

Data from the 2006 census on Canada's First Nations population counted 1,172,790 First Nations, Métis and Inuit people, representing 3.8% of Canada's total population. More than half the country's 1.2 million aboriginal people live off reserve. Aboriginal people were four times as likely as non-aboriginal people to live in a crowded dwelling and three times as likely to live in a dwelling in need of major repairs. Life expectancy for First Nations males is 7.4 years less and 5.2 years less for First Nations women compared to Canadian men and women respectively. There is also evidence to indicate that geographic location, as compared with Aboriginal identity, appears to have a large impact on health status and the use of physician services, with on-reserve Aboriginals reporting lower likelihood of having seen a physician. [79] The Study of Health Assessment and Risk Evaluation in Aboriginal Peoples (SHARE-AP) reported a higher frequency of cardiovascular disease (CVD) among Aboriginals in Canada and a greater burden of atherosclerosis when compared with Canadians of European ancestry. [80] As with other colonized people, there have been significant social, economic and cultural changes in the past decades which might accounted for an observed increase in hospitalization for coronary heart disease. [81] Given the increasing incidence of diabetes that accompanies the transition from traditional to urban lifestyles, [82,83] the incidence of CVD and therefore that of heart failure will likely also increase. There are very few data available that can directly guide the management of heart failure in the aboriginal population. In patients who have commenced dialysis in Alberta, Saskatchewan or Manitoba in Canada, the risk of death from heart failure was higher in Aboriginals than in Caucasians. [84] A recent report from the Australian Institute of Health and Welfare has indicated that heart failure is a major cause of illness and death among Aboriginal and Torres Strait Islander people. The prevalence of heart failure in Australian Aboriginals was nearly twice as high as in non-Aboriginal Australians [85].

When managing Aboriginal patients with heart failure, non-Aboriginal health care professionals need to understand how Aboriginal people interpret their illness and respond to treatment, and respect the logic and rationale of another system of thought where health is perceived as a harmonious order. They need to adapt their treatment plans and education programs to the cultural, social and economic circumstances and to recognize that many communities are geographically remote. Non-aboriginal health care workers caring Aboriginal patients with heart failure will likely need to adopt a holistic approach in offering advice and care for their patients, respecting local traditions and not to impose their own values. [86] Workers need to recognize the multigenerational legacies of colonization and the importance of local history; to respect traditional beliefs; and to acknowledge the role of the social determinants of health and, in many communities, inadequate resources. Health care workers should work in multidisciplinary teams and include community health representatives. They must be sensitive to cross-cultural care. Aboriginal patients might be operating in a second language and might not be comfortable questioning someone who is perceived to have greater power and knowledge.

Conclusion

In summary, the overview in this chapter demonstrates that there are important differences across ethnic minority groups in the etiologies of heart failure and how patients respond to treatment. However, most of the published studies are based on small sample sizes and suffer from other limitations. Given the increasing frequency of heart failure in these populations and an increasingly multiethnic world, additional studies on heart failure across different ethnic groups are needed, if these patients that originate different parts of the world are to have optimal management and outcomes. Furthermore, if one is to be successful in reducing the burden of heart failure and indeed heart disease at large, and if one is committed to providing the best care for all patients, then one must be cognizant of the healthcare disparities and if feasible take steps to narrow and eliminate gaps in care as a function of ethnicity. In this regard, the Canadian Cardiovascular Society has included a section on ethnicity and heart failure in its 2011 focused update.[55] Recommendations and practical tips on the management of patients with heart failure from the four largest ethnic minority groups in Canada are displayed on Table 1.

The Coalition to Reduce Racial and Ethnic Disparities in CV Outcomes (CREDO) launched by the American College of Cardiology [50], an initiative aimed to equip cardiologists and other healthcare providers treating cardiovascular disease the tools to examine disparities in practice and achieve a targeted reduction in these disparities through performance measure-based quality improvement, represent an exciting initial step.

Table 1. Ethnocultural considerations when managing patients with heart failure [55]

Population	Important risk factors for HF prevention	Language and ethnocultural considerations	Treatment
South Asian	Diabetes, obesity and metabolic syndrome	Mostly speak English. Family involvement in health care behavior is common	Evidence-based therapy from HF guidelines
Chinese	Hypertension*	Mostly speak Cantonese and Mandarin. Family involvement in health care behavior is common	Follow HF guidelines Be aware of the use of traditional Chinese medicines
Blacks	Hypertension	Almost all speak English apart from Quebec where French is prominent	Follow HF guidelines Consider adding nitrate hydralazine combination in those with severe HF
Aboriginals	Diabetes, obesity	Cree and Ojibwe are the main spoken languages Need to involve family and community representatives	Follow general HF guidelines

HF, heart failure; * Coronary heart disease, diabetes and obesity are emerging risk factors.

References

[1]   Statistics Canada. Canada's ethnocultural mosaic in 2006. *2006 Census of Canada* 2008.

[2]   Weinick RM, Jacobs EA, Stone LC, Ortega AN, Burstin H. Hispanic healthcare disparities: challenging the myth of a monolithic Hispanic population. *Med. Care* 2004;42:313-320.

[3]   Rideout E, Montemuro M. Hope, morale and adaptation in patients with chronic heart failure. *J. Adv. Nurs.* 1986;11:429-438.

[4]   Balsa AI, McGuire TG. Prejudice, clinical uncertainty and stereotyping as sources of health disparities. *J. Health Econ.* 2003;22:89-116.

[5]   Gerend MA, Pai M. Social determinants of Black-White disparities in breast cancer mortality: a review. *Cancer Epidemiol. Biomarkers Prev.* 2008;17:2913-2923.

[6]   Groman R, Ginsburg J. Racial and ethnic disparities in health care: a position paper of the American College of Physicians. *Ann. Intern. Med.* 2004;141:226-232.

[7]   Woolf SH, Johnson RE, Fryer GE, Jr., Rust G, Satcher D. The health impact of resolving racial disparities: an analysis of US mortality data. *Am. J. Public Health* 2008;98:S26-S28.

[8]   Mendez GF, Cowie MR. The epidemiological features of heart failure in developing countries: a review of the literature. *Int. J. Cardiol.* 2001;80:213-219.

[9]   Vivo RP, Krim SR, Cevik C, Witteles RM. Heart failure in Hispanics. *J. Am. Coll Cardiol.* 2009;53:1167-1175.

[10]   Yusuf S, Hawken S, Ounpuu S, Dans T, Avezum A, Lanas F, McQueen M, Budaj A, Pais P, Varigos J, Lisheng L. Effect of potentially modifiable risk factors associated with myocardial infarction in 52 countries (the INTERHEART study): case-control study. *Lancet* 2004;364:937-952.

[11]   Krauser DG, Chen AA, Tung R, Anwaruddin S, Baggish AL, Januzzi JL, Jr. Neither race nor gender influences the usefulness of amino-terminal pro-brain natriuretic peptide testing in dyspneic subjects: a ProBNP Investigation of Dyspnea in the Emergency Department (PRIDE) substudy. *J. Card Fail* 2006;12:452-457.

[12]   Ajayi AA, Balogun MO, Oycwo EA, Ladipo GO. Enalapril in African patients with congestive cardiac failure. *Br. J. Clin. Pharmacol.* 1989;27:400-403.

[13]   Sanderson JE, Chan SK, Yip G, Yeung LY, Chan KW, Raymond K, Woo KS. Beta-blockade in heart failure: a comparison of carvedilol with metoprolol. *J. Am. Coll Cardiol.* 1999;34:1522-1528.

[14]   Balarajan R. Ethnicity and health: the challenges ahead. *Ethn. Health* 1996;1:3-5.

[15]   Wild S, McKeigue P. Cross sectional analysis of mortality by country of birth in England and Wales, 1970-92. *BMJ* 1997;314:705-710.

[16]   Anand SS, Yusuf S, Vuksan V, Devanesen S, Teo KK, Montague PA, Kelemen L, Yi C, Lonn E, Gerstein H, Hegele RA, McQueen M. Differences in risk factors, atherosclerosis, and cardiovascular disease between ethnic groups in Canada: the Study of Health Assessment and Risk in Ethnic groups (SHARE). *Lancet* 2000;356:279-284.

[17]   Sheth T, Nair C, Nargundkar M, Anand S, Yusuf S. Cardiovascular and cancer mortality among Canadians of European, south Asian and Chinese origin from 1979 to 1993: an analysis of 1.2 million deaths. *CMAJ* 1999;161:132-138.

[18]   Blackledge HM, Newton J, Squire IB. Prognosis for South Asian and white patients newly admitted to hospital with heart failure in the United Kingdom: historical cohort study. *BMJ* 2003;327:526-531.

[19]   Newton JD, Blackledge HM, Squire IB. Ethnicity and variation in prognosis for patients newly hospitalised for heart failure: a matched historical cohort study. *Heart* 2005;91:1545-1550.

[20]   Singh N, Gupta M. Clinical characteristics of South Asian patients hospitalized with heart failure. *Ethn. Dis.* 2005;15:615-619.

[21]   Chow CM, Chu JY, Tu JV, Moe GW. Lack of awareness of heart disease and stroke among Chinese Canadians: results of a pilot study of the Chinese Canadian Cardiovascular Health Project. *Can. J. Cardiol.* 2008;24:623-628.

[22]   Sanderson JE, Tse TF. Heart failure: a global disease requiring a global response. *Heart* 2003;89:585-586.

[23]   Sanderson JE, Chan SK, Chan WW, Hung YT, Woo KS. The aetiology of heart failure in the Chinese population of Hong Kong--a prospective study of 730 consecutive patients. *Int. J. Cardiol.* 1995;51:29-35.

[24]   Yip GW, Ho PP, Woo KS, Sanderson JE. Comparison of frequencies of left ventricular systolic and diastolic heart failure in Chinese living in Hong Kong. *Am. J. Cardiol.* 1999;84:563-567.

[25]   Tso DK, Moe G. Cardiovascular disease in Chinese Canadians: a case-mix study from an urban tertiary care cardiology clinic. *Can. J. Cardiol.* 2002;18:861-869.

[26] Gu D, Reynolds K, Wu X, Chen J, Duan X, Reynolds RF, Whelton PK, He J. Prevalence of the metabolic syndrome and overweight among adults in China. *Lancet* 2005;365:1398-1405.

[27] Jiang H, Ge J. Epidemiology and clinical management of cardiomyopathies and heart failure in China. *Heart* 2009;95:1727-1731.

[28] Moe GW, Nemi E, Gupta M. Differences in the clinical profile of ethnic minority groups among patients with heart failure managed in specialized heart failure clinics. *Can. J. Cardiol.* 2011;26:93D.

[29] Guidelines for the diagnosis and management of chronic heart failure. *Zhonghua Xin Xue Guan Bing Za Zhi* 2007;35:1076-1095.

[30] Yip GW, Wang M, Wang T, Chan S, Fung JW, Yeung L, Yip T, Lau ST, Lau CP, Tang MO, Yu CM, Sanderson JE. The Hong Kong diastolic heart failure study: a randomised controlled trial of diuretics, irbesartan and ramipril on quality of life, exercise capacity, left ventricular global and regional function in heart failure with a normal ejection fraction. *Heart* 2008;94:573-580.

[31] Chan WK, Chan TY, Luk WK, Leung VK, Li TH, Critchley JA. A high incidence of cough in Chinese subjects treated with angiotensin converting enzyme inhibitors. *Eur. J. Clin. Pharmacol.* 1993;44:299-300.

[32] Woo J, Chan TY. A high incidence of cough associated with combination therapy of hypertension with isradipine and lisinopril in Chinese subjects. *Br. J. Clin. Pract.* 1991;45:178-180.

[33] Woo KS, Nicholls MG. High prevalence of persistent cough with angiotensin converting enzyme inhibitors in Chinese. *Br. J. Clin. Pharmacol.* 1995;40:141-144.

[34] 2001 Census:Ethnocultural Portrait, Ottawa, Statistics Canada. 2005. Ref Type: Data File.

[35] Ohkubo T, Chapman N, Neal B, Woodward M, Omae T, Chalmers J. Effects of an angiotensin-converting enzyme inhibitor-based regimen on pneumonia risk. *Am. J. Respir. Crit. Care Med.* 2004;169:1041-1045.

[36] Zhou HH, Koshakji RP, Silberstein DJ, Wilkinson GR, Wood AJ. Altered sensitivity to and clearance of propranolol in men of Chinese descent as compared with American whites. *N. Engl. J. Med.* 1989;320:565-570.

[37] Hunt SA, Abraham WT, Chin MH, Feldman AM, Francis GS, Ganiats TG, Jessup M, Konstam MA, Mancini DM, Michl K, Oates JA, Rahko PS, Silver MA, Stevenson LW, Yancy CW, Antman EM, Smith SC, Jr., Adams CD, Anderson JL, Faxon DP, Fuster V, Halperin JL, Hiratzka LF, Hunt SA, Jacobs AK, Nishimura R, Ornato JP, Page RL, Riegel B. ACC/AHA 2005 Guideline Update for the Diagnosis and Management of Chronic Heart Failure in the Adult--Summary Article: A Report of the American College of Cardiology/American Heart Association Task Force on Practice Guidelines (Writing Committee to Update the 2001 Guidelines for the Evaluation and Management of Heart Failure): Developed in Collaboration With the American College of Chest Physicians and the International Society for Heart and Lung Transplantation: Endorsed by the Heart Rhythm Society. *Circulation* 2005;112:1825-1852.

[38] Yancy CW. Heart failure in African Americans: a cardiovascular engima. *J. Card Fail* 2000;6:183-186.

[39] Afzal A, Ananthasubramaniam K, Sharma N, al-Malki Q, Ali AS, Jacobsen G, Jafri SM. Racial differences in patients with heart failure. *Clin. Cardiol.* 1999;22:791-794.

[40] Bibbins-Domingo K, Pletcher MJ, Lin F, Vittinghoff E, Gardin JM, Arynchyn A, Lewis CE, Williams OD, Hulley SB. Racial differences in incident heart failure among young adults. *N. Engl. J. Med.* 2009;360:1179-1190.

[41] Kalogeropoulos A, Georgiopoulou V, Kritchevsky SB, Psaty BM, Smith NL, Newman AB, Rodondi N, Satterfield S, Bauer DC, Bibbins-Domingo K, Smith AL, Wilson PW, Vasan RS, Harris TB, Butler J. Epidemiology of incident heart failure in a contemporary elderly cohort: the health, aging, and body composition study. *Arch. Intern. Med.* 2009;169:708-715.

[42] Chobanian AV, Bakris GL, Black HR, Cushman WC, Green LA, Izzo JL, Jr., Jones DW, Materson BJ, Oparil S, Wright JT, Jr., Roccella EJ. The Seventh Report of the Joint National Committee on Prevention, Detection, Evaluation, and Treatment of High Blood Pressure: the JNC 7 report. *JAMA* 2003;289:2560-2572.

[43] Dries DL, Exner DV, Gersh BJ, Cooper HA, Carson PE, Domanski MJ. Racial differences in the outcome of left ventricular dysfunction. *N. Engl. J. Med.* 1999;340:609-616.

[44] Alexander M, Grumbach K, Selby J, Brown AF, Washington E. Hospitalization for congestive heart failure. Explaining racial differences. *JAMA* 1995;274:1037-1042.

[45] Ghali JK, Kadakia S, Cooper R, Ferlinz J. Precipitating factors leading to decompensation of heart failure. Traits among urban blacks. *Arch. Intern. Med.* 1988;148:2013-2016.

[46] Evangelista LS, Ter-Galstanyan A, Moughrabi S, Moser DK. Anxiety and depression in ethnic minorities with chronic heart failure. *J. Card Fail* 2009;15:572-579.

[47] Saunders E. Hypertension in minorities: blacks. *Am. J. Hypertens* 1995;8:115s-119s.

[48] Exner DV, Dries DL, Domanski MJ, Cohn JN. Lesser response to angiotensin-converting-enzyme inhibitor therapy in black as compared with white patients with left ventricular dysfunction. *N. Engl. J. Med.* 2001;344:1351-1357.

[49] A trial of the beta-blocker bucindolol in patients with advanced chronic heart failure. *N. Engl. J. Med.* 2001;344:1659-1667.

[50] Yancy CW, Fowler MB, Colucci WS, Gilbert EM, Bristow MR, Cohn JN, Lukas MA, Young ST, Packer M. Race and the response to adrenergic blockade with carvedilol in patients with chronic heart failure. *N. Engl. J. Med.* 2001;344:1358-1365.

[51] Goldstein S, Deedwania P, Gottlieb S, Wikstrand J. Metoprolol CR/XL in black patients with heart failure (from the Metoprolol CR/XL randomized intervention trial in chronic heart failure). *Am. J. Cardiol.* 2003;92:478-480.

[52] Gottlieb SS, McCarter RJ, Vogel RA. Effect of beta-blockade on mortality among high-risk and low-risk patients after myocardial infarction. *N. Engl. J. Med.* 1998;339:489-497.

[53] Carson P, Ziesche S, Johnson G, Cohn JN. Racial differences in response to therapy for heart failure: analysis of the vasodilator-heart failure trials. Vasodilator-Heart Failure Trial Study Group. *J. Card Fail* 1999;5:178-187.

[54] Taylor AL, Ziesche S, Yancy C, Carson P, D'Agostino R, Jr., Ferdinand K, Taylor M, Adams K, Sabolinski M, Worcel M, Cohn JN. Combination of isosorbide dinitrate and hydralazine in blacks with heart failure. *N. Engl. J. Med.* 2004;351:2049-2057.

[55] Howlett JG, McKelvie RS, Costigan J, Ducharme A, Estrella-Holder E, Ezekowitz JA, Giannetti N, Haddad H, Heckman GA, Herd AM, Isaac D, Kouz S, Leblanc K, Liu P, Mann E, Moe GW, O'Meara E, Rajda M, Siu S, Stolee P, Swiggum E, Zeiroth S. The

2010 Canadian Cardiovascular Society guidelines for the diagnosis and management of heart failure update: Heart failure in ethnic minority populations, heart failure and pregnancy, disease management, and quality improvement/assurance programs. *Can. J. Cardiol.* 2010;26:185-202.

[56] Hunt SA, Abraham WT, Chin MH, Feldman AM, Francis GS, Ganiats TG, Jessup M, Konstam MA, Mancini DM, Michl K, Oates JA, Rahko PS, Silver MA, Stevenson LW, Yancy CW. 2009 Focused update incorporated into the ACC/AHA 2005 Guidelines for the Diagnosis and Management of Heart Failure in Adults A Report of the American College of Cardiology Foundation/American Heart Association Task Force on Practice Guidelines Developed in Collaboration With the International Society for Heart and Lung Transplantation. *J. Am. Coll Cardiol.* 2009;53:e1-e90.

[57] U.S. Census Bureau. Population Estimates. www.census.gov (last accessed January 19, 2011.

[58] Novello AC, Wise PH, Kleinman DV. Hispanic health: time for data, time for action. *JAMA* 1991;265:253-255.

[59] Alexander M, Grumbach K, Remy L, Rowell R, Massie BM. Congestive heart failure hospitalizations and survival in California: patterns according to race/ethnicity. *Am. Heart J.* 1999;137:919-927.

[60] Yeo KK, Li Z, Amsterdam E. Clinical characteristics and 30-day mortality among Caucasians, Hispanics, Asians, And African-Americans in the 2003 California coronary artery bypass graft surgery outcomes reporting program. *Am. J. Cardiol.* 2007;100:59-63.

[61] Minutello RM, Chou ET, Hong MK, Wong SC. Impact of race and ethnicity on inhospital outcomes after percutaneous coronary intervention (report from the 2000-2001 New York State Angioplasty Registry). *Am. Heart J.* 2006;151:164-167.

[62] Aronow WS, Ahn C, Kronzon I. Comparison of echocardiographic abnormalities in African-American, Hispanic, and white men and women aged >60 years. *Am. J. Cardiol.* 2001;87:1131-3, A10.

[63] Pawson IG, Martorell R, Mendoza FE. Prevalence of overweight and obesity in US Hispanic populations. *Am. J. Clin. Nutr.* 1991;53:1522S-1528S.

[64] Rosamond W, Flegal K, Furie K, Go A, Greenlund K, Haase N, Hailpern SM, Ho M, Howard V, Kissela B, Kittner S, Lloyd-Jones D, McDermott M, Meigs J, Moy C, Nichol G, O'Donnell C, Roger V, Sorlie P, Steinberger J, Thom T, Wilson M, Hong Y. Heart disease and stroke statistics--2008 update: a report from the American Heart Association Statistics Committee and Stroke Statistics Subcommittee. *Circulation* 2008;117:e25-146.

[65] Swenson CJ, Trepka MJ, Rewers MJ, Scarbro S, Hiatt WR, Hamman RF. Cardiovascular disease mortality in Hispanics and non-Hispanic whites. *Am. J. Epidemiol.* 2002;156:919-928.

[66] Liao Y, Cooper RS, Cao G, Kaufman JS, Long AE, McGee DL. Mortality from coronary heart disease and cardiovascular disease among adult U.S. Hispanics: findings from the National Health Interview Survey (1986 to 1994). *J. Am. Coll Cardiol.* 1997;30:1200-1205.

[67] Hunt KJ, Resendez RG, Williams K, Haffner SM, Stern MP, Hazuda HP. All-cause and cardiovascular mortality among Mexican-American and non-Hispanic White older

participants in the San Antonio Heart Study- evidence against the "Hispanic paradox". *Am. J. Epidemiol.* 2003;158:1048-1057.

[68] Becker TM, Wiggins CL, Key CR, Samet JM. Ethnic differences in mortality from acute rheumatic fever and chronic rheumatic heart disease in New Mexico, 1958-1982. *West J. Med.* 1989;150:46-50.

[69] DiGiorgi PL, Baumann FG, O'Leary AM, Schwartz CF, Grossi EA, Ribakove GH, Colvin SB, Galloway AC, Grau JB. Differences in mitral valve disease presentation and surgical treatment outcome between Hispanic and non-Hispanic patients. *Ethn. Dis.* 2008;18:306-310.

[70] Leiby DA, Rentas FJ, Nelson KE, Stambolis VA, Ness PM, Parnis C, McAllister HA, Jr., Yawn DH, Stumpf RJ, Kirchhoff LV. Evidence of Trypanosoma cruzi infection (Chagas' disease) among patients undergoing cardiac surgery. *Circulation* 2000;102:2978-2982.

[71] Schmunis GA. Epidemiology of Chagas disease in non-endemic countries: the role of international migration. *Mem. Inst. Oswaldo Cruz* 2007;102 Suppl 1:75-85.

[72] Milei J, Mautner B, Storino R, Sanchez JA, Ferrans VJ. Does Chagas' disease exist as an undiagnosed form of cardiomyopathy in the United States? *Am. Heart J.* 1992;123:1732-1735.

[73] Correa-de-Araujo R, Stevens B, Moy E, Nilasena D, Chesley F, McDermott K. Gender differences across racial and ethnic groups in the quality of care for acute myocardial infarction and heart failure associated with comorbidities. *Womens Health Issues* 2006;16:44-55.

[74] Albert NM, Fonarow GC, Abraham WT, Chiswell K, Stough WG, Gheorghiade M, Greenberg BH, O'Connor CM, Sun JL, Yancy CW, Young JB. Predictors of delivery of hospital-based heart failure patient education: a report from OPTIMIZE-HF. *J. Card Fail* 2007;13:189-198.

[75] Vivo RP, Krim SR, Cevik C, Witteles RM. Heart failure in Hispanics. *J. Am. Coll Cardiol.* 2009;53:1167-1175.

[76] Trevino FM, Moyer ME, Valdez RB, Stroup-Benham CA. Health insurance coverage and utilization of health services by Mexican Americans, mainland Puerto Ricans, and Cuban Americans. *JAMA* 1991;265:233-237.

[77] Bolen JC, Rhodes L, Powell-Griner EE, Bland SD, Holtzman D. State-specific prevalence of selected health behaviors, by race and ethnicity--Behavioral Risk Factor Surveillance System, 1997. *MMWR CDC Surveill Summ* 2000;49:1-60.

[78] DuBard CA, Garrett J, Gizlice Z. Effect of language on heart attack and stroke awareness among U.S. Hispanics. *Am. J. Prev. Med.* 2006;30:189-196.

[79] Newbold KB. Problems in search of solutions: health and Canadian aboriginals. *J. Community Health* 1998;23:59-73.

[80] Anand SS, Yusuf S, Jacobs R, Davis AD, Yi Q, Gerstein H, Montague PA, Lonn E. Risk factors, atherosclerosis, and cardiovascular disease among Aboriginal people in Canada: the Study of Health Assessment and Risk Evaluation in Aboriginal Peoples (SHARE-AP). *Lancet* 2001;358:1147-1153.

[81] Shah BR, Hux JE, Zinman B. Increasing rates of ischemic heart disease in the native population of Ontario, Canada. *Arch. Intern. Med.* 2000;160:1862-1866.

[82] Burrows NR, Geiss LS, Engelgau MM, Acton KJ. Prevalence of diabetes among Native Americans and Alaska Natives, 1990-1997: an increasing burden. *Diabetes Care* 2000;23:1786-1790.

[83] Fagot-Campagna A, Pettitt DJ, Engelgau MM, Burrows NR, Geiss LS, Valdez R, Beckles GL, Saaddine J, Gregg EW, Williamson DF, Narayan KM. Type 2 diabetes among North American children and adolescents: an epidemiologic review and a public health perspective. *J. Pediatr.* 2000;136:664-672.

[84] Tonelli M, Hemmelgarn B, Manns B, Pylypchuk G, Bohm C, Yeates K, Gourishankar S, Gill JS. Death and renal transplantation among Aboriginal people undergoing dialysis. *CMAJ* 2004;171:577-582.

[85] Australian Institute of Health and Welfare. Cardiovascular disease and its associated risk factors in Aboriginal and Torres Strait Islander peoples 2004-2005. Cardiovascular Disease Series Number 29 (www.aihw.gov.au/publications/index.cfm/title/10549 last accessed Jun 18 2009).

[86] Macaulay AC. Improving aboriginal health: How can health care professionals contribute? *Can. Fam. Physician* 2009;55:334-339.

Index

B

C

E

F

G

H

M

O

P

Q

R

S

T

U

V

W

X

Y

Z